ANAESTHESIA FOR MINIMALLY INVASIVE SURGERY

ANAESTHESIA FOR MINIMALLY INVASIVE SURGERY

By

Thomas Allen Crozier

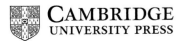

PUBLISHED BY THE PRESS SYNDICATE OF THE UNIVERSITY OF CAMBRIDGE
The Pitt Building, Trumpington Street, Cambridge, United Kingdom

CAMBRIDGE UNIVERSITY PRESS
The Edinburgh Building, Cambridge CB2 2RU, UK
40 West 20th Street, New York, NY 10011-4211, USA
477 Williamstown Road, Port Melbourne, VIC 3207, Australia
Ruiz de Alarcón 13, 28014 Madrid, Spain
Dock House, The Waterfront, Cape Town 8001, South Africa

http://www.cambridge.org

First published 2004

Printed in the United Kingdom at the University Press, Cambridge

Typeface: Ehrhardt 10/11pt   System: QuarkXpress®

A catalog record for this book is available from the British Library

Library of Congress Cataloging in Publication data

ISBN 1 841 10191 5

The publisher has used its best endeavors to ensure that the URLs
for external websites referred to in this book are correct and
active at the time of going to press. However, the publisher has
no responsibility for the websites and can make no guarantee
that a site will remain live or that the content is or will
remain appropriate.

Every effort has been made in preparing this book to provide accurate and
up-to-date information that is in accord with accepted standards and
practice at the time of publication. Nevertheless, the authors, editors and
publisher can make no warranties that the information contained herein is
totally free from error, not least because clinical standards are constantly
changing through research and regulation. The authors, editors and
publisher therefore disclaim all liability for direct or consequential
damages resulting from the use of material contained in this book. Readers
are strongly advised to pay careful attention to information provided by the
manufacturer of any drugs or equipment that they plan to use.

CONTENTS

PREFACE

The idea for this book was born during a workshop on anaesthesia for laparoscopic surgery, which I organized several years ago. What was intended for a regional audience of perhaps 250 anaesthetists at most, turned into an international event with the participants spilling out of the main lecture hall to view the presentations on video screens in adjacent halls. The overwhelming resonance of the workshop and the numerous requests for accompanying material was ample evidence of the need for a comprehensive treatise of the subject that merged experimental study data with clinical reality and the requirements of perioperative patient care.

This book is designed to fill the gap. It was clear that although laparoscopic procedures were the original focus of attention and should be given the most space, the scope of the book would have to be widened to include other minimally invasive surgical procedures, such as thoracic surgery, laser surgery of the upper airways or neurosurgery, that require adjustments and adaptations of routine anaesthetic management, or entail specific risks requiring specific precautions. These specialties are presented in separate chapters.

A format was chosen that starts with what the surgeon is actually doing to the patient, proceeds through an in-depth look at the patient's cardiopulmonary responses to the surgeon's manipulations, and then distils hands-on practical recommendations and guidelines for anaesthetic management from this basic information. These include tips on anaesthetic regimens derived from the application of recent pharmacokinetic and pharmacological research results to the clinical demands of minimally invasive operations. Special attention is given to the typical patient profile for selected operations; what to look for during their preoperative work-up, and what to watch for during and after surgery. With this synoptic foundation, the reader also has a better grasp of what goes awry during typical adverse events and complications, and how these can be prevented and treated.

The reader can easily choose just what depth of information is required for the task at hand, be it a how-to-do anaesthetic recipe or a fully-referenced detailed presentation. Important points are summarized in highlighted charts that allow the reader to find pertinent information at a glance, and numerous illustrations are included to enhance clarity.

FOREWORD

Minimally invasive surgery is increasingly popular with management in the drive to reduce hospital expenditure and especially the expense of patients' stay overnight in hospital after surgical procedures. Moreover, our patients can benefit enormously through reduced disturbance of their well-being and less interference with metabolic and other physiological processes. It has been made possible by amazing developments in surgical techniques such that conventional surgery for many procedures as we used to know them hardly exists today. Historically, advances in surgery were made possible through advances in anaesthesia; however, to some extent, at least, the boot is on the other foot because these advances in surgery through minimally invasive (so-called keyhole) techniques have demanded the refinement and development of existing anaesthetic techniques and the introduction of new drugs. Notably, these methods require keeping the patient safe at all times and returning the patient to full consciousness extremely rapidly, yet with freedom from pain, immediately the surgical procedure is completed.

Prof. Tom Crozier, with long-standing experience of this subject, writes from Göttingen – arguably the foremost centre of excellence of anaesthesia in Europe. Readers will note that, first and foremost, this is an essentially practical book. He defines the subject in terms of practicalities such that some often overlooked aspects, for example surgery of the upper aerodigestive tract, are included. This is eminently sensible in a book of this kind. In the early days of minimally invasive surgery some terrible disasters – unnoticed perforated bowel, massive haemorrhage from damaged vessels, gas embolism, etc. – befell some patients. Most often this was due to poor surgery by inexperienced surgeons; this hastened the need for absolutely continuous and complete monitoring of the patient by the anaesthetist on a beat-by-beat and breath-by-breath basis, surely the tenet of any form of first-class modern anaesthetic care. Fortunately, much of this surveillance can easily be carried out with modern patient monitoring equipment but it must be backed up by the attention of the attending anaesthetist and interpretation using all his vital senses.

Minimally invasive surgery continues to expand. However, now is a good time to consolidate and review anaesthetists' requirements in this area and Tom Crozier has included consideration of bariatric surgery, laser surgery, thoracic surgery and neurosurgery since these areas nowadays are tending to become minimally invasive. He has performed his task extremely well.

Anthony P Adams

Emeritus Professor of Anaesthetics in the University of London at Guy's, King's & St Thomas' Hospitals' School of Medicine; lately Editor-in-Chief, European Journal of Anaesthesiology.

London, UK
July 2004.

ACKNOWLEDGEMENTS

This book was made possible by the support and input of many friends and colleagues from many specialties, whose contributed time and resources greatly enriched the results. Without the initial enthusiasm, innovative activities and cooperation of members of the department of general surgery, particularly Dr Thomas Neufang, Dr Gerd Lepsien and Dr Olaf Horstmann, for the evolving techniques of laparoscopic surgery, my experience in the anaesthetic management of these operations would have been very limited, and several of our research projects would not have been possible. I must thank Dr Arnd Timmermann of the Department of Anaesthesiology, Emergency and Intensive Care Medicine, Dr Ralph Rödel of the Department of Otorhinolaryngology and Dr Hilmar Dörge of the Department of Cardiothoracic Surgery for contributing valuable photographic material.

Prof. Dietrich Kettler, chairman of our Department of Anaesthesiology, Emergency and Intensive Care Medicine, deserves honourable mention for providing research facilities and a creative environment in which this project could come to fruition.

Prof. Ulrich Braun, section head of our department and current president of the European Airway Management Society, provided me with a number of important tips on airway management in the course of many discussions.

I am particularly indebted to Prof. Wolfgang Steiner, chairman of our university's Department of Otorhinolaryngology, for his critical comments on the first draft of the chapter on laser surgery, and for the contribution of numerous illustrations for this chapter from his vast photographic archives.

I must extend my thanks to Prof. Michael Buchfelder, chairman of the Department of Neurosurgery and authority on endoscopic pituitary surgery, and his associate Dr Hans Ludwig, specialist for endoscopic neurosurgery, for their useful input on the topic of minimally invasive neurosurgery.

My colleagues in the Department of Anaesthesiology deserve particularly heartfelt mention for their interest in this project and their unspoken, amused tolerance of my preoccupation.

But above all, I am deeply grateful for the support, enthusiasm and patience of my wife, Chris, and our children, Jesse, Tristan, Julian and Hanna, who had to put up with a permanently distracted, frequently distraught, and repeatedly despairing family member during the final months running up to the manuscript deadline. Without them, this book would not have happened.

Göttingen,
July 22, 2004

The term *minimally invasive surgery* conjures up an image of innovation and cutting-edge technology that differs in a fundamental way from conventional surgical methods. Novel procedures have been introduced that have a spectrum of complications and contra-indications that differs distinctly from that of the conventional method and requires a modification of standard anaesthetic management. These, obviously, deserve to be dealt with in detail in a book on peri-operative management from the more comprehensive viewpoint of the anaesthetist. But all attempts at a general definition of which procedures should be included show how elusive the term actually is. If one takes it to describe procedures that do not require large incisions or extensive tissue destruction, it would include such diverse operations as circumcisions, cataract extractions or transurethral bladder surgery – none of which belong in this book. What then is the characteristic, the common denominator of what we generally refer to as "minimally invasive"? The answer lies in the context: minimally invasive does not refer to the magnitude of invasiveness as an absolute measure, but rather to the invasiveness compared with that of the conventional procedure. Add to this the element of novelty and a particular relevance for anaesthesia and one has a fairly good description of the scope of this book.

Minimally invasive surgery has virtually revolution-ized the surgical therapy of a large variety of diseases in the space of just a few years. While progress in the more spectacular surgical specialties, such as heart surgery, organ transplantation, or separating Siamese twins, captures the public imagination to a greater degree, these benefit only a small segment of the population. Endoscopic surgery, on the other hand, has changed the management of some of the most fre-quently performed surgical procedures, the most notable among these being gall bladder surgery. The continuing interest in endoscopic surgery is not only due to its aesthetic and cosmetic advantages, but also to the potentially smoother postoperative course, with fewer complications and a swifter return of the patient to his normal daily life. However, in order to exploit this potential to its fullest, perioperative anaesthetic management must adapt to the altered requirements of the new techniques.

Most, but not all, of these procedures are performed through small incisions with the aid of an endoscope. This has led some, particularly in the UK, to prefer the term "minimal access surgery". The endoscope most frequently used is the laparoscope, and the pro-cedures are sometimes referred to collectively as laparoscopic surgery, even though the operation site might be in the retroperitoneum or the mediastinum. Since these are the operations that started the present fascination with minimal invasiveness, and are also the ones whose anaesthetic management differ most from conventional operations, they shall be dealt with first in this introductory chapter.

Laparoscopy itself is not a new technique, but one that has been in use since the beginning of the 20th century, although it was mainly used only for diagnostic purposes. The urologist Georg Kelling examined the peritoneal cavity of a dog in 1901 with the aid of a cystoscope, and called the procedure "*koelioskopie*", the term by which it is still known in France.[1] In 1910, Jacobaeus described the first major series of such exam-inations in humans, in whom he studied both the peri-toneal and the thoracic cavities.[2] He coined the terms "Laparoskopie" and "Thorakoskopie" to describe the two techniques. Kalk improved the optical instruments and used two trocars instead of only one.[3] In 1938, Janos Veress introduced the insufflation needle that still bears his name (Figure 1.1).[4] The introduction of auto-matic insufflation devices resulted from the innovative

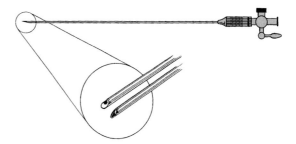

Figure 1.1 Details of the Veress needle. The round tip of the spring-loaded obturator is pushed back into the needle shaft while the needle tip is penetrating the abdominal wall. It springs forward as soon as the needle tip has cleared the peritoneum and protects against damage to the intestine or other viscera.

work of Karl Semm in the 1960s. Surgical working conditions were improved greatly by attaching a video camera to the endoscope and transmitting the view to a television monitor. This allowed the surgeon to stand in a normal position, and also made it possible to train several assistants simultaneously.

Gynaecologists, above all Semm and Lindemann, were the ones who pioneered the development of a technique with which intra-abdominal operations could be carried out without having to make a large abdominal incision.[5] This led to a marked increase in the number of laparoscopic operations in the 1970s, when laparoscopic ligation of the Fallopian tubes became a popular method of contraception.

The first laparoscopic cholecystectomy, which might be regarded as the birth of minimally invasive surgery as we understand it, was performed by Philippe Mouret in Lyons in March 1987. From this moment on, the technique spread worldwide, despite the controversy it ignited and the vigorous initial resistance from parts of the surgical establishment.[6–8] In time, other surgical specialties, such as urology, gynaecology and thoracic surgery, developed their own applications for the endoscopic technique and the cholecystectomy was joined by numerous other indications and operations.

One salient feature of the boom in laparoscopic surgery was the dramatic increase in the average duration of the operations due to the shift in the spectrum of surgical procedures. While the usual maximum duration of the typical diagnostic or sterilization procedure was less than 20 min, the average duration of laparoscopic operations is now 60–120 min, with some even lasting many hours. A second feature of the rapid expansion was that the indications widened to encompass a completely different patient population; whereas laparoscopic surgery had been formerly performed mainly on healthy young women, all age groups were now represented, from the hypotrophic, premature neonate to the nonagenarian. The method was also no longer restricted to large medical centres, but had spread with incredible speed on a broad front with even small- and medium-sized hospitals taking advantage of the new techniques. These factors meant that every anaesthetist was likely to be required to deal with laparoscopic operations of varying difficulty at some point.

Laparoscopic operations

In the short time since the first laparoscopic cholecystectomy was performed, development has advanced at such a rapid pace that there is now almost no surgical procedure that has not at least been attempted with endoscopic methods. Certain standard laparoscopic operations have become part of the repertoire of nearly every moderately well-equipped clinic. There is then the shifting group of laparoscopic operations that are routinely performed in specialized centres, and although no longer regarded as investigational, nevertheless require the experience of specialists. And then there is a continuously growing list of laparoscopic procedures that stand more or less at the cutting edge of medical science – some of which find their way into clinical routine, while others are dropped as not practicable. Laparoscopic operations routinely offered by many hospitals include cholecystectomy, appendectomy,[9,10] tubal ligation, treatment of ectopic pregnancies, minor urological operations and many others.[11,12] Other operations such as hernia repair, laparoscopically-assisted vaginal hysterectomy,[13–15] enucleation of myomas, ovarial cysts, etc.[16–20] have also become standard.

Some hospitals perform extensive abdominal and thoracic operations endoscopically, including major bowel resections, pancreatectomy, splenectomy and even oesophagectomy.[21–26] A wide range of urological operations such as nephrectomy,[27–29] adrenalectomy[24] or radical prostatectomy with retroperitoneal lymphadenectomy[30] are performed endoscopically. Paediatric urology is another field in which endoscopic operations are becoming very common.[31] Opinions

Table 1.1 Selected endoscopic operations	
Operation	**Where conducted**
Cholecystectomy	General hospitals
Hernia repair	
Appendectomy	
Tubal ligation	
Uterine myomas	
Cryptorchism, orchidopexy	
Ectopic pregnancy	
Oophorectomy etc.	
Colorectal surgery	Specialized centres
Gastric surgery	
Splenectomy	
Bariatric surgery	
Lung surgery	
Coronary artery surgery	
Thoracic sympathectomy	
Oesophagectomy	
Nephrectomy, kidney donor nephrectomy	
Adrenalectomy	
Radical prostatectomy	
Hepatic resection	
Retroperitoneal and pelvic lymphadenectomy etc.	

are divided regarding the question of whether laparoscopic surgery of malignant tumours is contraindicated,[30,32,33] while another controversy involves the question of whether laparoscopic surgery is contraindicated during pregnancy.[34–36] Obesity was once considered almost an absolute contraindication against laparoscopic surgery, but has now morphed into a strong indication.[37,38] Even weight reduction surgery in the morbidly obese is thought to have a lower total risk of serious complications when performed laparoscopically. Table 1.1 presents an overview of the range of endoscopically performed operations. This list is neither comprehensive nor final, as new techniques are constantly being added, and interventions regarded as investigational at best today, will have become routine operations tomorrow. The use of new techniques, such as the abdominal wall lift[39,40] or balloon dilators,[41] will help to avoid the problems associated with gas insufflation and increases of intra-abdominal pressure (IAP).[42]

Technical aspects of laparoscopic surgery

Laparoscopic operations are basically very standardized procedures that begin and end with a set sequence of events. A brief description of these phases will help to understand the contribution required of the anaesthetist and also to understand the pathology of a number of potentially lethal complications that can occur during laparoscopic surgery, most of which are caused by faulty surgical technique or malfunctioning equipment. These points will be taken up in more detail in the following chapters.

In the first step of the operation, the abdomen is inflating by leading gas into the abdominal cavity under pressure to create a pneumoperitoneum. This is sometimes referred to as a capnoperitoneum[43] in order to call attention to the particular problems that arise from using carbon dioxide (CO_2) as the insufflation gas (see Chapter 2). The surgeon lifts the ventral wall of the abdomen and introduces a specially designed safety needle through a small incision in the navel (Figure 1.2) for the initial inflation phase. The abdominal muscles must be well relaxed for this manoeuvre to succeed. This needle, known as a Veress needle after its inventor, is about 3–4 mm in diameter, and has a blunt, spring-loaded obturator that protrudes past the tip of the needle (see Figure 1.1). When the needle meets firm resistance, as for example when it is pushed through fascia or muscle, the tip of the obturator is pressed back, exposing the sharp tip of the needle. After the needle penetrates the

peritoneum, the obturator tip springs forward, preventing the needle from damaging the intestines or other intra-abdominal organs. Once the correct intraperitoneal position of the Veress needle has been confirmed, insufflation is started slowly and the patient is monitored closely. The gas flow rate is then increased and the abdomen inflated to a pressure of about 12 to 15 mmHg. IAP is kept constant with an electronically controlled insufflator (Figure 1.3) at a level sufficient to maintain optimal operating conditions for the surgeon (usually about 10–15 mmHg). Neuromuscular block must be sufficient during this period to keep the abdominal cavity compliant, and to prevent its being compressed by the return of muscular tension.

The typical adverse events that can happen during this phase of the operation is the insufflation of gas into preperitoneal tissue or directly into a blood vessel. The former is not infrequent, but is rarely serious, and requires no particular action on the part of the anaesthetist. Intravascular gas insufflation, on the other hand, can be extremely serious and requires rapid, deliberate action to avoid a lethal outcome (see Chapters 2 and 6).

When the abdomen has been sufficiently inflated, the Veress needle is removed and replaced with a larger trocar introduced through the same incision (Figure 1.4). The primary complication of this manoeuvre is injury to large vessels, such as the aorta or the iliac vessels,[44,45] or perforation of hollow viscera. Safety trocars with a sharp tip that retracts itself automatically once it has passed the peritoneum are now available. The obturator in the trocar is then removed and a laparoscope is introduced through the sleeve and used to guide the placing of the following trocars, the number and location of which vary according to the operation. The first trocar is used for intraoperative

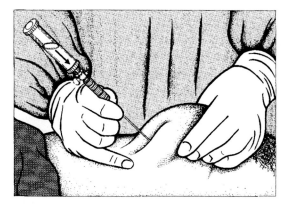

Figure 1.2 Blind introduction of the Veress needle.

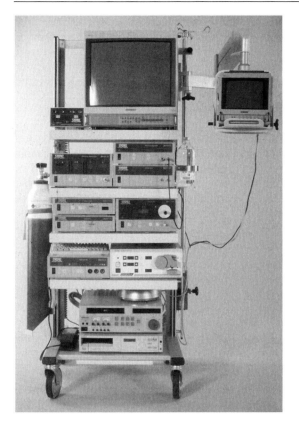

Figure 1.3 The basic mobile unit for laparoscopic surgery. The unit contains the insufflator for creating and maintaining a constant pressure in the body cavity, a bottle of pressurized CO_2, a peristaltic pump to irrigate and rinse the surgical field, a cold-light unit for illumination of the surgical field, a diathermy unit for coagulation and cutting, a video monitor for observing the operation and a video recorder for documentation.

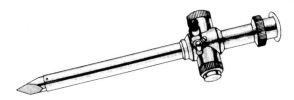

Figure 1.4 Trocar with sharp obturator.

insufflation and it can become dislodged with resulting insufflation of gas into preperitoneal tissues. The anaesthetist is frequently the first to notice this problem when end-tidal CO_2 concentrations start to rise.

Statistics on the mortality associated with laparoscopy are available from 1949 to the present. In the period from 1949 to 1977, when it was primarily a diagnostic

procedure, there was a mortality rate of 0.09% of a total of 265,900 laparoscopies performed. From 1983 to 1985, the rate had fallen to 0.024% of almost 250,000 operations.[46,47] In the US in the year 1977–1978, a mortality rate of 0.04% was registered for 750,000 sterilizations, which were carried out by laparoscopy as well as laparotomy. Of the cases resulting in death, 16 occurred in connection with laparoscopy, of which six were classified as anaesthetic complications. Even for the very short surgical procedures evaluated in this study, the risk of death was low but not negligible, considering that the patients were healthy and young. The expanding range of indications with operations having an order of magnitude increase in duration, and the inclusion of patients from extreme age groups and high-risk patients with serious pre-existing pathologies will obviously increase the risk of morbidity and mortality. The realization of this fact should act as a clear warning against incautiously equating minimal invasiveness of the operation with minimal risk to the patient, and should induce the anaesthetist to do his or her utmost to contribute towards minimizing this risk. The most important factors that the anaesthetist has to take into account during laparoscopic operations are the pathophysiological changes due to gas insufflation, the risk of intravascular gas injection and the occasionally extreme position of the patient.

There are other entire groups of minimally invasive operations that are not performed by laparoscopy and thus are not associated with the problems of the pneumoperitoneum and CO_2 insufflation. They will be described in detail in their respective chapters and are therefore only mentioned shortly at this point. Among these are thoracoscopic surgery, minimal access cardiac and coronary surgery, endoscopic laser surgery of the aerodigestive tract and endoscopic neurosurgery. Thoracoscopic operations differ less from their conventional counterparts than the laparoscopic operations do from theirs, and anaesthetic management will not require the same extent of adaptive modifications. The peripheral lung is easily accessible with an endoscope, and thoracoscopic operations, such as wedge resection or lobectomy, ablation of blebs and others have become common.[48–50] The mediastinum can be approached either by the traditional suprasternal access or through the pleural cavity after allowing the lung to collapse.[51,52] Cardiac and coronary artery surgery can be considered minimally invasive if they avoid using a midline sternotomy or extracorporeal circulation, the two factors that contribute most to the invasiveness of the conventional methods.[53] Endoscopic laser surgery of the aerodigestive tract allows operations that are not possible by any other means.[54] Tissue trauma can be extensive when considered in relation to the narrow anatomy of the larynx, but postoperative recovery is rapid and usually uneventful. Endoscopic and microsurgical procedures in neurosurgery are truly much less invasive than their conventional counterparts and do not generally require any modification of anaesthetic management.

The following chapters will deal with important anaesthesiological aspects of modern minimally invasive surgery, be it endoscopic surgery of the abdomen or thorax, endoscopic laser surgery of the larynx and adjacent structures, or endoscopic neurosurgery. They are designed to offer the anaesthetist the specialized theoretical and practical knowledge which he or she needs to meet the particular challenges of these operations, and to provide competent anaesthetic care with optimal risk reduction for the patient.

References

1. Kelling G. Über Oesophagoskopie, Gastroskopie und Koelioskopie. *Munchen Med Wochenschr* 1901; **49**: 21–31.
2. Jacobaeus HC. Über die Möglichkeit die Zystoskopie bei Untersuchung seröser Höhlungen anzuwenden. *München Med Wochenschr* 1910; **57**: 2090–2098.
3. Kalk H. Erfahrungen mit der Laparoskopie. *Z klin Med* 1929; **111**: 303–319.
4. Veress J. Neues Instrument zur Ausführung von Brust-oder Bauchpunktionen und Pneumothoraxbehandlung. *Dtsch Med Wochenschr* 1938; **41**: 1480–1483.
5. Semm K. *Pelviskopie und Hysteroskopie*. Stuttgart: Schattauer Verlag, 1976.
6. Keith RG. Laparoscopic cholecystectomy: let us control the virus. *Can J Surg* 1990; **33**: 435–436.
7. Miller TA. Laparoscopic cholecystectomy: passing fancy or legitimate treatment option? *Gastroenterology* 1990; **99**: 1527–1529.
8. Tompkins RK. Laparoscopic cholecystectomy. Threat or opportunity? *Arch Surg* 1990; **125**: 1245.
9. Nowzaradan Y, Westmoreland J, McCarver CT, Harris RJ. Laparoscopic appendectomy for acute appendicitis: indications and current use. *J Laparoendosc Surg* 1991; **1**: 247–257.
10. Pier A, Gotz F, Bacher C. Laparoscopic appendectomy in 625 cases: from innovation to routine. *Surg Laparosc Endosc* 1991; **1**: 8–13.
11. Fahlenkamp D, Raatz D, Schonberger B. Laparoskopische Diagnose und Therapie des Kryptorchismus. *Urologe A* 1992; **31**: 328–332.
12. Jarow JP, Assimos DG, Pittaway DE. Effectiveness of laparoscopic varicocelectomy. *Urology* 1993; **42**: 544–547.
13. Gill F, Wierrani F, Grunberger W. Die pelviskopische Hysterektomie – eine prospektive Vergleichsstudie über 40 Fälle [Pelviscopic hysterectomy – a prospective comparative study of 40 cases]. *Geburtshilfe Frauenheilkd* 1992; **52**: 681–683.
14. Semm K. Hysterektomie per laparotomiam oder per pelviskopiam. Ein neuer Weg ohne Kolpotomie durch CASH [Hysterectomy via laparotomy or pelviscopy. A new CASH method without colpotomy]. *Geburtshilfe Frauenheilkd* 1991; **51**: 996–1003.
15. Daniell JF, Kurtz BR, McTavish G *et al.* Laparoscopically assisted vaginal hysterectomy. The initial Nashville, Tennessee, experience. *J Reprod Med* 1993; **38**: 537–542.
16. Chatwani A, Yazigi R, Amin-Hanjani S. Operative laparoscopy in the management of tubal ectopic pregnancy. *J Laparoendosc Surg* 1992; **2**: 319–324.
17. Lehmann-Willenbrock E, Mecke H, Semm K. Pelviskopische Ovarialchirurgie–eine retrospektive Untersuchung von 1016 operierten Zysten. *Geburtshilfe Frauenheilkd* 1991; **51**: 280–287.
18. Mettler L, Caesar G, Neunzling S, Semm K. Stellenwert der endoskopischen Ovar-Chirurgie – kritische Analyse von 626 pelviskopisch operierten Ovarialzysten an der Universitats-Frauenklinik Kiel 1990–1991 [Value of endoscopic ovarian surgery – critical analysis of 626 pelviscopically operated ovarian cysts at the Kiel University Gynecologic Clinic 1990–1991]. *Geburtshilfe Frauenheilkd* 1993; **53**: 253–257.
19. Neeser E, Hirsch HA. Diagnostische und therapeutische Eingriffe bei Extrauteringraviditat [Diagnostic and therapeutic interventions in extrauterine pregnancy]. *Geburtshilfe Frauenheilkd* 1987; **47**: 149–153.
20. Nezhat F, Winer W, Nezhat C. Salpingectomy via laparoscopy: a new surgical approach. *J Laparoendosc Surg* 1991; **1**: 91–95.
21. Law WL, Chu KW, Tung PH. Laparoscopic colorectal resection: a safe option for elderly patients. *J Am Coll Surg* 2002; **195**: 768–773.
22. Cuschieri SA, Jakimowicz JJ. Laparoscopic pancreatic resections. *Semin Laparosc Surg* 1998; **5**: 168–179.
23. Rescorla FJ, Engum SA, West KW, Tres Scherer III LR, Rouse TM, Grosfeld JL. Laparoscopic splenectomy has become the gold standard in children. *Am Surg* 2002; **68**: 297–301.
24. Heslin MJ, Winzeler AH, Weingarten JO, Diethelm AG, Urist MM, Bland KI. Laparoscopic adrenalectomy and splenectomy are safe and reduce hospital stay and charges. *Am Surg* 2003; **69**: 377–381.
25. Collard JM, Lengele B, Otte JB, Kestens PJ. En bloc and standard esophagectomies by thoracoscopy. *Ann Thorac Surg* 1993; **56**: 675–679.
26. Gossot D, Fourquier P, Celerier M. Thoracoscopic esophagectomy: technique and initial results. *Ann Thorac Surg* 1993; **56**: 667–670.
27. Hensman C, Lionel G, Hewett P, Rao MM. Laparoscopic live donor nephrectomy: the preliminary experience. *Aust NZ J Surg* 1999; **69**: 365–368.
28. Clayman RV, Kavoussi LR, Figenshau RS, Chandhoke PS, Albala DM. Laparoscopic nephroureterectomy: initial clinical case report. *J Laparoendosc Surg* 1991; **1**: 343–349.
29. Kavoussi LR, Kerbl K, Capelouto CC, McDougall EM, Clayman RV. Laparoscopic nephrectomy for renal neoplasms. *Urology* 1993; **42**: 603–609.

30. Rassweiler J, Tsivian A, Kumar AV *et al.* Oncological safety of laparoscopic surgery for urological malignancy: experience with more than 1000 operations. *J Urol* 2003; **169**: 2072–2075.

31. Peters CA. Laparoscopy in pediatric urology. *Curr Opin Urol* 2004; **14**: 67–73.

32. Ordemann J, Jacobi CA, Schwenk W, Stosslein R, Muller JM. Cellular and humoral inflammatory response after laparoscopic and conventional colorectal resections. *Surg Endosc* 2001; **15**: 600–608.

33. Wexner SD, Cohen SM. Port site metastases after laparoscopic colorectal surgery for cure of malignancy. *Br J Surg* 1995; **82**: 295–298.

34. Reedy MB, Kallen B, Kuehl TJ. Laparoscopy during pregnancy: a study of five fetal outcome parameters with use of the Swedish Health Registry. *Am J Obstet Gynecol* 1997; **177**: 673–679.

35. Al-Fozan H, Tulandi T. Safety and risks of laparoscopy in pregnancy. *Curr Opin Obstet Gynecol* 2002; **14**: 375–379.

36. Oelsner G, Stockheim D, Soriano D *et al.* Pregnancy outcome after laparoscopy or laparotomy in pregnancy. *J Am Assoc Gynecol Laparosc* 2003; **10**: 200–204.

37. Gadacz TR, Talamini MA. Traditional versus laparoscopic cholecystectomy. *Am J Surg* 1991; **161**: 336–338.

38. Miles RH, Carballo RE, Prinz RA *et al.* Laparoscopy: the preferred method of cholecystectomy in the morbidly obese. *Surgery* 1992; **112**: 818–822.

39. Paolucci V, Gutt CN, Schaeff B, Encke A. Gasless laparoscopy in abdominal surgery. *Surg Endosc* 1995; **9**: 497–500.

40. Volz J, Volz E, Koster S, Weiss M, Wischnik A, Melchert F. Pelviskopisches Operieren ohne Pneumoperitoneum? Eine neue Methode und ihre Auswirkungen auf die Narkose. *Geburtshilfe Frauenheilkd* 1993; **53**: 258–260.

41. Kieturakis MJ, Nguyen DT, Vargas H, Fogarty TJ, Klein SR. Balloon dissection facilitated laparoscopic extraperitoneal hernioplasty. *Am J Surg* 1994; **168**: 603–607.

42. Andersson L, Lindberg G, Bringman S, Ramel S, Anderberg B, Odeberg Wernerman S. Pneumoperitoneum versus abdominal wall lift: effects on central haemodynamics and intrathoracic pressure during laparoscopic cholecystectomy. *Acta Anaesthesiol Scand* 2003; **47**: 838–846.

43. Blobner M, Felber AR, Hosl P, Gogler S, Schneck HJ, Jelen Esselborn S. Auswirkungen des Kapnoperitoneums auf den postoperativen Kohlendioxidhaushalt. *Anaesthesist* 1994; **43**: 718–722.

44. Bacourt F, Mercier F. Plaies de l'aorte abdominale au cours des laparoscopies [Injuries to the abdominal aorta during laparoscopy]. *Chirurgie* 1993; **119**: 457–461.

45. Apelgren KN, Scheeres DE. Aortic injury. A catastrophic complication of laparoscopic cholecystectomy. *Surg Endosc* 1994; **8**: 689–691.

46. Riedel HH, Lehmann Willenbrock E, Conrad P, Semm K. German pelviscopic statistics for the years 1978–1982. *Endoscopy* 1986; **18**: 219–222.

47. Riedel HH, Lehmann Willenbrock E, Mecke H, Semm K. The frequency distribution of various pelviscopic (laparoscopic) operations, including complications rates – statistics of the Federal Republic of Germany in the years 1983–1985. *Zentralbl Gynakol* 1989; **111**: 78–91.

48. Kirby TJ, Rice TW. Thoracoscopic lobectomy. *Ann Thorac Surg* 1993; **56**: 784–786.

49. Inderbitzi R, Furrer M, Klaiber C, Ris HB, Striffeler H, Althaus U. Thoracoscopic wedge resection. *Surg Endosc* 1992; **6**: 189–192.

50. Hazelrigg SR, Landreneau RJ, Mack M *et al.* Thoracoscopic stapled resection for spontaneous pneumothorax. *J Thorac Cardiovasc Surg* 1993; **105**: 389–392.

51. Fiocco M, Krasna MJ. Thoracoscopic lymph node dissection in the staging of esophageal carcinoma. *J Laparoendosc Surg* 1992; **2**: 111–115.

52. Facciolo F, Sposi A, Catarci M, Della-Rocca G, Carboni M, Ricci C. Thoracoscopic resection of mediastinal cystic schwannoma. *Surg Endosc* 1993; **7**: 447–449.

53. Detter C, Reichenspurner H, Boehm DH *et al.* Minimally invasive direct coronary artery bypass grafting (MIDCAB) and off-pump coronary artery bypass grafting (OPCAB): two techniques for beating heart surgery. *Heart Surg Forum* 2002; **5**: 157–162.

54. Steiner W, Ambrosch P. *Endoscopic Laser Surgery of the Upper Aerodigestive Tract: With Special Emphasis on Cancer Surgery.* 2nd edition. New York: Thieme Medical Publisher, 2001.

The physiological consequences of laparoscopic–endoscopic surgery are primarily due to the effects of increased intra-abdominal pressure (IAP) and the systemic absorption of the insufflated gas. The magnitude of these changes is modulated by the position of the patient and the choice of insufflation gas.

Operations in the peritoneum, uterus or bladder require active expansion of the pre-existing cavity by the application of exogenous pressure. This is usually unnecessary for thoracoscopy, where the self-retracting tendency of the lungs is exploited and reinflation of the lungs is prevented by a selective ventilation, such as with a double-lumen endotracheal tube. In operations on organs surrounded by connective tissue, such as in the retroperitoneum (nephrectomy, adrenalectomy, lymphadenectomy), the groin (hernia repair), or in the mediastinum, an artificial cavity must be created with insufflated gas or with the aid of a dilation balloon. The specific effects of these measures will occur in addition to the already ongoing changes resulting from anaesthesia and surgery.

Circulation

During laparoscopic surgery, the circulation undergoes typical changes of cardiac output (CO), blood pressure, venous pressure and cardiac filling pressures that are the result of the complex interactions between anaesthesia, patient position, pressure changes in the body cavities and neuroendocrine reactions. Depending on the circumstances, the effects of these factors can either reinforce each other or they can cancel each other out.

Increased IAP and the patient's position (supine, head-down Trendelenburg, or head-up reverse Trendelenburg) are – given constant arterial carbon dioxide (CO_2) tension – the main determinants governing circulatory changes during laparoscopy. These two factors must be considered separately, since they can either reinforce or oppose each other, depending on body position. If ventilation is not adjusted properly, CO_2 retention will occur causing initial stimulation and then, ultimately, depression of the circulation, depending on the extent of the resulting hypercapnia and acidosis (see the following text).

Cholecystectomy is one of the most common laparoscopic operations, and a discussion of the effects of laparoscopic surgery on the circulation should be begin with this operation that is typically performed with the patient in the reverse Trendelenburg, head-up position. Joris and co-workers[1] describe the typical haemodynamic course of a laparoscopic cholecystectomy in healthy patients in a 15–30° head-up position. After induction of anaesthesia in the supine patient, there is usually a parallel reduction of CO and mean arterial pressure (MAP). Changing from the supine to the reverse Trendelenburg position induces a further fall in blood pressure and CO accompanied by a decrease in right and left ventricular filling pressures, measured as right atrial pressure (RAP) and pulmonary capillary wedge pressure (PCWP).[2]

Inflating the abdomen with the patient in this position causes an initial increase in MAP, RAP and PCWP with a decrease in CO. Systemic blood pressure gradually returns to the baseline level at anaesthesia induction, RAP and PCWP increase to above their initial levels, while CO decreases still further. There is a sharp rise in peripheral systemic vascular resistance (SVR), which is partly responsible for the observed increase in blood pressure. The changes in MAP and central venous pressure (CVP) are significantly less when the abdominal cavity is expanded with an external lift and not by increasing IAP.[3,4]

This situation lasts only for about 15–20 min, after which CO returns to the baseline level before insufflation, blood pressure remains constant, and SVR decreases slightly, while RAP and PCWP still remain elevated. Since the reduction of CO lasts only such a short time, it may be easily missed if measurements are not timed properly. This could be a reason for the contradictory results of various studies. Figure 2.1 summarizes the behaviour of CO in the studies of Joris *et al.*[1] and Reid *et al.*[5] The reasons for the gradual normalization of CO are not entirely clear. Some authors see it secondary to a reduction in afterload, while others consider positive inotropic effects subsequent to sympathetic nervous system activation by absorbed CO_2 to be the decisive factor. As described in more detail below, CO does not recover if nitrous oxide (N_2O) rather than CO_2 is used for insufflation.

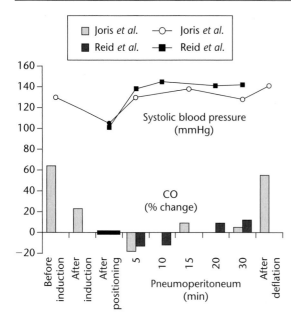

Figure 2.1 Postoperative CO changes after laparoscopic cholecystectomy. Relative changes after induction of anaesthesia and positioning of patient as well as at various times after begin of pneumoperitoneum (PP) are shown. For ease of comparing the two studies the value determined after the patient had been positioned was defined as 100%.[1,5]

This argues in favour of hypercapnia-induced activation of the sympathetic nervous system as the force driving haemodynamic normalization.

The increases in RAP and wedge pressure measured against atmosphere are the consequence of increased IAP, an increase which is transmitted into the thorax.[4] This should not automatically be assumed to reflect a rise in cardiac filling, since in the Trendelenburg position, intrathoracic pressure increases to an equal or even greater extent, so that effective transmural atrial pressures may even decrease[4] (Table 2.1). This is supported by the echocardiographic study of Cunningham et al.,[6] which shows a decrease in end-diastolic left ventricular volume. In the head-up position, gravity-induced reduction of venous return causes the initial decrease in CO. Increasing IAP during pneumoperitoneum reduces blood flow in the inferior vena cava with venous congestion and blood pooling in the lower extremities and a further reduction in cardiac filling volumes (Figure 2.2).[7,8] A more recent model uses the Starling resistor concept to explain the behaviour of pressures and blood flow in the intrathoracic and intra-abdominal inferior vena cava.[9] Elevated IAP in patients with ascites is known to cause narrowing of the cephalad portion of the intra-abdominal vena cava,[10] and this is also observed during pneumoperitoneum.[11] Increasing IAP in

Table 2.1 Changes in right atrial filling pressures in animal studies and in patients after creation of pneumoperitoneum under different conditions. There is a consistent reduction of transmural pressures that reflects reduced cardiac filling

A. Studies in dogs after creation of pneumoperitoneum with CO_2 or N_2O with different IAP[a]

Duration (min)	0	5	10	15	20	25
IAP (mmHg)	0	20	20	30	40	0
Right atrial pressure (RAP)						
CO_2	6.5 ± 3	12.5 ± 7	14.3 ± 8	14.6 ± 9	15.9 ± 11	6.0 ± 3
N_2O	6.0 ± 3	13.1 ± 7	13.0 ± 9	14.1 ± 8	16.8 ± 11	6.4 ± 3
Intrathoracic pressure						
CO_2	3.8 ± 2	11.6 ± 6	12.8 ± 5	14.0 ± 6	15.1 ± 7	3.9 ± 2
N_2O	3.8 ± 2	11.6 ± 6	12.2 ± 7	13.1 ± 9	15.9 ± 10	4.5 ± 2
Transmural atrial pressure (RAP_{tm})						
CO_2	2.7 ± 1.2	0.9 ± 0.5	1.5 ± 0.9	0.6 ± 0.3	0.9 ± 0.5	2.1 ± 1.2
N_2O	2.2 ± 1.1	2.1 ± 1.1	0.8 ± 0.3	1.0 ± 0.5	0.9 ± 0.4	1.9 ± 0.9

B. Patients in reverse Trendelenburg position and CO_2 pneumoperitoneum with constant IAP of 14 mmHg.[b] Intrathoracic pressure increased (ΔITP) during the study

Duration (min)	0	5	15	30	0
RAP	5.0	11.0	10.0	10.0	8
ΔITP	0	9.4	9.6	8.7	0
RAP_{tm}	5	1.6	0.4	1.3	8

[a] Adapted from Ivankovich et al.[26]

[b] Adapted from Joris et al.[1]

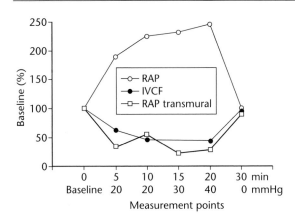

Figure 2.2 Changes of IAP and blood flow in the inferior vena cava (IVCF). RAP increases with increasing IAP (abscissa). However, transmural filling pressure (RAP$_{tm}$) decreases significantly, while IVCF is also reduced. (Adapted from Ref [26].)

study animals by the intraperitoneal instillation of normal saline solution established a pressure gradient between the intra- and extrathoracic portions of the inferior vena cava.[12] Clinical studies in patients undergoing laparoscopic cholecystectomy showed that increasing IAP also increases the pressure gradient between intrathoracic and intra-abdominal vena cava pressures.[9] A rise in IAP as occurs during pneumoperitoneum will impair venous return through the inferior vena cava. Blood flow into the thorax will cease whenever transmural pressure across the wall of the vein falls to zero or below. Evidence that this actually occurs is given by the observation that blood flow in the femoral vein is slowed and ceases intermittently in patients undergoing laparoscopic cholecystectomy.[13,14]

Reduction of cardiac filling is seen as the primary cause of reduced CO. This view is supported by observations in animal experiments, in which CO changed only slightly in normovolaemic animals, but fell markedly when they were hypovolaemic. In over-infused, hypervolaemic animals, on the other hand, CO increased by ca. 50% over the baseline values.[15] On the other hand, Gentili and co-workers presented circumstantial echocardiographic evidence suggesting myocardial dysfunction during laparoscopy in children.[16] During moderate pressure pneumoperitoneum with an IAP of 10 mmHg or less, left ventricular end-diastolic volume increased without the concomitant increase of left ventricular ejection fraction that one might expect according to the Frank–Starling mechanism. Body position itself has an important influence on CO. In animal studies, the head-up position caused a further decrease in CO, while the Trendelenburg position led to a partial normalization.[17] The interdependent factors governing

the circulatory effects of CO_2 pneumoperitoneum in the head-up position are shown schematically in Figure 2.3.

Pneumoperitoneum has been shown to induce or to worsen valvular regurgitation.[18] Increased SVR during pneumoperitoneum, preoperative hydration and head-down positioning are thought to be causal factors.

The situation in the Trendelenburg position with increased IAP differs from that in the head-up position, and the circulatory responses deviate in several important aspects from those described so far. The forces of gravity and IAP that act synergistically in the head-up position to reduce cardiac filling, oppose each other in the head-down position. In the Trendelenburg position, CO either remains constant or can even increase.[19–21] Kelman reports, for example, that the IAP of 15 mmHg normally used for pneumoperitoneum caused an increase in CO, and that CO only decreased when IAP was elevated to 40 mmHg or higher.[19] One of the reasons for the lack of CO reduction is that transmural atrial pressures (RAP$_{tm}$, LAP$_{tm}$) remain unchanged or even increase slightly (Table 1.2) during insufflation with an IAP of 15–20 mmHg in the head-down position, and there was thus no reduction of left ventricular end-diastolic volume.[6]

On the other hand, Lenz et al.[22] and Johannsen et al.[23] reported a decrease in CO of approximately 20%, even though RAP$_{tm}$ remained constant. These contradictory results, however, might be due to methodological short-comings, since CO was measured in these studies by bioimpedance, a method that might have a systematic error under the given study conditions. The bioimpedance method measures changes in a high-frequency signal applied to the thorax with electrodes on the upper and lower thorax aperture. Given a constant thorax geometry, changes in the signal reflect changes in the impedance (Z) assumed to be due to fluctuations in intrathoracic blood volume. Stroke volume (SV) is calculated from the cyclic impedance changes by applying the function

$$SV = f(\mathrm{L}^3)\frac{\mathrm{d}Z}{\mathrm{d}t}Z_0^{-1}$$

or, with older systems, with the function

$$SV = f\left[\left(\frac{L}{Z_0}\right)^2\left(\frac{\mathrm{d}Z}{\mathrm{d}t}\right)_{min}\right]$$

The distance between the upper and lower electrodes (L) enters into the calculation to the third or second power, so that minor deviations in the distance between the electrodes result in large errors. For example, a 6% decrease in L results in a 17% reduction in the calculated SV. A deviation of this magnitude is conceivable

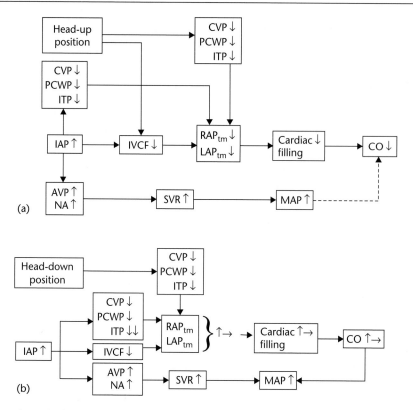

Figure 2.3 Haemodynamic changes during pneumoperitoneum with CO_2: (a) in head-up reverse Trendelenburg position, or (b) in head-down Trendelenburg position. T: Trendelenburg position; rT: reverse Trendelenburg head-up position; ITP: intrathoracic pressure; AVP: vasopressin; NA: norepinephrine; $\uparrow$increase; $\downarrow$decrease; $\uparrow\rightarrow$ no change or only slight increase. (For abbreviation see text.)

in the head-down position and with increased IAP, since the combined effects of gravity and pneumoperitoneum would widen the lower thorax aperture and would thus bring the upper and lower electrodes closer together. Moreover, the basic impedance of the thorax, Z_0, will also be altered to an unknown degree by the shift of diaphragm, liver, spleen and other abdominal organs into the measurement area. Using only a very low IAP (5–8 mmHg) and taking the altered baseline impedance into the equation, as in the study by Ekman et al.,[24] the bioimpedance method yields results similar to those of the dye dilution method. This problem is perhaps not as relevant in the head-up position, since the effects of gravity and the pneumoperitoneum tend to balance each other out.[25]

The blood pressure and peripheral vascular resistance responses to inflation of the abdomen with CO_2 are the same whether the patient is in a supine position, head-down Trendelenburg position or in a head-up position, despite the fact that the change in CO is totally different. This suggests that neuroendocrine stress responses with increased plasma concentrations of norepinephrine, vasopressin and renin–angiotensin, and consequently elevated SVR and not changes in stroke volume are responsible for blood pressure changes (see Section on stress reactions).

Cardiovascular changes during pneumoperitoneum are not only due to the increased IAP, but are also caused by the systemic effects of the absorbed CO_2 and the vegetative reactions to peritoneal irritation. The studies cited so far only investigated the cardiovascular effects of CO_2 as insufflation gas, but using N_2O for inflation instead of CO_2 changes the pattern of cardiovascular effects. Comparing the results of these studies helps to delineate the causative factors.

Ivankovich and co-workers directly compared the haemodynamic changes induced by a pneumoperitoneum with either CO_2 or N_2O in dogs.[26] Although they described the changes as essentially identical, they did observe that after 20 min at an IAP of 20 mmHg CO had decreased by 57% with CO_2 and by only 47% with N_2O, while vascular resistance had increased by 148% with CO_2 and only by 93% with N_2O (Table 2.2).

Table 2.2 Haemodynamic effects of pneumoperitoneum using either CO_2 or N_2O as insufflation gas

Author	Position	Gas	ΔCVP (% or mmHg)	ΔCO (%)	ΔMAP (%)	ΔSVR (%)
Ivankovich dogs[26]	Supine	CO_2	–	−57	+11	+148
		N_2O	–	−47	+7	+93
Rademaker[27]	Head-up	CO_2	−50 (6 → 3)	−31	0	+45
		N_2O	−40 (5 → 3)	−40	−33	+12
Marshall[20,28]	Head-down	CO_2	+38 (8 → 11)	−0.7	+26	+25
		N_2O	+25 (8 → 10)	−23	+17	+49

Changes are given between baseline values after induction of anaesthesia and the value in the described position after creating the pneumoperitoneum.
Note: Changes in CVP (ΔCVP) do not necessary indicate a change in right atrial filling pressure.

Unfortunately, the authors did not test their data for statistical significance.

The results of a comparative study by Rademaker et al.[27] on patients undergoing cholecystectomy carry more weight. They observed a reduction of CO in both the CO_2 as well as the N_2O group, but when the patients were in the reverse Trendelenburg position, the reduction in the group with N_2O was significantly greater. At the same time, MAP and SVR were markedly higher in the CO_2 group (Table 2.2).

Marshall et al. made similar observations using dye dilution in patients in the Trendelenburg position.[20,28] CO exhibited a varying response during inflation with CO_2: it increased in two patients, decreased in two patients and remained constant in three patients. During inflation with N_2O, CO decreased in all patients by approximately 23% (Table 2.2). Blood pressure rose in both groups but the increase was greater in the CO_2 group (26%) than in the N_2O group (17%).

One can see from the results of these studies that using CO_2 as the insufflation gas can partially alleviate the negative effects of increased IAP on CO. This might be due in part to the stimulatory effects of absorbed CO_2 on the sympathetic nervous system, since there was no attempt to maintain normocapnia in any of the studies.[29] However, a different study claims to have found no effect of normocapnia or hypercapnia on blood pressure behaviour.[30]

Predicting the cardiovascular effects of absorbed CO_2 is hampered by the fact that it exerts manifold effects on various segments of the circulation itself and on regulatory functions. Some of these effects directly oppose one another and some act synergistically. CO_2 with acidaemia can reduce myocardial contractility,[31] but in the intact organism this is more than compensated for by the CO_2-induced activation of the

sympathetic nervous system with increases of heart rate, vascular resistance and CO.[32–34] Figure 2.4 gives a synopsis of these interactions. A study in children showed that pneumoperitoneum without hypercapnia caused left ventricular regional wall movement abnormalities.[35]

An increase in SVR, often combined with a coincident increase in MAP is a constant observation in virtually all investigations, while simultaneously measured CO exhibited no consistent relationship with blood pressure. The clinical relevance of this fact is that during laparoscopy one cannot make any inferences about the cardiac pump function or perfusion from the arterial blood pressure. An increase in afterload also has the inherent risk of precipitating cardial decompensation in patients with congestive heart failure. Intravenous nitroglycerine has been used to decrease SVR during laparoscopy and restore haemodynamic function.[36,37]

The consistently occurring blood pressure increase that is usually accompanied by tachycardia, indicates an increase in myocardial oxygen consumption ($M\dot{V}O_2$).[38] The marked rise in the concentration of circulating catecholamines is associated with an increase in the inotropic state of the myocardium and an further increase of $M\dot{V}O_2$. The combination of these factors can compromise patients at cardiovascular risk. Circulatory collapse and dysrhythmias also deserve mention as relevant adverse cardiovascular events. These can be interpreted as resulting either from the activation of the sympathetic nervous system or from a vagal reaction to peritoneal stretching and intra-abdominal manipulation combined with reduced venous return.[39–41]

A study in cardiac transplant patients undergoing laparoscopic cholecystectomy is interesting, despite the small number of patients.[42] These patients did not have an increase in MAP or SVR after inflation of the abdomen, but only an increase of CVP. CO returned

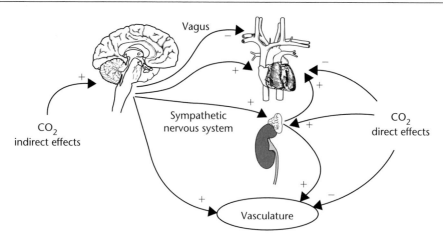

Figure 2.4 Direct and indirect cardiovascular effects of CO_2 absorbed during laparoscopic surgery. CO_2 has a negative inotropic effect on the myocardium, stimulates adrenal medullary catecholamine release and cause vasodilation. These direct effects are cancelled out to a large extent by indirect effects, such as stimulation of the sympathetic nervous system and inhibition of parasympathetic innervation.

to normal after inflation and remained constant at preoperative levels. These observations were basically corroborated by another study.[43] Case reports have also shown that laparoscopic surgery is uneventful in heart transplant recipients.[44,45]

Note Inflating the abdomen with CO_2 typically causes an increase in peripheral vascular resistance and a compression of the atria with a reduction of cardiac filling. The initial response to this is:

- Increase in arterial blood pressure
- Decrease in CO
- Increase in CVP
- Increase in left ventricular wall tension
- Increase in $M\dot{V}O_2$

Note The position of the patient can either enhance or diminish the effect on CO:

- Transient decrease with gradual recovery in reverse Trendelenburg position (e.g. during cholecystectomy and other upper abdominal operations)
- No change or slight increase in Trendelenburg position (e.g. during gynaecological or urological operations, transperitoneal hernia repair)

Note Increased abdominal pressure causes congestion and stasis in the veins of the legs, particularly with the patient in the reverse Trendelenburg position.

This leads to: Risk of deep vein thrombosis and requires rapid postoperative mobilization and thrombosis prophylaxis.

Regional blood flow

Increased IAP not only influences global haemodynamics but interferes also with the blood flow to individual organs. Alterations of regional perfusion can cause problems independent of total blood flow, such as impairing organ function or altering drug delivery and disposal.

Studies with transcranial Doppler sonography (TCD) showed that CO_2 pneumoperitoneum increased blood flow velocity in the middle cerebral artery.[46] This was probably not due to the increase in IAP but to a rise in arterial CO_2 tension, since other authors could not confirm an effect of increased IAP on cerebral blood flow when arterial CO_2 tension was kept constant.[47,48] A further study demonstrated that arterial PCO_2 was directly correlated with cerebral blood flow.[49]

Increasing IAP by insufflating CO_2 markedly reduces blood flow in the portal vein, hepatic artery and superior mesenteric artery,[50] although in one study, flow in the hepatic artery remained unchanged.[51] Inflating with helium (He) causes a more marked decrease in hepatic blood flow than CO_2.[52] The sum effect was a reduction in indocyanine green clearance.[53] Intestinal mucosal perfusion is reduced as well and possible mucosal ischaemia is suggested by the decrease of intramural pH in the jejunum.[54,55] A more recent study suggests that insufflated CO_2 enhances splanchnic blood flow up to an inflation pressure of 16 mmHg.[56] One recent study showed that hepatic blood flow can be affected to a degree that impairs hepatocyte integrity depending on the nature of the operation and patient position. Laparoscopic cholecystectomy caused greater postoperative increases in alcohol dehydrogenase, glutathione S-transferase, aspartate aminotransferase and alanine aminotransferase than laparoscopic colectomy reflecting significant hepatic hypoperfusion during cholecystectomy.[57]

The data on the effects of laparoscopy on renal function show that urine output, renal blood flow and creatinine clearance are reduced during pneumoperitoneum.[55,58,59] One study suggested that it was not elevated IAP *per se* that it is responsible for the observed effects on urine flow, but that intraperitoneal cooling might possibly also be involved, since the changes were not observed when warm gas was used for insufflation.[60] This does not seem likely in view of the results of numerous other investigations that give strong evidence that pressure itself and not the insufflated CO_2 or its temperature is the probable trigger. In one animal study, renal function deteriorated when IAP was increased with an inflatable bag inserted into the peritoneal cavity,[61] and in another, renal blood flow and diuresis were both significantly reduced by directly compressing the kidney to a pressure of 15 mmHg.[62] Some clinical studies showed only inconsistent effects on renal function of patients: urine output and creatinine clearance were reduced in only 60% of the patients, and either not affected at all or even increased in the others,[63] but the most common observation is that increased abdominal pressure significantly reduces urine output and can even cause anuria.[64]

The primary effect of increased IAP is a decrease in renal venous blood flow that can persist after pressure is released.[65] Renal cortical perfusion also decreases during pneumoperitoneum.[66] This reduction in renal blood flow is the most likely cause of the increased plasma renin activity seen with laparoscopy (see below). Urine O_2 tension decreases when abdominal expansion is achieved by gas inflation but not when the abdominal wall is lifted mechanically.[64] The fall in urine O_2 tension is a consequence of renal vasoconstriction.[67,68] Increased urinary levels of N-acetyl-beta-D-glucosaminidase have been described,[55,69] which reflect significant renal parenchymal hypoxia with tubular damage that can ultimately lead to acute tubular necrosis and acute renal failure in the predisposed patient. There is a direct relationship between reduced renal blood flow, decreased urine O_2 tension and the observed reduction in creatinine clearance[63,70] as was demonstrated in patients undergoing cardiac surgery.[71] Some suggest that supporting urine flow with the use of diuretics or low-dose dopamine might be beneficial,[70] but the currently available data are not sufficient to generally recommend this.[65]

The observed reductions in renal and hepatic perfusion can affect the elimination of drugs used for anaesthesia, for example, by reducing their clearance. It is conceivable that the half-lives of both hepatically as well as renally eliminated substances could be prolonged by laparoscopic surgery. Reduced indocyanine green clearance during pneumoperitoneum supports this assumption.[53]

The effect of CO_2 pneumoperitoneum on uterine blood flow is of particular importance whenever laparoscopic surgery is to be performed during pregnancy. In gravid ewes, CO_2 pneumoperitoneum significantly reduced uterine blood flow, increased maternal and foetal CO_2 tensions and caused maternal and foetal acidosis.[72] A different study showed that uterine blood flow remained unaffected if partial pressure of CO_2 in arterial blood (P_aCO_2) was kept constant.[73] Contrary to these results, He pneumoperitoneum reduced uterine blood flow without altering arterial CO_2 tension or blood pH, indicating that pressure is an independent factor.[74] Hypercapnia is known to independently reduce uterine blood flow[75] and the combination of IAP and elevated P_aCO_2 might enhance the deleterious effects on the foetus.

> **Note** The increased pressure in the pneumoperitoneum induces a reduction of splanchnic and renal blood flow.
>
> Clinical consequences:
>
> - Reduction of hepatic perfusion might prolong half-life of drugs eliminated by the liver
> - Reduction of creatinine clearance and urine flow might reduce the clearance of drugs that are eliminated through the kidneys

Insufflation gas

The choice of the gas used for insufflation is an important factor affecting the safety of laparoscopic procedures and determining the character of the physiological consequences. Once practitioners had realized that the use of room air for insufflation carried a high risk of fatal gas embolism, a large number of gases, including O_2, CO_2, He and N_2O were investigated as possible alternatives, and also employed in the clinical setting. None of the gases were found to be ideal, and each represented a compromise. The choice of a particular gas will depend on the risk–benefit assessment of the individual advantages, disadvantages and adverse effects. The details required for this decision will be sketched in the following paragraphs.

Factors influencing the choice of insufflation gas are physicochemical properties, such as solubility, diffusibility and flammability, as well as the pharmacological effects after systemic uptake. Solubility determines how much of the insufflated gas can be absorbed by the body and how it behaves once in solution. Diffusibility is a characteristic that determines how fast the gas can follow a concentration gradient from one compartment to another. In the case of pneumoperitoneum one must keep in mind that the gas passes from a gas phase to a liquid phase and not through a membrane from one gas phase to another. This is particularly important when considering He, N_2O and CO_2. He is highly diffusible owing to the small size of its single atom, but it enters the liquid phase only slowly since it is poorly soluble. N_2O and CO_2 are much larger molecules, but both have markedly higher diffusion coefficients due to their greater solubility (Table 2.3). What is the most important determinant of safety in an insufflation gas?

Room air, a mixture of nitrogen, oxygen, argon and other gases, is dangerous when used as an insufflation gas. All of the component gases are poorly soluble, and should air enter the venous system directly, as can happen during insufflation, the ensuing intravascular bubbles will not dissolve, but will collect in the right heart and the pulmonary circulation. The small amount of

20–50 ml is sufficient to cause a fatal gas embolism. The same applies for the even less soluble He (Table 2.3). The primary requirement of an insufflation gas is thus high solubility. Although diffusibility itself is not an important factor, the product of diffusibility and solubility is thought to give a better indication of the relative risk of a gas than solubility alone.[76,77]

N_2O and CO_2 have a much higher solubility in blood and inadvertent intravascular application is thus much less dangerous than with the gases mentioned above. Systemic absorption of N_2O does not cause the derangement of acid–base status as seen with CO_2, but there are other problems associated with its use. One of these is the risk of intra-abdominal fire or explosion that has been repeatedly described with its use.[78–81] N_2O is not flammable itself but it supports the combustion of other materials, such as methane or hydrogen sulphide that can escape into the peritoneal cavity from the intestinal lumen through small, inapparent lesions to the bowel (Table 2.4).

CO_2 was substituted for air as insufflation gas towards the end of the 1940s, mainly by the German gynaecologists Lindemann and Semm, since it offers a number of advantages over the alternative gases, foremost among them being its high solubility in blood.[82–84] This results from the fact that most of the CO_2 in blood is not in simple solution, but has been reversibly converted into bicarbonate ions reducing CO_2 partial pressure. An additional factor is its binding to haemoglobin. Studies on spontaneously breathing dogs have shown that 50–100 ml/min of CO_2 can be injected directly into the femoral vein without cardiovascular consequences.[83] However, the choice of anaesthetic, such as the use of N_2O can markedly reduce the amount of CO_2 that is tolerated.[85] This must be taken into account during operations with a high risk of intravascular gas entrainment. The advantages of CO_2 as insufflation gas are its excellent solubility in blood and its rapid uptake from cavities (Table 2.3). On the other hand, CO_2 is not pharmacologically inert after

Table 2.3 Physicochemical properties of insufflation gases

Gas	Solubility coefficient (ml gas per ml H_2O at 760 mmHg)	Relative solubility ($O_2 = 1$)	Relative diffusion coefficient ($O_2 = 1$)
CO_2	0.57	24.0	20.5
N_2O	0.47	16.3	14.0
O_2	0.024	1.0	1.0
N_2	0.012	0.52	0.55
He	0.008	0.37	1.05

Table 2.4 Biochemical and pharmacological properties and risk profile of insufflation gases

	Biochemical effects	Pharmacological effects	Risk of embolism	Supports combustion
CO_2	Acidosis	Activation of SNS, direct circulatory depression, pain	−(+)	−
N_2O	Inert	Narcosis	−(+)	+
O_2	Inert	Inert	+	++
N_2	Inert	Inert	++	−
He	Inert	Inert	++	−

SNS: sympathetic nervous system.

systemic uptake. CO_2 absorption raises P_aCO_2 and causes a respiratory acidosis that must be compensated for by increasing alveolar ventilation (see below).

Uptake of insufflated CO_2

CO_2 absorption is a further consistent characteristic of laparoscopic surgery that has an impact both on physiological consequences as well as on the management of anaesthesia.[86,87] One study found a high CO_2 tension in the epigastric veins draining the peritoneum, gives additional support to the assumption that CO_2 uptake from the abdominal cavity actually is responsible for the observed increase in arterial CO_2 tension.[88] It causes respiratory acidosis, predisposes to cardiac dysrhythmias and has to be eliminated by increasing minute ventilation.

There are approximately 120 l of CO_2 stored in the body,[89] most of it in the form of carbonates in the bones or dissolved in lipids. Aqueous solutions contain circa 500 ml CO_2 per litre. CO_2 stores can be divided into three compartments – fast, intermediate and slow – that differ in their equilibration times. Blood and organs with high blood flow, such as the brain, liver and kidneys constitute the fast compartment, while the intermediate compartment comprises muscle and less well-perfused parenchymal organs. The CO_2 tension in the fast compartment lies only slightly higher than partial pressure of CO_2 in alveolar gas (P_ACO_2) and rapidly follows any change in arterial P_aCO_2. The intermediate compartment is relatively large and less sensitive to fluctuations of arterial CO_2 tension – acute hyper- or hypoventilation has little effect on CO_2 tension in the muscles. These two compartments have a total storage capacity of approximately 2 ml of CO_2 per kg body weight and mmHg P_aCO_2 in a normal individual.[90–92] This means that the uptake of 2 ml of CO_2 per kg will raise arterial CO_2 tension by 1 mmHg

$$\left.\begin{array}{c} CO_2 \text{ storage} \\ \text{capacity} \end{array}\right\} = \frac{ml\, CO_2}{(kg\ body\ weight)(mmHg\ P_aCO_2)}$$

Adipose tissue, bones and other tissues with low blood flow comprise the slow compartment. The storage capacity of this compartment is approximately 10 ml $CO_2 kg^{-1} mmHg^{-1} P_aCO_2$. The slow compartment is in close contact with the fast compartment, but transfer of CO_2 between them is slow. This is due to the low blood flow in adipose tissue, while in bones the limiting factor is the conversion of CO_2 to hydroxyapatite and vice versa.

Due to its high diffusion coefficient CO_2 can easily pass from gas-filled cavities into the blood (and vice

versa). The speed with which absorption takes place depends on the absorbing surface. Uptake through the thick, smooth and relatively poorly perfused peritoneum is slower than from loose connective tissue.[93–95] The amount of gas absorbed has a decisive influence on the manner and magnitude of the physiological consequences.

Despite high solubility and ease of tissue penetration, only a fraction of the insufflated CO_2 is absorbed from the abdominal cavity. The amount can be estimated using data typical for laparoscopic operations. Approximately 5 l of CO_2 are required to create the pneumoperitoneum. Using the formula for the CO_2 storage capacity given above shows that this volume of CO_2 would acutely raise the arterial CO_2 tension of a 60 kg patient from 40 to 82 mmHg. In reality, P_aCO_2 increases only about 9 mmHg during a 10–30 min operation in a patient ventilated mechanically with a constant minute volume. This represents the uptake of approximately 1080 ml.

This is a rough estimate of CO_2 uptake using the average storage capacity of the fast and intermediate compartments in a patient with constant alveolar ventilation. A more accurate determination can be made using indirect calorimetry to measure the increase in the volume of CO_2 eliminated through the lungs during CO_2 insufflation. During the measurements, arterial CO_2 tensions must be kept constant to ensure that absorbed CO_2 is completely eliminated and not allowed to enter the storage compartments. This requirement is crucial since CO_2 uptake will be underestimated considerably if a relevant amount of the absorbed CO_2 is stored (as evidenced by an increasing P_aCO_2 or partial pressure of CO_2 at end-tidal ($P_{et}CO_2$)) then. A constant P_aCO_2 reflects the fulfilment of this requirement, although in most studies arterial tension is not measured directly, and end-tidal CO_2 concentrations ($P_{et}CO_2$) are used as a surrogate parameter.

One obtains the rate of CO_2 absorption ($\dot{V}CO_{2\,absorb}$) by subtracting the endogenous CO_2 production ($\dot{V}CO_{2\,endog}$) from the total exhaled CO_2 ($\dot{V}CO_{2\,total}$) (Equation (2.1)):

$$\dot{V}CO_{2\,absorb} = \dot{V}CO_{2\,total} - \dot{V}CO_{2\,endog} \quad (2.1)$$

Endogenous CO_2 production can be continuously calculated from total body O_2 uptake ($\dot{V}O_2$) using the respiratory quotient (R):

$$\dot{V}CO_{2\,endog} = \dot{V}O_2 R \quad (2.2)$$

Table 2.5 CO_2 output und O_2 uptake (ml min^{-1})

Author	CO_2 output			ΔCO_2	O_2 uptake	
	Preoperative	Intraoperative	Maximum		Preoperative	Intraoperative
Lewis et al.[97]	102	126	–	24	–	–
Blobner et al.[101]	145–180	179–222	–	–	–	–
Kazama et al.[87]	110 ± 24	163 ± 26	–	54 ± 16	129 ± 26	142 ± 26
Luiz et al.[108]	156 ± 24	216 ± 35	–	–	206 ± 15	211 ± 23
Mullett et al.[93]						
Intraperitoneal	132	176	–	–	–	–
Extraperitoneal	133	207	–	–	–	–
Puri and Singh[199]	3.6 ± 0.51 (ml kg^{-1})	4.4 ± 0.56 (ml kg^{-1})	–	–	–	–
Seed et al.[96]	135	151	–	16	–	–
Sumpf et al.[95]						
Extraperitoneal	161.0	331.9	788	153.4	226.9	250.9
Transperitoneal	154.4	222.2	300.2	59.2	220.4	232.0
Tan et al.[200]	146 ± 20	183 ± 17	–	42.1 ± 17	169 ± 13	164 ± 18
Weyland et al.[98]	138 ± 29	212 ± 50	361	–	201	

Older studies give an average CO_2 uptake of 20 ml min^{-1}.[96,97] These data were gathered during short diagnostic laparoscopic procedures without regard to maintaining endogenous CO_2 stores at a constant level. More recent studies, in which care was taken to keep P_aCO_2 constant, give much a higher uptake (Table 2.5) and have helped deepen our understanding of the physiological and physical events during CO_2 uptake.[87,95,98]

CO_2 uptake from the abdominal cavity does not proceed at a constant rate, but is a function of capillary perfusion in the peritoneum and the prevailing pressure gradient. CO_2 uptake initially increases with rising IAP, but there is indirect evidence that further increasing IAP reduces capillary perfusion and decreases the rate of CO_2 absorption.[99–101] The rate of CO_2 absorption during laparoscopic cholecystectomy varies widely from patient to patient and can be increased by a factor of three over baseline values (Table 2.5). The absorption rate can also vary widely during the course of the operation as shown in Figure 2.5.

One consistent observation is that CO_2 uptake depends on the tissue surface that is in contact with the gas phase, and therefore to a large degree on the type of operation.[93,94] Absorption is low during laparoscopic operations without further damage to the smooth, tough and relatively thick peritoneum. Opening the peritoneum for dissection into the surrounding connective tissue, or even the creation of artificial cavities as for nephrectomy or preperitoneal herniotomy, can enlarge the exposed surface area and enable a higher absorption rate.[94,102,103] The increase in CO_2 uptake over baseline during an uncomplicated transperitoneal laparoscopic herniotomy ranges between 55% and 70%.[93,95,104] The highest absorption rate is seen during extraperitoneal procedures complicated by subcutaneous emphysema, since the absorbing surface area is very large and the tissue thickness through which the gas has to diffuse is shorter (Figure 2.6).[93,95,105–107] Chiche and co-workers found that CO_2 elimination was only 16.9% above baseline in patients without subcutaneous emphysema, while this complication caused an increase to 70%.[105] We found an increase in CO_2 uptake of more than 500 ml min^{-1} in patients with extensive subcutaneous emphysema during extraperitoneal hernia repair, which corresponds to a relative increase of 250% compared to patients without emphysema[95] (Table 2.5).

The absorbed CO_2 must be eliminated by increasing alveolar ventilation, since large P_aCO_2 increases cause considerable pH and electrolyte shifts. The latter are associated with an increased incidence of cardiovascular complications such as hypertension and cardiac dysrhythmias. The relative increase in ventilation that was necessary to maintain normocapnia varied between 0% and 145% in one study. The corresponding mean absolute increase in minute volume was 14–16 l min^{-1}.[98,108] Debois and co-workers observed that ventilation had to be increased by an average of 30% during laparoscopic cholecystectomy, while an increase of 55% was required during endoscopic hernia repair.[104] Our own data show that ventilation has to be increased by more than 400% in patients with extensive subcutaneous emphysema. The corresponding absolute value of minute volume was 30 l min^{-1}.[95]

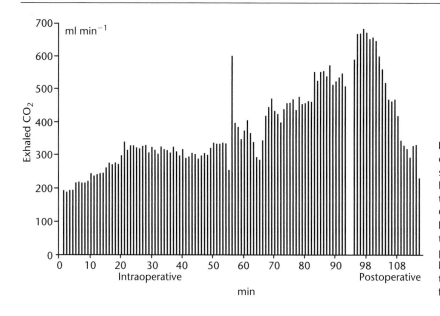

Figure 2.5 CO_2 absorption during the course of laparoscopic extraperitoneal inguinal hernioplasty. One can easily see that the amount of absorbed CO_2 does not remain constant, but increases during the operation. The highest values are seen postoperatively and are probably due to the extensive subcutaneous emphysema. (Adapted from Ref [95].)

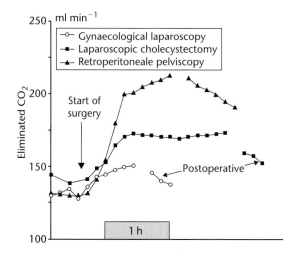

Figure 2.6 The magnitude of CO_2 absorption depends on operation site. (Adapted from Ref [93].) The gynaecological laparoscopy were short diagnostic or operative procedures, such as tubal ligation. The pelviscopic operations were retroperitoneal lymphadenectomy. Arterial CO_2 tensions were not kept constant so the actual amount of CO_2 uptake might be significantly higher.

It is important to be aware of the expected magnitude of CO_2 uptake, since the increase in alveolar ventilation required to maintain normocapnia might not be possible in patients with severely compromised lung function. This is an aspect that cannot be ignored, considering the number of elderly patients with chronic obstructive lung disease (COLD) who might present for laparoscopic surgery. It must be taken into

account when drawing up the list of possible contraindications for laparoscopic surgery.

There is a constant risk of hypercapnia in the spontaneously breathing patient, as is shown in Table 2.6. This is not entirely due to suppression of ventilatory drive by the anaesthetic as the data obtained using N_2O as insufflation gas show. But mechanical ventilation alone does not guard against hypercapnia if is not adapted to the rate of CO_2 absorption.

Thermocautery and laser surgery produce high intra-abdominal concentrations of carbon monoxide. This can be absorbed from the peritoneum and induce relevant levels of carboxyhaemoglobin.[109,110]

Note

- CO_2 absorption varies widely, both between patients as well as during a single operation
- It is greatest during surgery outside the borders of anatomically defined cavities with insufflation of gas into loose connective tissue (e.g. lymphadenectomy, herniotomy, nephrectomy)
- Minute ventilation required to maintain normocapnia during these operations can increase by more than $20\,l\,min^{-1}$
- Capnometric or blood gas monitoring is indispensable in order to detect the P_aCO_2 increase and to adapt ventilation

Clinical conclusion

- Patients with compromised pulmonary function and reduced ventilatory reserve (e.g. COLD or after lung resection) are at a higher risk

Table 2.6 Changes of P_aCO_2 and P_aO_2 during pneumoperitoneum with N_2O or CO_2

Mode of ventilation	Author	Gas	F_IO_2	ΔP_aCO_2 (mmHg)	ΔP_aO_2 (mmHg)
Spontaneous breathing	Baratz and Karis[195]	CO_2	0.99	4.8	−20
	Hodgson et al.[196]	CO_2	–	7.0	–
	Lewis et al.[97]	CO_2	0.98	4.6	–
	Scott and Julian[41]	CO_2	–	17.6	–
		N_2O	–	5.9	–
	Kenefick et al.[119]	CO_2	0.35	10.0	−29
Mechanical ventilation	Alexander and Brown[197]	CO_2	–	8.7	−24
		N_2O	–	−2.4	−28
	Baratz and Karis[195]	CO_2	0.99	1.1	−32
	Hodgson et al.[196]	CO_2	–	10.1	–
	Kelman et al.[19]	CO_2	0.3	8.4	3
	Motew et al.[21]	CO_2	0.5	12.1	−6
	Magno et al.[198]	CO_2	0.3	9.0	−9
		N_2O	0.3	−1.0	−13

ΔP_aCO_2 and ΔP_aO_2 denote changes of the respective partial pressures between beginning and end of gas insufflation.

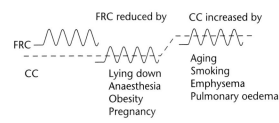

Figure 2.7 Numerous conditions can bring the FRC within the range of CC, either by reducing FRC or by increasing CC.

RESPIRATION

Gas exchange

Every operation in general anaesthesia is associated with characteristic intra- and postoperative alterations of lung function. Functional residual capacity (FRC) and total compliance (C_{tot}) decrease by an average of 20% and dead-space ventilation (V_D/V_T) increases immediately after induction of anaesthesia. The magnitude of FRC reduction depends on the patient's build and can be 50% in adipose patients.[111] Even a moderate reduction of FRC can cause arterial O_2 desaturation in patients with increased closing capacity (CC), such as cigarette smokers and patients with COLD (Figure 2.7). These changes are associated with the cessation of spontaneous breathing and institution of mechanical ventilation.[112–114] The ultimate causes are a disturbance of the normal ventilation–perfusion relationship, the loss of dorsobasal diaphragm motion and the changes in intrathoracic pressures. The ventilation–perfusion relationship is shifted in wide areas of the lungs (Figure 2.8), leading to reduced

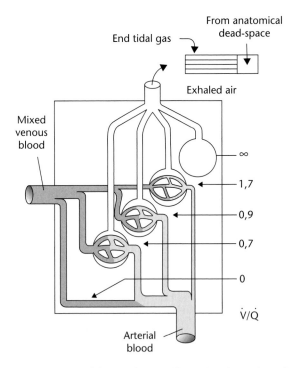

Figure 2.8 Schematic diagram illustrating the variety of ventilation–perfusion ratios ($\dot{V}/\dot{Q}$) present in the lung. V_D/V_T occurs in alveoli with a high $\dot{V}/\dot{Q}$ ratio, whereas venous admixture occurs in alveoli with a $\dot{V}/\dot{Q}$ ratio below unity. A $\dot{V}/\dot{Q}$ of zero indicates shunt perfusion.

ventilation of the well-perfused basal regions with an increase in shunt perfusion (Q_S/Q_T), while the well-ventilated but poorly perfused superior regions (West zone I) are responsible for the increase in V_D/V_T

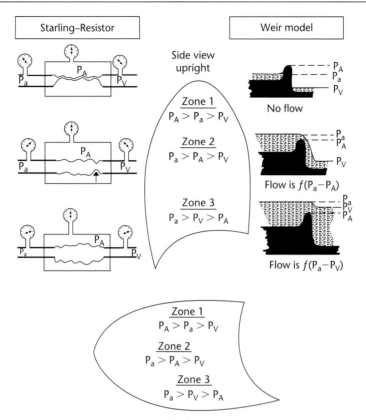

Figure 2.9 The influence of gravity and the prevailing pressures in the lungs and pulmonary vessels lead to the development of areas with differing perfusion, which were divided by West into the zones 1–3. In zone 1, which is located in the apical portions of the lung in the upright subject or in the uppermost portions in the recumbent patient, alveolar pressure (P_A) is higher than the pressure in the pulmonary capillaries (P_a). The capillaries collapse and blood flow ceases. In zone 2, blood flows as long as P_a is higher than P_A, and stops intermittently during the cardiac cycle or due to increased alveolar pressure during mechanical ventilation. In zone 3, which is in the dependent portions of the lungs, pulmonary venous pressure (P_V) is higher than P_A, so that the capillaries never collapse and blood flow is continuous. (Modified from West *et al. J Appl Physiol* 1964; **19**: 713–724.) Changes in blood pressure or intrathoracic pressure influence the distribution of the zones; increasing vascular filling and blood pressure reduces the extent of areas with zone 1 characteristics, and thus V_D/V_T whereas increasing intrathoracic pressure (e.g. during pneumoperitoneum) will increase P_A and V_D/V_T.

mentioned above (Figure 2.9). Dorsobasal atelectatic areas develop immediately after induction of anaesthesia that can be seen in computerized tomography scans.[112,114] The resulting alterations of pulmonary function are seen clinically as a decrease in arterial O_2 and CO_2 tensions as well as an increase in airway pressure (P_{AW}) during mechanical ventilation. These factors are obviously effective during laparoscopic or thoracoscopic operations, and can be intensified by the increase in IAP, head-down position or one-lung ventilation.[99,115–117]

Available data indicate that pneumoperitoneum causes a further reduction of FRC (Table 2.6).[115,118,119] One would expect an effect of this nature under the influence of elevated IAP with cephalad shift of the diaphragm.[116,117] Applying constant positive P_{AW} can largely prevent the FRC reduction,[120,121] an observation that has great practical value for the management of anaesthesia, since it improves gas exchange and oxygenation.[121,122]

The changes observed in infants during pneumoperitoneum differ from those in adults. These patients rely nearly completely on diaphragm motion for ventilation due to the horizontal position of their ribs. Even slight increases of IAP can cause a sharp drop in arterial O_2 saturation that requires positive end-expiratory pressure of nearly the same magnitude as IAP for compensation.[123]

Intraoperative pulmonary function

C_{tot} of the chest and lungs falls markedly after creation of the pneumoperitoneum, with the thoracic component decreasing more than the pulmonary one.[115,118,124,125] In patients without lung pathology, creating a pneumoperitoneum in the supine patient induces a 43% drop in C_{tot}, which remains unchanged when the patient is brought into a reverse Trendelenburg position.[126] This position improves compliance and oxygenation in obese patients and patients with COLD.[127,128] When the abdomen is inflated after the patient has been brought into the head-up position the C_{tot} reduction is also between 32% and 48%.[129,130] There is a large body of evidence that abdominal inflation and not patient position is responsible for the compliance reduction.[124,126,131] The change is also independent of the duration of the pneumoperitoneum and is rapidly reversible after IAP has been released.[130] The changes in American Society of Anaesthesiologists (ASA) III and IV patients are similar to those in their healthy counterparts with a compliance decrease of approximately 40%[132] (Table 2.7).

The clinical correlate of reduced compliance is the rise in P_{AW} at otherwise unchanged respirator settings. Plateau pressure increases between 45% and 75%.[108,130,132,133] The combination of low compliance and increased minute volume can lead to unacceptably high P_{AW} and necessitate termination of the operation or conversion to an open procedure. A sudden, sharp increase in P_{AW} should alert the anaesthetist to the possibility of a complication such as a pneumothorax.[105,134]

Essentially the same respiratory changes are seen during thoracoscopy as during thoracotomy, which are a considerable increase of shunt perfusion and a reduction of vital capacity (VC). This can impede the necessary increase in minute ventilation. The effects of extraperitoneal endoscopic procedures on lung function are probably much less impressive.

> **Note** Pneumoperitoneum induces a reduction of compliance, an increase of pulmonary shunt perfusion and V_D/V_T and the development of basal pulmonary atelectases.
>
> The clinical consequences are:
>
> - P_{AW} increase (cave barotrauma)
> - Total minute ventilation has to be increased just in order to keep alveolar constant
> - Arterial O_2 desaturation (PEEP ventilation recommended, pulse oximetry required)

Postoperative pulmonary function

Laparoscopic surgery is thought to compromise lung function to a lesser degree than conventional open procedures.[135–138] While the intraoperative alterations of lung function depend primarily on the patient's position and the ventilatory mode (spontaneous vs. controlled), the postoperative changes are governed by the incision and the surgical site – upper vs. lower abdomen and intraperitoneal vs. extraperitoneal. After upper abdominal and thoracic surgery, there is a prolonged reduction of VC, forced expiratory volume (FEV_1) and FRC.[111] Reduced VC prevents effective coughing and periodic deep breathing (sighing), FRC can fall below CC, the lung volume at which airway closure begins (Figure 2.7). This causes an increase of venous admixture and is responsible for late postoperative hypoxaemia.[139] These changes are not observed after lower abdominal or body surface surgery, or at least not in this magnitude and duration. Lung function is restricted by incision pain and increased tension of the abdominal wall muscles as well as by a reflex inhibition of inspiratory diaphragm motion.[140–142] The I:E relationship is shifted towards expiration, the ventilatory contribution of the diaphragm is sharply reduced and there is a shift from abdominal to rib-cage breathing (Figure 2.10).[143] Ventilatory minute volume

Table 2.7 Changes in thoracic and pulmonary compliance induced by pneumoperitoneum

Author	Compliance (ml/cmH$_2$O)			
	Position	Baseline value	After positioning	With pneumo-peritoneum
Drummond[115]	HD	60	61	44	−27%
Johannsen[23]	HD	50	42	30	−40%
Kendall[124]	HU	55	–	28	−49% (thorax)
		102	–	62	−39% (lung)
Luiz[108]	HU	Absolute values not given			−40%
Weyland[98]	Supine	60	–	40	−33%

HD: head-down position; HU: head-up position.

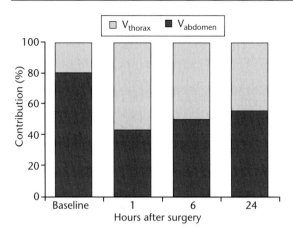

Figure 2.10 The incisional wound pain of laparoscopic cholecystectomy causes a reflectory inhibition of diaphragm activity with a change in the relative contributions of abdominal and rib-cage breathing that is detectable 24 h after surgery. (Adapted from Ref [143].)

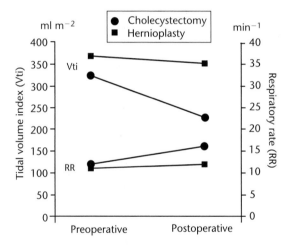

Figure 2.11 The postoperative respiratory changes of tidal volume and respiratory rate depend on the intra-abdominal location of the surgical site. Tidal volume exhibits a greater decrease following laparoscopic cholecystectomy than after hernioplasty. Respiratory rate increases to a greater degree after cholecystectomy. (Adapted from Ref [141].)

remains constant but tidal volume is reduced by 30% and respiratory rate is increased (Figure 2.11). These effects are observed after laparoscopic surgery, but depend on the intraperitoneal localization of the operation site. Laparoscopic hernia repair and cholecystectomy have virtually identical trocar insertion sites but the two operations can have very different effects on postoperative diaphragm function.[141,144] The effects

are not due to a residual pneumoperitoneum.[145] A greater degree of respiratory impairment is seen following more extensive laparoscopic operations in the lower abdomen and pelvis, such as laparoscopic-assisted vaginal hysterectomy or laparoscopic-assisted prostatectomy.[146]

VC is reduced by approximately 24% during the first 24 h after laparoscopic cholecystectomy, but by 52% in the same period following the conventional procedures (Table 2.8). It returns to normal after 2 or 3 days after the laparoscopic operation, while it remains depressed for a much longer period after the open operation.[137,147] Recovery of VC is delayed in older patients (Figure 2.12).[148] Our own data show that VC was reduced by 19% on the first postoperative day, but that this had resolved on day two.

Twenty-four hours after surgery, FRC is reduced by 8% after laparoscopic cholecystectomy compared to 27% after the conventional technique. The impairment is much more short-lived after the minimally invasive procedure, and resolves within 3 days, while FRC is still reduced by 23% at this time following the open procedure (Figure 2.13).[137] Other authors report similar findings.[149] The magnitude of arterial O_2 desaturation parallels FRC reduction, and postoperative hypoxaemia is much less severe following laparoscopic operations.

Pneumonia is the most serious pulmonary complication of laparotomy. It can develop on the basis of an intraoperative atelectasis perpetuated by impaired deep breathing and abolishment of effective coughing. The incidence described in the literature varies between 10% and 70% depending on how it is defined in the individual study. It depends on the surgical incision – upper or lower abdomen, midline vs. transverse vs. subcostal – and the diagnostic criteria employed – clinical symptoms, blood gases or radiographic signs. Hypoxaemia is a regular postoperative feature even without clinical evidence of pneumonia. Pulmonary infiltrates are seen in up to 90% of all patients following conventional cholecystectomy, while the incidence was only 40% after the corresponding laparoscopic procedure (Figure 2.14).[136] Only 10% of the patients with laparoscopic cholecystectomy developed segmental atelectasis.[136,149] An elevated right hemidiaphragm is a common observation.[144] A study in our hospital revealed a 50% incidence of pneumonia in patients with abdomino-thoracic oesophagus resection.[150] Pneumonia was defined as the presence of pulmonary infiltrates in chest X-ray and elevated body temperature later than 24 h after surgery. The presence of this complication prolonged the median duration of intensive care from 8 to 15 days. Pneumonia is one of

Table 2.8 Changes in lung function 24 h after laparoscopic (LC) or conventional open cholecystectomy (OC)

Parameter	LC (%)	OC (%)	P	Source
FVC	−21	−50	<0.05	Schauer[136]
	−28	−44	<0.05	Williams[201]
	−26	−48	<0.05	Frazee[202]
	−20	−45	<0.05	Putensen-Himmer[137]
	−42	−71	<0.05	Rademaker[170]
	−13	n.s.		Johnson[149]
	−25	n.s.		Rotbøll Nielsen[203]
	−23	n.s.		Beebe[146]
Mean FVC	**−24**	**−52**		
FEV$_1$	−24	−55	<0.05	Schauer[136]
	−24	−45	<0.05	Williams[201]
	−28	−47	<0.05	Frazee[202]
	−16	−43	<0.05	Putensen-Himmer[137]
	−22	n.s.		Rotbøll Nielsen[203]
	−26	n.s.		Beebe[146]
Mean FEV$_1$	**−23**	**−48**		
TLC	−8	−22	<0.05	Schauer[136]
	−17	n.s.		Rotbøll Nielsen[203]
MVV	−22	−52	<0.05	Schauer[136]
FEF$_{max}$	−19	−57	<0.05	Williams[201]
	−33	n.s.		Beebe[146]
FEF$_{25-75}$	−19	−47	n.s.	Frazee[202]
FRC	−15	−27	n.s.*	Putensen-Himmer[137]
	−7	n.s.		Johnson[149]
	−8	n.s.		Rotbøll Nielsen[203]
Mean FRC	**−8**	**−27**		

OC: open cholecystectomy; LC: laparoscopic cholecystectomy; FVC: forced vital capacity; FEV$_1$: one second volume; TLC: total lung capacity; MVV: maximal voluntary ventilation; FEF$_{max}$: maximal expiratory flow; FEF$_{25-75}$: maximal flow between 25% und 75% of expiration; n.s.: not studied.
*FRC was also reduced to a significantly greater degree in the open cholecystectomy group at 6 and also at 72 h after surgery (see also Figure 2.13).

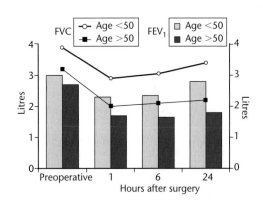

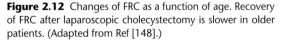

Figure 2.12 Changes of FRC as a function of age. Recovery of FRC after laparoscopic cholecystectomy is slower in older patients. (Adapted from Ref [148].)

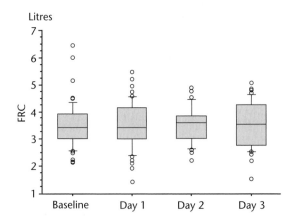

Figure 2.13 FRC is changed only slightly following laparoscopic cholecystectomy (Hamo and Crozier, unpublished data). The contrasts with the marked FRC reduction seen after the open procedure (see Table 2.8).

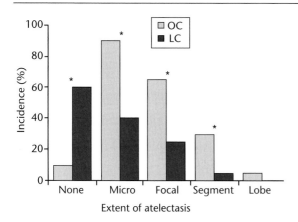

Figure 2.14 The incidence of pulmonary atelectasis detectable in chest radiogram is significantly lower after laparoscopic (LC) than after open cholecystectomy (OC). This finding is relevant for the incidence of postoperative pneumonia. (Adapted from Ref [136] and [149].)

the main causes of postoperative morbidity and mortality along with anastomotic leak and sepsis. All available data suggest that the incidence of pulmonary complications is greatly reduced after laparoscopic cholecystectomy and also suggest an advantage of the laparoscopic over the open approach for patients with pre-existing pulmonary pathology. The probability of an uneventful postoperative course usually outweighs the intraoperative problems.

Note

- Postoperative impairment of pulmonary function is significantly less after laparoscopy than after laparotomy
- Arterial O_2 desaturation is less severe after laparoscopic operations
- The incidence of atelectases and pneumonia is lower after laparoscopic operations

---

Intracranial pressure during laparoscopy

The safety of laparoscopic surgery in patients with elevated intracranial pressure (ICP) or closed head injuries is controversial. Pneumoperitoneum has been shown in numerous animal studies to increase ICP, independent of arterial CO_2 tension.[11,151,152] Studies in children with ventriculoperitoneal shunts demonstrated that inflating the abdomen immediately increased intraventricular pressure by up to 25 mmHg.[153] When performed in patients with closed head injuries, laparoscopy can increase intracranial

pressure from normal values to over 60 mmHg, and this increase can persist even after IAP has been released.[154] Symptoms of increased intracranial pressure, such as headache and nausea, are seen significantly more often after laparoscopic surgery than after open procedures.[155] The cause of the ICP increase is thought to be venous congestion and increased pressure in the sagittal sinus, lumbar cistern and the dural sleeves of spinal nerve roots leading to impaired cerebrospinal fluid absorption.[11,156] A mechanical abdominal wall retractor could be an alternative to pneumoperitoneum in patients at risk of ICP increases, since animal studies have shown that ICP does not increase during laparoscopy when a gasless abdominal wall lift device is employed.[157,158]

Neuroendocrine and immunological reactions to laparoscopic surgery

The rapid adoption of laparoscopic techniques has made the prospective, randomized comparison of laparoscopic operations with their conventional counterparts almost no longer possible. One would expect that the small incisions of laparoscopic surgery would induce only minor increases in the circulating concentrations of the typical stress indicators, such as epinephrine, norepinephrine, cortisol and blood glucose or the neuroendocrine hormones, such as vasopressin, adrenocorticotropin (ACTH) and prolactin. The results of the available comparative studies reveal a certain discordance in the reactions of the various neuroendocrine stress parameters. But expectation and reality do not coincide – numerous studies have shown that perioperative endocrine stress responses to laparoscopic surgery does not differ relevantly from conventional open surgery laparoscopy.[135,159–163]

Simply inflating the abdomen increases circulating plasma concentrations of catecholamines, ACTH, cortisol and vasopressin.[164–166] Increasing IAP and CO_2 absorption activates the sympathetic nervous system and stimulates the secretion of catecholamines from the adrenal medulla.[167,168] The reduction of renal perfusion stimulates the release of renin from the kidneys.[169] Cortisol, ACTH, β-endorphin, interleukin-6, and blood glucose increase during surgery (Figure 2.15) while the plasma concentrations of insulin and glucagon remain unchanged.[161,162,165,170–172] Our data confirm these findings. In a study comparing the time course of hormone concentrations during abdominal hysterectomy and laparoscopic cholecystectomy, we observed comparable increases of cortisol, epinephrine and norepinephrine that indicate a similar degree

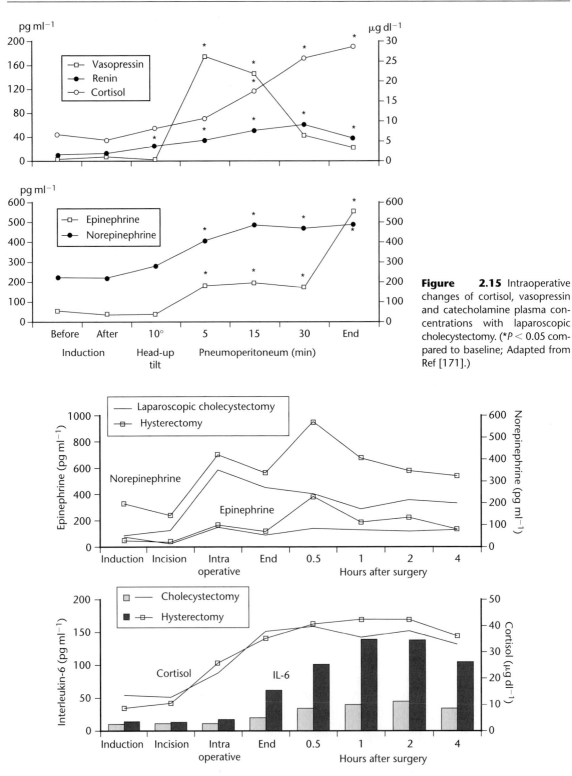

Figure   2.15 Intraoperative changes of cortisol, vasopressin and catecholamine plasma concentrations with laparoscopic cholecystectomy. (*$P < 0.05$ compared to baseline; Adapted from Ref [171].)

Figure 2.16 Perioperative changes of typical endocrine and inflammatory stress parameters interleukin-6 plasma concentrations seen with laparoscopic cholecystectomy compared to a conventional abdominal operation of medium invasiveness (hysterectomy) (Crozier *et al.*, unpublished data).

of intraoperative stress. However, the concentrations of these hormones decreased postoperatively more rapidly after the laparoscopic operation (Figure 2.16). Plasma concentrations of atrial natriuretic hormone remained unchanged despite increased PCWP.[173]

The perioperative time courses of catecholamines, cortisol, vasopressin and blood glucose are virtually

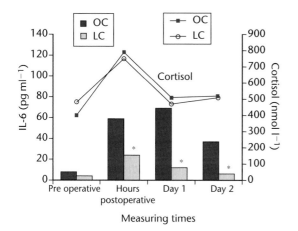

Measuring times

Figure 2.17 The less traumatic nature of laparoscopic surgery compared to the conventional procedure is reflected in the reduced increases of interleukin-6 (IL-6) (*$P < 0.05$ from baseline). Cortisol concentrations are essentially the same after both techniques.

the same with laparoscopic or open cholecystectomy.[135,169,170] In some studies, catecholamine responses were even more pronounced after laparoscopic operations.[165] The temporal coincidence suggests a causal relationship between the rapid increase of plasma renin activity and vasopressin and norepinephrine plasma concentrations and the concomitant blood pressure increase. A positive correlation between vasopressin concentrations and MAP was documented in one study.[174] However, in other studies comparing pneumoperitoneum with gasless mechanical wall lift, the increase in vasopressin plasma concentrations were virtually identical in both groups, but MAP was significantly lower in the wall lift group.[64,169] Pneumoperitoneum is considered a possible independent stimulus for catecholamine secretion during surgery for the resection of phaeochromocytoma.[175]

Open and laparoscopic operations do differ in the behaviour of indicators of tissue trauma, such as C-reactive protein, erythrocyte sedimentation rate and leucocytes: changes of these parameters are attenuated following laparoscopic surgery.[135,159–161,163] This might be due to the lower plasma concentrations of interleukin-6 following minimally invasive operations (Figure 2.17 and Table 2.9).[135,163] The significance of interleukin-6 as a stress parameter is seen in its pivotal importance in the acute phase reaction and postoperative catabolism. The more rapid reconvalescence after laparoscopic surgery is likely to be due

Table 2.9 Synopsis of the endocrine, metabolic and immunological reactions to the stress of open or laparoscopic cholecystectomy

Parameter	Donald et al.[165]	Mealy et al.[162]	Joris et al.[135,171]	Mansour et al.[172]	Rademaker et al.[170]	Dionigi et al.[161]
Epinephrine	O = L	–	(O = L)*	–	–	–
Norepinephrine	L > O	–	(O = L)*	–	–	–
VMA	–	L > O	–	–	–	–
Cortisol	(O = L)†	O = L	O = L	O = L	O = L	O > L
ACTH	O > L	–	–	–	–	–
Prolactin	–	–	–	–	–	O > L
Vasopressin	O > L	–	–	–	–	–
Insulin	–	–	–	O = L	–	–
Glucagon	–	–	–	O = L	–	–
Blood glucose	–	–	–	O = L	O = L	–
IL-6	–	–	O > L	–	–	–
CRP	–	O > L	O > L	–	–	O > L
Leukocyte count	–	–	O > L	–	–	–
CD3-decrease	–	–	–	–	–	O > L
OKDR-decrease	–	–	–	–	–	O > L

O: open cholecystectomy; L: laparoscopic cholecystectomy; VMA: Vanillin mandelic acid; CRP: C-reactive protein; CD3-lympocyte count: total number of circulating T-lymphocytes; OKDR-count: number of activated lymphocytes in peripheral blood.

*The first blood sample 4 h postoperatively may have been too late to detect intraoperative changes.

†Cortisol concentrations were similar in both groups, but returned to normal more rapidly in the laparoscopy group.

to the lower intensity of acute phase reactions that persist into the postoperative period.

One can only speculate on the reason for the lack of any spectacular difference in the classic endocrine stress reactions between minimally invasive operations and their conventional counterparts. One might hypothesize that the adrenergic and adrenocortical reactions have a threshold that is lower than the stimulus arising from IAP increase or manipulations on the liver hilus. The afferent limb of the reflex loop might possibly run through the vagus or phrenic nerves, since the initial increases in the blood concentrations of cortisol and glucose are not blocked by thoracic epidural anaesthesia.[170] There is evidence that elevated IAP alone is responsible for part of the endocrine stress reaction, since the increase of both plasma renin activity and norepinephrine plasma concentrations is attenuated when a mechanical abdominal wall lift is used to enlarge the abdominal cavity instead of gas insufflation.[169]

Transient immunosuppression is observed following a wide variety of injuries and surgical operations, and its magnitude depends to a certain extent on the extent of the tissue trauma. Immunosuppression is particularly important in tumour surgery, since it encourages tumour growth[176] and enhance the risk of metastases. Laparoscopy has a smaller effect on immunological parameter than laparotomy. This has been documented in animal studies, in which the delayed type hypersensitivity to various, intradermally injected antigens was retained after laparoscopy, but diminished following laparotomy.[177,178] Total leukocyte count is higher in patients following an open cholecystectomy, but the total T-lymphocyte count (CD3 cells) and the activated-lymphocyte count (OKDR cells) was significantly reduced.[161,179]

Differences of this sort might be responsible for the results of an animal study in which tumour cells were inoculated intradermally into mice subsequently subjected to either midline laparotomy or to abdominal inflation.[180] Tumour were established more easily and grew more aggressively in the laparotomy group. Seventy per cent of these animals, but none of those in the laparoscopy group had intradermal tumours on day 14. There might also be a connection between the choice of insufflation gas, the degree of immunosuppression and tumour growth. Animals studies have shown that abdominal insufflation with air or laparotomy inhibits phagocytosis of Candida albicans cells by peritoneal macrophages to a greater degree than when CO_2 is used for inflation.[181] Recurrence of experimentally induced hepatocellular carcinoma was more frequent after partial hepatectomy in a murine

model when the operation was performed as open laparotomy or laparoscopically with a room air pneumoperitoneum than when He or CO_2 were used to inflate the abdomen.[182]

> **Note**
> - Laparoscopic surgery induces a marked endocrine stress reaction
> - The reduction of tissue trauma with laparoscopic operations is reflected in a reduction of the inflammatory response as attenuated changes of C-reactive protein, interleukin-6, leukocyte count, erythrocyte sedimentation rate and total T-lymphocyte count
> - Laparoscopy causes less immunosuppression than laparotomy

Temperature loss

During laparotomy, a drop in body temperature occurs regularly due to radiant and evaporative heat losses from the open abdomen in combination with the anaesthetic-induced impairment of thermoregulatory mechanisms. Unintentional hypothermia should be avoided since it can cause postoperative myocardial ischaemia and angina[183] as well as enhance postoperative tumour growth.[184] Hypothermia does not occur if the patient is completely draped and the wound is small as in eye or otorhinolaryngological surgery. The situation is similar during laparoscopic surgery, and yet unexpected, and occasionally significant cooling is observed in nearly a third of all patients.[185,186] The reason for this is likely to be the gas flow through the abdominal cavity. An argument in favour of this explanation is the correlation of temperature drop and volume of insufflated gas. Body temperature decreases by $0.3°C/50l$ of insufflated gas.[186] The ultimate causative factor could be the heat required for the intra-abdominal evaporation of water to moisten the gas, or that required to bring the room temperature gas to body temperature. The results of one study suggest that warming the insufflation gas to 30°C will prevent intraoperative hypothermia during laparoscopy,[187] although this is contradicted by a different study.[188] Let us perform a simple calculation to assess the probability of this being correct.

The amount of heat required to bring the insufflated gas to body temperature can be calculated approximately with Equation (2.3):

$$\Delta Q = \frac{C_{PCO_2}(37 - \text{gas temperature in } °C)V_{insuff}}{MV_i}$$

(2.3)

where ΔQ is the heat loss of the body in calories; C_{PCO_2} is the molar heat capacity of CO_2 under constant pressure at room temperature and is equal to 8.97 cal/$^{\circ}$C and mole CO_2; V_{insuff} is the volume of insufflated gas in litres and MV_i is the mole volume of an ideal gas at 293°K (~ 24.0 l).

The resulting temperature decrease ΔT is a function of the heat capacity and the mass of the body (Equation (2.4)). The heat capacity is approximately 0.83 kcal/$^{\circ}$C and kg:

$$\Delta T = \frac{\Delta Q(\text{kcal})/0.83\ (\text{kcal}^{\circ}\text{C}^{-1}\ \text{kg}^{-1})}{\text{body mass (kg)}} \quad (2.4)$$

With an initial gas temperature of 20°C, an insufflated gas volume of 50 l and a body mass of 75 kg, the calculated heat loss would be 318 cal which would cause the body temperature to decrease by 0.005°C.

This temperature change is far from the observed value of approximately -0.3°C/50 l.[186] Even if the gas left the trocar under pressure and cooled adiabatically to -10°C, the temperature drop that this would induce in the body would only be about 0.015°C. It is obvious that gas warming alone does not explain the observations, and that other factors must be acting to cause the change in body temperature.

Large amounts of heat can be lost through evaporation of water from the surface of abdominal organs, and the continuous flow of dry gas will augment this process. If this was the cause, then moistening the insufflation gas should prevent intraoperative hypothermia. This was shown to be the case in animal studies.[189,190] The contribution of humidified insufflation gas to intraoperative normothermia in adequately draped and externally warmed patients was found to be minimal in one study.[191] Humidifying the insufflation gas and applying external warming to the patient will prevent unintentional intraoperative hypothermia during laparoscopic surgery.[192–194]

Note

- Monitoring body temperature is recommended, since significant hypothermia can occur during laparoscopic surgery
- Appropriate preventive measures such as humidifying the insufflation gas, forced air heating or heating blankets should be taken in patients with an increased risk of cardiovascular complications or those undergoing laparoscopic tumour surgery

References

1. Joris JL, Noirot DP, Legrand MJ, Jacquet NJ, Lamy ML. Hemodynamic changes during laparoscopic cholecystectomy. *Anesth Analg* 1993; **76**: 1067–1071.
2. Galizia G, Prizio G, Lieto E *et al.* Hemodynamic and pulmonary changes during open, carbon dioxide pneumoperitoneum and abdominal wall-lifting cholecystectomy. A prospective, randomized study. *Surg Endosc* 2001; **15**: 477–483.
3. Lindgren L, Koivusalo A-M, Kellokumpu I. Conventional pneumoperitoneum compared with abdominal wall lift for laparoscopic cholecystectomy. *Br J Anaesth* 1995; **75**: 567–572.
4. Andersson L, Lindberg G, Bringman S, Ramel S, Anderberg B, Odeberg Wernerman S. Pneumoperitoneum versus abdominal wall lift: effects on central haemodynamics and intrathoracic pressure during laparoscopic cholecystectomy. *Acta Anaesthesiol Scand* 2003; **47**: 838–846.
5. Reid CW, Martineau RJ, Hull KA, Miller DR. Haemodynamic consequences of abdominal insufflation with CO_2 during laparoscopic cholecystectomy. *Can J Anaesth* 1992; **39**: A132.
6. Cunningham AJ, Turner J, Rosenbaum S, Rafferty T. Transoesophageal echocardiographic assessment of haemodynamic function during laparoscopic cholecystectomy. *Br J Anaesth* 1993; **70**: 621–625.
7. Beebe DS, McNevin MP, Crain JM *et al.* Evidence of venous stasis after abdominal insufflation for laparoscopic cholecystectomy. *Surg Gynecol Obstet* 1993; **176**: 443–447.
8. Millard JA, Hill BB, Cook PS, Fenoglio ME, Stahlgren LH. Intermittent sequential pneumatic compression in prevention of venous stasis associated with pneumoperitoneum during laparoscopic cholecystectomy. *Arch Surg* 1993; **128**: 914–918.
9. Giebler RM, Behrends M, Steffens T, Walz MK, Peitgen K, Peters J. Intraperitoneal and retroperitoneal carbon dioxide insufflation evoke different effects on caval vein pressure gradients in humans: evidence for the Starling resistor concept of abdominal venous return. *Anesthesiology* 2000; **92**: 1568–1580.
10. Wachsberg RH, Sebastiano LLS, Levine CD. Narrowing of the upper abdominal inferior vena cava in patients with elevated intraabdominal pressure. *Abdom Imaging* 1998; **23**: 99–102.
11. Rosenthal RJ, Friedman RL, Chidambaram A *et al.* Effects of hyperventilation and hypoventilation on P_aCO_2 and intracranial pressure during acute elevations of intraabdominal pressure with CO_2 peritoneum: large animal observations. *J Am Coll Surg* 1998; **187**: 32–38.
12. Takata M, Wise RA, Robotham JL. Effects of abdominal pressure on venous return: abdominal vascular zone conditions. *J Appl Physiol* 1990; **69**: 1961–1972.
13. Jorgensen JO, Lalak NJ, North L, Hanel K, Hunt DR, Morris DL. Venous stasis during laparoscopic cholecystectomy. *Surg Laparosc Endosc* 1994; **4**: 128–133.

14. Goodale RL, Beebe DS, McNevin MP, Boyle R. Hemodynamic, respiratory, and metabolic effects of laparoscopic cholecystectomy. *Am J Surg* 1993; **166**: 533–537.

15. Kashtan J, Green JF, Parsons EQ, Holcroft JW. Hemodynamic effects of increased abdominal pressure. *J Surg Res* 1981; **30**: 249–255.

16. Gentili A, Iannettone CM, Pigna A, Landuzzi V, Lima M, Baroncini S. Cardiocirculatory changes during videolaparoscopy in children: an echocardiographic study. *Paediatr Anaesth* 2000; **10**: 399–406.

17. Williams MD, Murr PC. Laparoscopic insufflation of the abdomen depresses cardiopulmonary function. *Surg Endosc* 1993; **7**: 12–16.

18. Fahy BG, Hasnain JU, Flowers JL, Plotkin JS, Odonkor P, Ferguson MK. Transesophageal echocardiographic detection of gas embolism and cardiac valvular dysfunction during laparoscopic nephrectomy. *Anesth Analg* 1999; **88**: 500–504.

19. Kelman GR, Swapp GH, Smith I, Benzie RJ, Gordon NLM. Cardiac output and arterial blood–gas tension during laparoscopy. *Br J Anaesth* 1972; **44**: 1155–1159.

20. Marshall RL, Jebson PJR, Davie IT, Scott DB. Circulatory effects of carbon dioxide insufflation of the peritoneal cavity for laparoscopy. *Br J Anaesth* 1972; **44**: 680–684.

21. Motew M, Ivankovich AD, Bieniarz J, Albrecht RF, Zahed B, Scommegna A. Cardiovascular effects and acid–base and blood gas changes during laparoscopy. *Am J Obstet Gynec* 1973; **115**: 1002–1012.

22. Lenz RJ, Thomas TA, Wilkins DG. Cardiovascular changes during laparoscopy. Studies of stroke volume and cardiac output using impedance cardiography. *Anaesthesia* 1976; **31**: 4–12.

23. Johannsen G, Andersen M, Juhl B. The effect of general anaesthesia on the haemodynamic events during laparoscopy with CO₂-insufflation. *Acta Anaesthesiol Scand* 1989; **33**: 132–136.

24. Ekman LG, Abrahamsson J, Biber B, Forssman I, Milson I, Sjöqvist BA. Hemodynamic changes during laparoscopy with positive end-expiratory pressure ventilation. *Acta Anaesthesiol Scand* 1988; **32**: 447–453.

25. Critchley LAH, Critchley JAJH, Gin T. Haemodynamic changes in patients undergoing laparoscopic cholecystectomy: measurement by transthoracic electrical bioimpedance. *Br J Anaesth* 1993; **70**: 681–683.

26. Ivankovich AD, Miletich DJ, Albrecht RF, Heyman HJ, Bonnet RF. Cardiovascular effects of intraperitoneal insufflation with carbon dioxide and nitrous oxide in the dog. *Anesthesiology* 1975; **42**: 281–287.

27. Rademaker BMP, Odoom JA, deWit LT, Kalkman CJ, ten Brink SA, Ringers J. Haemodynamic effects of pneumoperitoneum for laparoscopic surgery: a comparison of CO₂ with N₂O insufflation. *Eur J Anaesthesiol* 1994; **11**: 301–306.

28. Marshall RL, Jebson PJ, Davie IT, Scott DB. Circulatory effects of peritoneal insufflation with nitrous oxide. *Br J Anaesth* 1972; **44**: 1183–1187.

29. Liu SY, Leighton T, Davis I, Klein S, Lippmann M, Bongard F. Prospective analysis of cardiopulmonary responses to laparoscopic cholecystectomy. *J Laparoendosc Surg* 1991; **1**: 241–246.

30. Huang SJ, Lee CY, Yeh FC, Chang CL. Hypercarbia is not the determinant factor of systemic arterial hypertension during carboperitoneum in laparoscopy. *Ma Tsui Hsueh Tsa Chi* 1991; **29**: 592–595.

31. Irwin MG, Ng JK. Transoesophageal acoustic quantification for evaluation of cardiac function during laparoscopic surgery. *Anaesthesia* 2001; **56**: 623–629.

32. Prys-Roberts C, Kelman GR, Greenbaum R, Robinson RH. Circulatory influences of artificial ventilation during nitrous oxide anaesthesia in man. II. Results: the relative influence of mean intrathoracic pressure and arterial carbon dioxide tension. *Br J Anaesth* 1967; **39**: 533–548.

33. Dorsay DA, Greene FL, Baysinger CL. Hemodynamic changes during laparoscopic cholecystectomy monitored with transesophageal echocardiography. *Surg Endosc* 1995; **9**: 128–133.

34. De Waal EE, Kalkman CJ. Haemodynamic changes during low-pressure carbon dioxide pneumoperitoneum in young children. *Paediatr Anaesth* 2003; **13**: 18–25.

35. Huettemann E, Sakka SG, Petrat G, Schier F, Reinhart K. Left ventricular regional wall motion abnormalities during pneumoperitoneum in children. *Br J Anaesth* 2003; **90**: 733–736.

36. Hein HAT, Joshi GP, Ramsay MAE *et al.* Hemodynamic changes during laparoscopic cholecystectomy in patients with severe cardiac disease. *J Clin Anaesth* 1997; **9**: 261–265.

37. Feig BW, Berger DH, Dougherty TB *et al.* Pharmacologic intervention can reestablish baseline hemodynamic parameters during laparoscopy. *Surgery* 1994; **116**: 733–741.

38. Hoeft A, Sonntag H, Stephan H, Kettler D. The influence of anesthesia on myocardial oxygen utilization efficiency in patients undergoing coronary bypass surgery. *Anesth Analg* 1994; **78**: 857–866.

39. Harris SN, Ballantyne GH, Luther MA, Perrino ACJ. Alterations of cardiovascular performance during laparoscopic colectomy: a combined hemodynamic and echocardiographic analysis. *Anesth Analg* 1996; **83**: 482–487.

40. Myles PS. Bradyarrhythmias and laparoscopy: a prospective study of heart rate changes with laparoscopy. *Aust NZ J Obstet Gynaecol* 1991; **31**: 171–173.

41. Scott DB, Julian DG. Observations on cardiac arrhythmias during laparoscopy. *Br Med J* 1972; **12**: 411–413.

42. Morris JJ, Perkins SR, Hein HAT, Ramsay MAE, Arnold J. Physiologic alterations during laparoscopic cholecystectomy in cardiac transplant patients. *Anesth Analg* 1995; **80**: S329.

43. Joshi GP, Hein HA, Ramsay MA, Foreman ML. Hemodynamic response to anesthesia and pneumoperitoneum in orthotopic cardiac transplant recipients. *Anesthesiology* 1996; **85**: 929–933.

44. Detry O, Defraigne JO, Chiche JD *et al.* Laparoscopic-assisted colectomy in heart transplant recipients. *Clin Trans* 1996; **10**: 191–194.

45. Menegaux F, Huraux C, Jordi Galais P *et al.* Lithiase biliaire chez le transplante cardiaque [Cholelithiasis in

heart transplant patients]. *Ann Chir* 2000; **125**: 832–837.

46. Fujii Y, Tanaka H, Tsuruoka S, Toyooka H, Amaha K. Middle cerebral arterial blood flow velocity increases during laparoscopic cholecystectomy. *Anesth Analg* 1994; **78**: 80–83.

47. Granry JC, Monrigal C, Jacob JP, Monrigal JP. Cerebral blood flow velocities (CBFV) during anaesthesia for gynaecological laparoscopic surgery. *Br J Anaesth* 1993; **70**: A32.

48. Colomina MJ, Godet C, Pellise F, Bago J, Villanueva C. Transcranial Doppler monitoring during laparoscopic anterior lumbar interbody fusion. *Anesth Analg* 2003; **97**: 1675–1679.

49. Papadimitriou LS, Livanios SH, Moka EG, Demesticha TD, Papadimitriou JD. Cerebral blood flow velocity alterations, under two different carbon dioxide management strategies, during sevoflurane anesthesia in gynecological laparoscopic surgery. *Neurol Res* 2003; **25**: 361–369.

50. Junghans T, Bohm B, Grundel K, Schwenk W, Muller JM. Does pneumoperitoneum with different gases, body positions, and intraperitoneal pressures influence renal and hepatic blood flow? *Surgery* 1997; **121**: 206–211.

51. Ishizaki Y, Bandai Y, Shimomura K, Abe H, Ohtomo Y, Idezuki Y. Changes in splanchnic blood flow and cardiovascular effects following peritoneal insufflation of carbon dioxide. *Surg Endosc* 1993; **7**: 420–423.

52. Sala-Blanch X, Fontanals J, Martinez-PAlli G *et al.* Effects of carbon dioxide vs helium pneumoperitoneum on hepatic blood flow. *Surg Endosc* 1998; **12**: 1121–1125.

53. Tunon MJ, Gonzalez P, Jorquera F, Llorente A, Gonzalo Orden M, Gonzalez Gallego J. Liver blood flow changes during laparoscopic surgery in pigs. A study of hepatic indocyanine green removal. *Surg Endosc* 1999; **13**: 668–672.

54. Kotzampassi K, Kapanidis N, Kazamias P, Eleftheriadis E. Hemodynamic events in the peritoneal environment during pneumoperitoneum in dogs. *Surg Endosc* 1993; **7**: 494–499.

55. Koivusalo AM, Kellokumpu I, Ristkari S, Lindgren L. Splanchnic and renal deterioration during and after laparoscopic cholecystectomy: a comparison of the carbon dioxide pneumoperitoneum and the abdominal wall lift method. *Anesth Analg* 1997; **85**: 886–891.

56. Blobner M, Bogdanski R, Kochs E, Henke J, Findeis A, Jelen Esselborn S. Effects of intraabdominally insufflated carbon dioxide and elevated intraabdominal pressure on splanchnic circulation: an experimental study in pigs. *Anesthesiology* 1998; **89**: 475–482.

57. Kotake Y, Takeda J, Matsumoto M, Tagawa M, Kikuchi H. Subclinical hepatic dysfunction in laparoscopic cholecystectomy and laparoscopic colectomy. *Br J Anaesth* 2001; **87**: 774–777.

58. Lindberg F, Bergqvist D, Bjorck M, Rasmussen I. Renal hemodynamics during carbon dioxide pneumoperitoneum: an experimental study in pigs. *Surg Endosc* 2003; **17**: 480–484.

59. Cisek LJ, Gobet RM, Peters CA. Pneumoperitoneum produces reversible renal dysfunction in animals with normal and chronically reduced renal function. *J Endourol* 1998; **12**: 95–100.

60. Bäcklund M, Kellokumpu I, Scheinin T, von Smitten K, Lindgren L. Warm CO_2 insufflation for laparoscopic surgery. *Eur J Anaesthesiol* 1996; **13**: 159.

61. Harman PK, Kron IL, McLachlan HD, Freedlender AE, Nolan SP. Elevated intra-abdominal pressure and renal function. *Ann Surg* 1982; **196**: 594–597.

62. Razvi HA, Fields D, Vargas JC, Vaughan EJ, Vukasin A, Sosa RE. Oliguria during laparoscopic surgery: evidence for direct renal parenchymal compression as an etiologic factor. *J Endourol* 1996; **10**: 1–4.

63. Kubota K, Kajiura N, Teruya M *et al.* Alterations in respiratory function and hemodynamics during laparoscopic cholecystectomy under pneumoperitoneum. *Surg Endosc* 1993; **7**: 500–504.

64. Koivusalo AM, Kellokumpu I, Scheinin M, Tikkanen I, Makisalo H, Lindgren L. A comparison of gasless mechanical and conventional carbon dioxide pneumoperitoneum methods for laparoscopic cholecystectomy. *Anesth Analg* 1998; **86**: 153–158.

65. McDougall EM, Monk TG, Wolf Jr. JS *et al.* The effect of prolonged pneumoperitoneum on renal function in an animal model. *J Am Coll Surg* 1996; **182**: 317–328.

66. Chiu AW, Chang LS, Birkett DH, Babayan RK. The impact of pneumoperitoneum, pneumoretroperitoneum, and gasless laparoscopy on the systemic and renal hemodynamics. *J Am Coll Surg* 1995; **181**: 397–406.

67. Leonhardt KO, Landes RR. Oxygen tension of the urine and renal structures. Preliminary report of clinical findings. *N Engl J Med* 1963; **269**: 115–121.

68. Kainuma M, Kimura N, Shimada Y. Effect of acute changes in renal arterial blood flow on urine oxygen tension in dogs. *Crit Care Med* 1990; **18**: 309–312.

69. Laisalmi M, Koivusalo AM, Valta P, Tikkanen I, Lindgren L. Clonidine provides opioid-sparing effect, stable hemodynamics, and renal integrity during laparoscopic cholecystectomy. *Surg Endosc* 2001; **15**: 1331–1335.

70. Perez J, Taura P, Rueda J *et al.* Role of dopamine in renal dysfunction during laparoscopic surgery. *Surg Endosc* 2002; **16**: 1297–1301.

71. Kainuma M, Yamada M, Miyake T. Continuous urine oxygen tension monitoring in patients undergoing cardiac surgery. *J Cardiothorac Vasc Anesth* 1996; **10**: 603–608.

72. Curet MJ, Vogt DA, Schob O, Qualls C, Izquierdo LA, Zucker KA. Effects of CO_2 pneumoperitoneum in pregnant ewes. *J Surg Res* 1996; **63**: 339–344.

73. Cruz AM, Southerland LC, Duke T, Townsend HG, Ferguson JG, Crone LA. Intraabdominal carbon dioxide insufflation in the pregnant ewe. Uterine blood flow, intraamniotic pressure, and cardiopulmonary effects. *Anesthesiology* 1996; **85**: 1395–1402.

74. Curet MJ, Weber DM, Sae A, Lopez J. Effects of helium pneumoperitoneum in pregnant ewes. *Surg Endosc* 2001; **15**: 710–714.

75. Walker AM, Oakes GK, Ehrenkranz R, McLaughlin M, Chez RA. Effects of hypercapnia on uterine and umbilical circulations in conscious pregnant sheep. *J Appl Physiol* 1976; **41**: 727–733.

76. Loring SH, Butler JP. Gas exchange in body cavities. In: Fishman AP (Ed.), *Handbook of Physiology, Section 3: The Respiratory System*. Bethesda: American Physiological Society, 1987; pp. 283–295.

77. Verstappen FT, Bernards JA, Kreuzer F. Effects of pulmonary gas embolism on circulation and respiration in the dog: I. Effects on circulation. *Pflugers Arch* 1977; **368**: 89–96.

78. Robinson JS, Thompson JM, Wood AW. Laparoscopy explosion hazards nitrous oxide. *Br Med J* 1975; **3**: 764–765.

79. Neuman GG, Sidebotham G, Negolanu E *et al*. Laparoscopy explosion hazards with nitrous oxide. *Anesthesiology* 1993; **78**: 875–879.

80. El-Kady AA, Abd-El-Razek M. Intraperitoneal explosion during female sterilization by laparoscopic electrocoagulation. *Int J Gynaecol Obstet* 1976; **14**: 487–488.

81. Drummond GB, Scott DB. Laparoscopy explosion hazards with nitrous oxide. *Br Med J* 1976; **1**: 586.

82. Palmer R. Instrumentation et téchnique de la coelioscopie gynécologique. *Gynéc Obstét* 1947; **46**: 420–427.

83. Lindemann HJ, Gallinat A. Physikalische und physiologische Grundlagen der CO_2-Hysteroskopie. *Geburtsh Frauenheilk* 1976; **36**: 729–737.

84. Semm K. Pelviskopie und Hysteroskopie. Stuttgart: Schattauer Verlag, 1976.

85. Steffey EP, Johnson BH, Eger EI. Nitrous oxide intensifies the pulmonary arterial pressure response to venous injection of carbon dioxide in the dog. *Anesthesiology* 1980; **52**: 52–55.

86. Voigt E. Notwendigkeit der endexpiratorischen CO_2-Kontrolle während laparoskopischer Sterilisation in Allgemeinnarkose mit kontrollierter Beatmung. *Anaesthesist* 1978; **27**: 219–222.

87. Kazama T, Ikeda L, Kato T, Kikura M. Carbon dioxide output in laparoscopic cholecystectomy. *Br J Anaesth* 1996; **76**: 530–535.

88. Weiss M, Krieter H, Volz J, Albrecht DM, van Akern K. Hemodynamics and acid–base balance during inflation with CO_2 or air at different pressures for laparoscopic surgery in a porcine model. *Anesth Analg* 1995; **80**: S549.

89. Nunn JF. Nunn's Applied Respiratory Physiology, 4th edition. London: Butterworth-Heinemann; 1993.

90. Fahri LE. Gas stores of the body. In: Fenn WO, Rahn H (Eds), *Section 3: Respiration I*. Washington, DC: American Physiological Society, 1964; pp. 873–885.

91. Haffor AS, Bartels RL, Kirby TE, Hamlin RL, Kunz AL. Carbon dioxide storage capacity of endurance and sprint-trained athletes in exercise. *Arch Int Physiol Biochim* 1987; **95**: 81–90.

92. Wurst H, Schulte-Steinberg H, Finsterer U. Zur Frage der CO_2-Speicherung bei laparoskopischer Cholezystektomie mit CO_2-Peritoneum. *Anaesthesist* 1995; **44**: 147–153.

93. Mullett CE, Viale JP, Sagnard PE *et al*. Pulmonary CO_2 elimination during surgical procedures using intra- or extraperitoneal CO_2 insufflation. *Anesth Analg* 1993; **76**: 622–626.

94. Liem MS, Kallewaard JW, de Smet AM, van Vroonhoven TJ. Does hypercarbia develop faster during laparoscopic herniorrhaphy than during laparoscopic cholecystectomy? Assessment with continuous blood gas monitoring. *Anesth Analg* 1995; **81**: 1243–1249.

95. Sumpf E, Crozier TA, Ahrens D, Brauer A, Neufang T, Braun U. Carbon dioxide absorption during extraperitoneal and transperitoneal endoscopic hernioplasty. *Anesth Analg* 2000; **91**: 589–595.

96. Seed RF, Shakespeare TF, Muldoon MJ. Carbon dioxide homeostasis during anaesthesia for laparoscopy. *Anaesthesia* 1970; **25**: 223–231.

97. Lewis DG, Ryder W, Burn N, Wheldon JT, Tacchi D. Laparoscopy – an investigation during spontaneous ventilation with halothane. *Br J Anaesth* 1972; **44**: 685–691.

98. Weyland W, Crozier TA, Bräuer A *et al*. Anästhesiologische Besonderheiten der operativen Phase bei laparoskopischen Operationen. *Zentralbl Chir* 1993; **118**: 582–587.

99. Lister DR, Rudston Brown B, Warriner CB, McEwen J, Chan M, Walley KR. Carbon dioxide absorption is not linearly related to intraperitoneal carbon dioxide insufflation pressure in pigs. *Anesthesiology* 1994; **80**: 129–136.

100. Blobner M, Bogdanski R, Jelen Esselborn S, Henke J, Erhard W, Kochs E. [Visceral resorption of intra-abdominal insufflated carbon dioxide in swine]. *Anästhesiol Intensivmed Notfallmed Schmerzther* 1999; **34**: 94–99.

101. Blobner M, Felber AR, Gogler S *et al*. Zur Resorption von Kohlendioxid aus dem Pneumoperitoneum bei laparoskopischen Cholezystektomien [The absorption of carbon dioxide from the pneumoperitoneum in laparoscopic cholecystectomy]. *Anaesthesist* 1993; **42**: 288–294.

102. Kazama T, Ikeda K, Sanjo Y. Comparative carbon dioxide output through injured and noninjured peritoneum during laparoscopic procedures. *J Clin Monit Comput* 1998; **14**: 171–176.

103. Streich B, Decailliot F, Perney C, Duvaldestin P. Increased carbon dioxide absorption during retroperitoneal laparoscopy. *Br J Anaesth* 2003; **91**: 793–796.

104. Debois P, Sabbe MB, Wouters P, Vandermeersch E, Van Aken H. Carbon dioxide adsorption during laparoscopic cholecystectomy and inguinal hernia repair. *Eur J Anaesthesiol* 1996; **13**: 191–197.

105. Chiche JD, Joris J, Lamy M. Respiratory changes induced by subcutaneous emphysema during laparoscopic fundoplication. *Br J Anaesth* 1994; **72 (Suppl)**: A37.

106. Wurst H, Finsterer U. CO_2-Emphysem bei laparoskopischer Chirurgie: Veränderungen der pulmonalen CO_2-Elimination [Carbon dioxide emphysema during laparoscopic surgery. Changes in pulmonary carbon dioxide elimination]. *Anaesthesist* 1994; **43**: 466–468.

107. Glascock JM, Winfield HN, Lund GO, Donovan JF, Ping ST, Griffiths DL. Carbon dioxide homeostasis during transperitoneal or extraperitoneal laparoscopic pelvic lymphadenectomy: a real-time intraoperative comparison. *J Endourol* 1996; **10**: 319–323.

108. Luiz T, Huber T, Hartung HJ. Veränderungen der Ventilation während laparoskopischer Cholezystektomie [Ventilatory changes during laparoscopic cholecystectomy]. *Anaesthesist* 1992; **41**: 520–526.

109. Esper E, Russell TE, Coy B, Duke BEr, Max MH, Coil JA. Transperitoneal absorption of thermocautery-induced carbon monoxide formation during laparoscopic cholecystectomy. *Surg Laparosc Endosc* 1994; **4**: 333–335.

110. Ott DE. Carboxyhemoglobinemia due to peritoneal smoke absorption from laser tissue combustion at laparoscopy. *J Clin Laser Med Surg* 1998; **16**: 309–315.

111. Wahba RW. Perioperative functional residual capacity. *Can J Anaesth* 1991; **38**: 384–400.

112. Strandberg A, Tokics L, Brismar B, Lundquist H, Hedenstierna G. Atelectasis during anaesthesia and in the postoperative period. *Acta Anaesthesiol Scand* 1986; **30**: 154–158.

113. Hedenstierna G. Gas exchange during anaesthesia. *Br J Anaesth* 1990; **64**: 507–514.

114. Brismar B, Hedenstierna G, Lundquist H, Strandberg Å, Svensson L, Tokics L. Pulmonary densities during anesthesia with muscular relaxation – a proposal of atelectasis. *Anesthesiology* 1985; **62**: 422–428.

115. Drummond GB, Martin LV. Pressure volume relationships in the lung during laparoscopy. *Br J Anaesth* 1978; **50**: 261–266.

116. Hong SK, Cerretelli J, Cruz C, Rahn H. Mechanics of respiration during submersion in water. *J Appl Physiol* 1969; **27**: 535–538.

117. Marini JJ, Tyler ML, Hudson LD, Davis BS, Huseby JS. Influence of head-dependent positions on lung volume and oxygen saturation in chronic air-flow obstruction. *Am Rev Respir Dis* 1984; **129**: 101–105.

118. Pelosi P, Foti G, Cereda M, Vicardi P, Gattinoni L. Effects of carbon dioxide insufflation for laparoscopic cholecystectomy on the respiratory system. *Anaesthesia* 1996; **51**: 744–749.

119. Kenefick JP, Leader A, Maltby JR, Taylor PJ. Laparoscopy: blood-gas values and minor sequelae associated with 3 techniques based on isoflurane. *Br J Anaesth* 1987; **59**: 189–195.

120. Rehder K, Wenthe FM, Sessler. Function of each lung during mechanical ventilation with ZEEP and with PEEP in man anesthetized with thiopental-meperidine. *Anesthesiology* 1973; **39**: 597–606.

121. Tokics L, Hedenstierna G, Strandberg A, Brismar B, Lundquist H. Lung collapse and gas exchange during general anesthesia: effects of spontaneous breathing, muscle paralysis and positive end-expiratory pressure. *Anesthesiology* 1987; **66**: 157–167.

122. Loeckinger A, Kleinsasser A, Hoermann C, Gassner M, Keller C, Lindner KH. Inert gas exchange during pneumoperitoneum at incremental values of positive end-expiratory pressure. *Anesth Analg* 2000; **90**: 466–471.

123. Pighin G, Crozier TA, Weyland W, Ludtke FE, Kettler D. Anasthesiologische Besonderheiten bei laparoskopischen Operationen im Sauglingsalter. *Zentralbl Chir* 1993; **118**: 628–630.

124. Kendall AP, Bhatt S, Oh TE. Pulmonary consequences of carbon dioxide insufflation for laparoscopic cholecystectomies. *Anaesthesia* 1995; **50**: 286–289.

125. Casati A, Comotti L, Tommasino C *et al*. Effects of pneumoperitoneum and reverse Trendelenburg position on cardiopulmonary function in morbidly obese patients receiving laparoscopic gastric banding. *Eur J Anaesthesiol* 2000; **17**: 300–305.

126. Feinstein H, Ghouri A. Changes in pulmonary mechanics during laparoscopic cholecystectomy. *Anesth Analg* 1993; **76**: S102.

127. Perilli V, Sollazzi L, Bozza P *et al*. The effects of the reverse trendelenburg position on respiratory mechanics and blood gases in morbidly obese patients during bariatric surgery. *Anesth Analg* 2000; **91**: 1520–1525.

128. Salihoglu Z, Demiroluk S, Dikmen Y. Respiratory mechanics in morbid obese patients with chronic obstructive pulmonary disease and hypertension during pneumoperitoneum. *Eur J Anaesthesiol* 2003; **20**: 658–661.

129. Mäkinen MT. Dynamic lung compliance during laparoscopic cholecystectomy. *Anesth Analg* 1994; **78**: S261.

130. Monk TG, Weldon BC, Lemon D. Alterations in pulmonary function during laparoscopic surgery. *Anesth Analg* 1993; **76**: S274.

131. Grissom TE, Gootos PJ, Brown TR. Pulmonary compliance is not affected by changes in position during laparoscopic surgery. *Anesthesiology* 1993; **79**: A261.

132. Fox LG, Hein HAT, Gawey BJ, Hellman CL, Ramsay MAE. Physiologic alterations during laparoscopic cholecystectomy in ASA III & IV patients. *Anesthesiology* 1993; **79**: A55.

133. Feig BW, Berger DH, Dougherty TB, *et al*. Pulmonary effects of CO_2 abdominal insufflation (CAI) during laparoscopy in high-risk patients. *Anesth Analg* 1994; **78**: S108.

134. Togal T, Gulhas N, Cicek M, Teksan H, Ersoy O. Carbon dioxide pneumothorax during laparoscopic surgery. *Surg Endosc* 2002; **16**: 1242.

135. Joris J, Cigarini I, Legrand M *et al*. Metabolic and respiratory changes after cholecystectomy performed via laparotomy or laparoscopy. *Br J Anaesth* 1992; **69**: 341–345.

136. Schauer PR, Luna J, Ghiatas AA, Glen ME, Warren JM, Sirinek KR. Pulmonary function after laparoscopic cholecystectomy. *Surgery* 1993; **114**: 389–397.

137. Putensen-Himmer G, Putensen C, Lammer H, Lingau W, Aigner F, Benzer H. Comparison of postoperative respiratory function after laparoscopy or open laparotomy for cholecystectomy. *Anesthesiology* 1992; **77**: 675–680.

138. Nguyen NT, Lee SL, Goldman C *et al*. Comparison of pulmonary function and postoperative pain after laparoscopic versus open gastric bypass: a randomized trial. *J Am Coll Surg* 2001; **192**: 469–476.

139. Braun U, Voigt E. Die Rolle von ventilatorischen Verteilungsstörungen bei der späten postoperativen Hypoxämie nach Oberbauchlaparotomien. *Anaesthesist* 1978; **27**: 163–171.

140. Ford GT, Rosenal TW, Clergue F, Whitelaw WA. Respiratory physiology in upper abdominal surgery. *Clin Chest Med* 1993; **14**: 237–252.

141. Erice F, Fox GS, Salib YM, Romano E, Meakins JL, Magder SA. Diaphragmatic function before and after

laparosopic cholecystectomy. *Anesthesiology* 1993; **79**: 966–975.

142. Ayoub J, Cohendy R, Prioux J *et al*. Diaphragm movement before and after cholecystectomy: a sonographic study. *Anesth Analg* 2001; **92**: 755–761.

143. Sharma R, Clergue F, Jansson E, Reiz S. Diaphragmatic function after laparoscopic cholecystectomy (abstract). *Br J Anaesth* 1994; **72(Suppl 1)**: A34.

144. Couture JG, Chartrand D, Gagner M, Bellemare F. Diaphragmatic and abdominal muscle activity after endoscopic cholecystectomy. *Anesth Analg* 1994; **78**: 733–739.

145. Benhamou D, Simonneau G, Poynard T, Goldman M, Chaput JC, Duroux P. Diaphragm function is not impaired by pneumoperitoneum after laparoscopy. *Arch Surg* 1993; **128**: 430–432.

146. Beebe DS, Roettger RD, Tran P, Belani KG, Gilmour IJ, Goodale RL. Evidence of impaired pulmonary function after lower abdominal laparoscopic surgery. *Anesth Analg* 1995; **80**: S35.

147. Craig DB. Postoperative recovery of pulmonary function. *Anesth Analg* 1981; **60**: 46–52.

148. Tousigant G, Wiesel S, Laporta D, Sigman H. The effect of age on recovery of pulmonary function after laparoscopic cholecystectomy. *Anesth Analg* 1992; **74**: S321.

149. Johnson D, Litwin D, Osachoff J *et al*. Postoperative respiratory function after laparoscopic cholecystectomy. *Surg Laparosc Endosc* 1992; **2**: 221–226.

150. Crozier TA, Sydow M, Siewert JR, Braun U. Postoperative pulmonary complication rate and long-term changes in respiratory function following esophagectomy with esophagogastrostomy. *Acta Anaesthesiol Scand* 1992; **36**: 10–15.

151. Schob OM, Allen DC, Benzel E *et al*. A comparison of the pathophysiologic effects of carbon dioxide, nitrous oxide, and helium pneumoperitoneum on intracranial pressure. *Am J Surg* 1996; **172**: 248–253.

152. Ben Haim M, Mandeli J, Friedman RL, Rosenthal RJ. Mechanisms of systemic hypertension during acute elevation of intraabdominal pressure. *J Surg Res* 2000; **91**: 101–105.

153. Uzzo RG, Bilsky M, Mininberg DT, Poppas DP. Laparoscopic surgery in children with ventriculoperitoneal shunts: effect of pneumoperitoneum on intracranial pressure – preliminary experience. *Urology* 1997; **49**: 753–757.

154. Mobbs RJ, Yang MO. The dangers of diagnostic laparoscopy in the head injured patient. *J Clin Neurosci* 2002; **9**: 592–593.

155. Cooke SJ, Paterson-Brown S. Associated between laparoscopic abdominal surgery and postoperative symptoms of raised intracranial pressure. *Surg Endosc* 2001; **15**: 723–725.

156. Halvorsen AJ, Barrett WL, Iglesias AR, Lee WT, Garber SM, Sackier JM. Decreased cerebrospinal fluid absorption during abdominal insufflation. *Surg Endosc* 1999; **13**: 797–800.

157. Este-McDonald JR, Josephs LG, Birkett DH, Hirsch EF. Changes in intracranial pressure associated with apnumic retractors. *Arch Surg* 1995; **130**: 362–365.

158. Moncure M, Salem R, Moncure K *et al*. Central nervous system metabolic and physiologic effects of laparoscopy. *Am Surg* 1999; **65**: 168–172.

159. Zengin K, Taskin M, Sakoglu N, Salihoglu Z, Demiroluk S, Uzun H. Systemic inflammatory response after laparoscopic and open application of adjustable banding for morbidly obese patients. *Obes Surg* 2002; **12**: 276–279.

160. Rorarius MG, Kujansuu E, Baer GA *et al*. Laparoscopically assisted vaginal and abdominal hysterectomy: comparison of postoperative pain, fatigue and systemic response. A case–control study. *Eur J Anaesthesiol* 2001; **18**: 530–539.

161. Dionigi R, Dominioni L, Benevento A *et al*. Effects of surgical trauma of laparoscopic vs. open cholecystectomy. *Hepatogastroenterology* 1994; **41**: 471–476.

162. Mealy K, Gallagher H, Barry M, Lennon F, Traynor O, Hyland J. Physiological and metabolic responses to open and laparoscopic cholecystectomy. *Br J Surg* 1992; **79**: 1061–1064.

163. Kristiansson M, Saraste L, Soop M, Sundqvist KG, Thörne A. Diminished interleukin-6 and C-reactive protein responses to laparoscopic versus open cholecystectomy. *Acta Anaesthesiol Scand* 1999; **43**: 146–152.

164. Solis-Herruzo JA, Castellano G, Larrodera L *et al*. Plasma arginine vasopressin concentration during laparoscopy. *Hepatogastroenterology* 1989; **36**: 499–503.

165. Donald RA, Perry EG, Wittert GA *et al*. The plasma ACTH, AVP, CRH and catecholamine responses to conventional and laparoscopic cholecystectomy. *Clin Endocrinol Oxf* 1993; **38**: 609–615.

166. Marana E, Scambia G, Maussier ML *et al*. Neuroendocrine stress response in patients undergoing benign ovarian cyst surgery by laparoscopy, mini-laparotomy, and laparotomy. *J Am Assoc Gynecol Laparosc* 2003; **10**: 159–165.

167. Millar RA. Plasma adrenaline and noradrenaline during diffusion respiration. *J Physiol* 1960; **150**: 79–90.

168. Sechzer PH, Egbert LD, Linde HW, Cooper DY, Dripps RD, Price HL. Effect of CO_2 inhalation of arterial pressure, E.C.G. and plasma catecholamines and 17-OH corticosteroids in normal man. *J Appl Physiol* 1960; **15**: 454–463.

169. Koivusalo AM, Kellokumpu I, Scheinin M, Tikkanen I, Halme L, Lindgren L. Randomized comparison of the neuroendocrine response to laparoscopic cholecystectomy using either conventional or abdominal wall lift techniques. *Br J Surg* 1996; **83**: 1532–1536.

170. Rademaker BM, Ringers J, Odoom JA, de-Wit LT, Kalkman CJ, Oosting J. Pulmonary function and stress response after laparoscopic cholecystectomy: comparison with subcostal incision and influence of thoracic epidural analgesia. *Anesth Analg* 1992; **75**: 381–385.

171. Joris J, Lamy M. Neuroendocrine changes during pneumoperitoneum for laparoscopic cholecystectomy. *Br J Anaesth* 1993; **70**: A33.

172. Mansour MA, Stiegmann GV, Yamamoto M, Berguer R. Neuroendocrine stress response after minimally invasive surgery in pigs. *Surg Endosc* 1992; **6**: 294–297.

173. Hirvonen EA, Nuutinen LS, Vuolteenaho O. Hormonal responses and cardiac filling pressures in head-up or head-down position and pneumoperitoneum in patients undergoing operative laparoscopy. *Br J Anaesth* 1997; **78**: 128–133.

174. Walder A, Aitkenhead AR. Role of vasopressin in the haemodynamic response to laparoscopic cholecystectomy. *Br J Anaesth* 1997; **78**: 264–266.

175. Joris J, Hamoir EE, Hartstein GM *et al.* Hemodynamic changes and catecholamine release during laparoscopic adrenalectomy for pheochromocytoma. *Anesth Analg* 1999; **88**: 16–21.

176. Allendorf JD, Bessler M, Kayton ML, Whelan RL, Treat MR, Nowygrod R. Tumor growth after laparotomy or laparoscopy. A preliminary study. *Surg Endosc* 1995; **9**: 49–52.

177. Trokel MJ, Bessler M, Treat MR, Whelan RL, Nowygrod R. Preservation of immune response after laparoscopy. *Surg Endosc* 1994; **8**: 1385–1387.

178. Bessler M, Whelan RL, Halverson A, Treat MR, Nowygrod R. Is immune function better preserved after laparoscopic versus open colon resection? *Surg Endosc* 1994; **8**: 881–883.

179. Halevy A, Lin G, Gold Deutsch R *et al.* Comparison of serum C-reactive protein concentrations for laparoscopic versus open cholecystectomy. *Surg Endosc* 1995; **9**: 280–282.

180. Allendorf JD, Bessler M, Kayton ML *et al.* Increased tumor establishment and growth after laparotomy vs. laparoscopy in a murine model. *Arch Surg* 1995; **130**: 649–653.

181. Watson RW, Redmond HP, McCarthy J, Burke PE, Bouchier Hayes D. Exposure of the peritoneal cavity to air regulates early inflammatory responses to surgery in a murine model. *Br J Surg* 1995; **82**: 1060–1065.

182. Schmeding M, Schwalbach P, Reinshagen S, Autschbach F, Benner A, Kuntz C. Helium pneumoperitoneum reduces tumor recurrence after curative laparoscopic liver resection in rats in a tumor-bearing small animal model. *Surg Endosc* 2003; **17**: 951–959.

183. Frank SM, Beattie C, Christopherson R *et al.* Unintentional hypothermia is associated with postoperative myocardial ischemia. The Perioperative Ischemia Randomized Anesthesia Trial Study Group. *Anesthesiology* 1993; **78**: 468–476.

184. Nduka CC, Puttick M, Coates P, Yong L, Peck D, Darzi A. Intraperitoneal hypothermia during surgery enhances postoperative tumor growth. *Surg Endosc* 2002; **16**: 611–615.

185. Rose DK, Cohen MM, Soutter DI. Laparoscopic cholecystectomy: the anaesthetist's point of view. *Can J Anaesth* 1992; **39**: 809–815.

186. Ott DE. Laparoscopic hypothermia. *J Laparoendosc Surg* 1991; **1**: 127–131.

187. Ott DE. Correction of laparoscopic insufflation hypothermia. *J Laparoendosc Surg* 1991; **1**: 183–186.

188. Nelskyla K, Yli-Hankala A, Sjoberg J, Korhonen I, Korttila K. Warming of insufflation gas during laparoscopic hysterectomy: effect on body temperature and the autonomic nervous system. *Acta Anaesthesiol Scand* 1999; **43**: 974–978.

189. Bessell JR, Ludbrook G, Millard SH, Baxter PS, Ubhi SS, Maddern GJ. Humidified gas prevents hypothermia induced by laparoscopic insufflation: a randomized controlled study in a pig model. *Surg Endosc* 1999; **13**: 101–105.

190. Mouton WG, Bessell JR, Pfitzner J, Dymock RB, Brealey J, Maddern GJ. A randomized controlled trial to determine the effects of humidified carbon dioxide insufflation during thoracoscopy. *Surg Endosc* 1999; **13**: 382–385.

191. Nguyen NT, Furdui G, Fleming NW *et al.* Effect of heated and humidified carbon dioxide gas on core temperature and postoperative pain: a randomized trial. *Surg Endosc* 2002; **16**: 1050–1054.

192. Matsuzaki Y, Matsukawa T, Ohki K, Yamamoto Y, Nakamura M, Oshibuchi T. Warming by resistive heating maintains perioperative normothermia as well as forced air heating. *Br J Anaesth* 2003; **90**: 689–691.

193. Weyland W, Fritz U, Fabian S *et al.* Postoperative Wärmetherapie im Aufwachraum. Ein Vergleich von radiativer und konvektiver Wärmezufuhr. *Anaesthesist* 1994; **43**: 648–657.

194. Weyland W, Weyland A, Hellige G *et al.* Efficiency of a new radiant heater for postoperative rewarming. *Acta Anaesthesiol Scand* 1994; **38**: 601–606.

195. Baratz RA, Karis JH. Blood gas studies during laparoscopy under general anesthesia. *Anesthesiology* 1969; **30**: 463–464.

196. Hodgson C, McClelland RMA, Newton JR. Some effects of the peritoneal insufflation of carbon dioxide at laparoscopy. *Anaesthesia* 1970; **25**: 382–390.

197. Alexander GD, Brown WM. Physiologic alterations during pelvic laparoscopy. *Am J Obstet Gynecol* 1969; **105**: 1078–1081.

198. Magno R, Medegard A, Bengtsson R, Tronstad SE. Acid–base balance during laparoscopy. *Acta Obstet Gynecol Scand* 1979; **58**: 81–85.

199. Puri GD, Singh H. Ventilatory effects of laparoscopy under general anaesthesia. *Br J Anaesth* 1992; **68**: 211–213.

200. Tan PL, Lee TL, Tweed EA. Carbon dioxide absorption and gas exchange during pelvic laparoscopy. *Canad J Anaesth* 1992; **39**: 677–681.

201. Williams MD, Sulentich SM, Murr PC. Laparoscopic cholecystectomy produces less postoperative restriction of pulmonary function than open cholecystectomy. *Surg Endosc* 1993; **7**: 489–492.

202. Frazee RC, Roberts JW, Okeson GC *et al.* Open versus laparoscopic cholecystectomy. A comparison of postoperative pulmonary function. *Ann Surg* 1991; **213**: 651–653.

203. Rotbøll Nielsen P, Brushøj J, Sonnenschein C. Pulmonary function after laparoscopic cholecystectomy. *Br J Anaesth* 1994; **72(Suppl 1)**: A36.

The positioning of the patient for laparoscopic surgery, and the positions of the surgeon, assistants and scrub nurses differ in many ways from conventional operations. These differences must be taken into account when preparing the patient for anaesthesia, since they frequently interfere with routine management and impair the anaesthetist's access to the patient's head and extremities. A simple example in point is the positioning for a laparoscopic herniotomy. In the conventional procedure, the surgeon stands at the level of the groin, and the anaesthetist has unimpeded access to the arms and head. For the laparoscopic procedure, on the other hand, the surgeon stands at the patient's head in order to guide the instruments from above, into the hernial orifice. One or even both of the patient's arms are positioned at his side, his head is almost completely covered and the operating table is brought into a steep Trendelenburg position. The result of this is that the anaesthetist has difficulties in accessing the venous cannulae and the endotracheal tube, as well as monitoring the patient's skin colour and pupils. At the same time, there is a higher risk of endotracheal tube movement relative to the carina with endobronchial intubation,[1–4] without the anaesthetist being unable to confirm or correct it (Figure 3.1).

Preparing the patient

Preparing the patient for anaesthesia – from selecting the venous cannulation site, to the choice of endotracheal tube and the monitoring modes – must take the above-mentioned set of problems and risks as well as the particular routine of the individual hospital into account. For the anaesthetist, it is important to retain access to at least one of the patient's arms and to the head and endotracheal tube. Unfortunately, this is not always possible, either because it would interfere with the operation, or simply because that is just the way things are done. In some hospitals, for example, the video monitor for laparoscopic cholecystectomy and other upper abdominal procedures is mounted on a bridge that spans the patient's head. Both of the patient's arms are positioned at his side, and access to his head in the event of an emergency is nearly impossible impeded (Figure 3.2).

One arm is all one needs for venous access, but if both arms are fixed at the patient's sides, one can either connect an extension with an access port to a catheter in a peripheral vein, or one can cannulate the external jugular vein, which usually remains fairly accessible even when the patient is completely draped. In more extensive operations, and especially with older patients, the use of a central venous catheter might be indicated in any case. Infusion lines from the syringe pumps for intravenous anaesthetics should be connected as closely as possible to the catheter to avoid infusion dead-space.

When the patient's head is covered with drapes, particular care must be taken to protect the eyes from abrasions and other injuries. This is usually done by taping the eyelids shut with a strip of non-irritating surgical adhesive tape (e.g. Leukosilk®). This does not always prevent corneal abrasions,[5] but not taking this kind of precaution might be construed as negligence. We do not use eye ointment in our institution, since the patients complain of postoperative visual impairment caused by corneal oedema or conjunctivitis. If there is any danger of the patient's eyes being exposed to pressure (e.g. members of the surgical team leaning on the patient's head), plastic eye protectors can be applied (Figure 3.3).

The position of the endotracheal tube and the presence of bilateral breath sounds must be confirmed by careful auscultation after intubation, and then checked at regular intervals during the operation, since the tube can migrate into an endobronchial position.[1–4] A double-lumen endotracheal tube, usually a left-sided tube, is usually required for thoracoscopic operations to allow one-lung ventilation with collapse of the lung on the affected side.

When the patient is in a steep head-down position, padded shoulder supports must be used to prevent him from slipping. These should not be attached either too far laterally or too far medially, so as to avoid damage to the brachial plexus, a common complication of the Trendelenburg position (see Chapter 6). For the same reason, the patient should not be fastened by the wrists.[6,7]

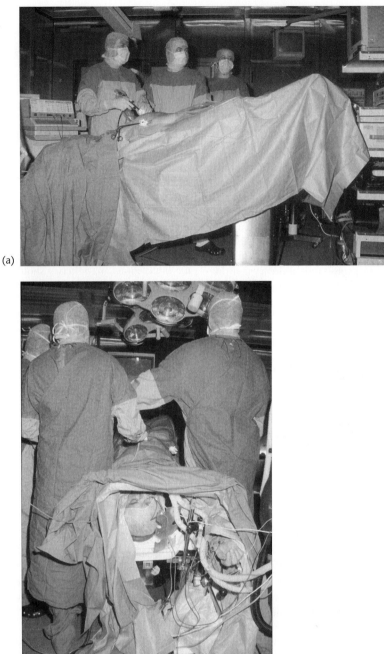

(a)

(b)

Figure 3.1 Patient undergoing laparoscopic hernioplasty. (a) One recognizes the Trendelenburg position with the patient's head completely covered and towards the left of the picture, and the inflated abdomen. (b) The patient as seen by the anaesthetist. One arm is positioned above the patient's head to facilitate access to the venous cannula.

It is not necessary to insert a urinary catheter for cholecystectomy, or for any other upper abdominal procedure of short duration.[8] Voiding the bladder before the operation ensures adequate surgical access, and only three out of 50 patients require a single postoperative catheterization. However, the situation is different with laparoscopic hernia repair or other lower abdominal and pelvic

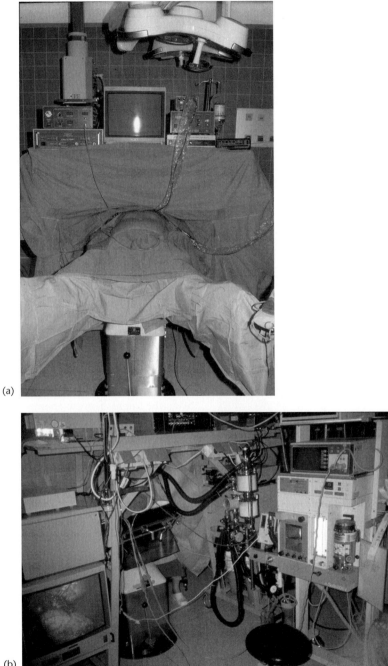

(a)

(b)

Figure 3.2 Monitor support bridge used for laparoscopic cholecystectomy and other upper abdominal procedures. (a) Surgeon's view. (b) Anaesthetist's view.

operations. A distended bladder can impede surgical progress during these procedures, and can increase the risk of injury to the bladder when inserting the trocars.

The indication for inserting a central venous catheter is based, first of all, on the clinical status of the patient, as well as on the invasiveness of the surgical procedure. An indwelling arterial catheter for invasive

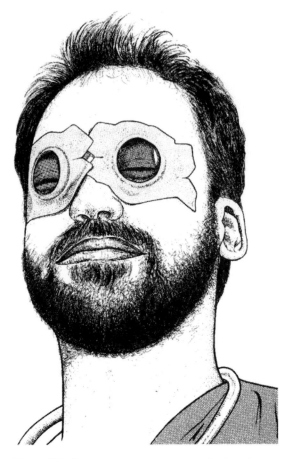

Figure 3.3 Eye protectors to prevent mechanical damage to the eyes or corneal abrasions.

blood pressure monitoring is indicated for patients with increased cardiac risk. It can provide useful information for the management of patients with severe pulmonary impairment, and for coping with difficult respiratory situations (see Chapter 4).

Note   The patient's arms are often fastened at his sides for laparoscopic procedures:

- Attach non-compliant extension lines to the venous and arterial catheters
- Consider catheterization of the jugular vein (external or internal)

The head is often completely covered:

- Protect the eyes from mechanical injury
- Secure endotracheal tube against dislocation
- Check position of endotracheal tube frequently

Consider urinary catheterization for lower abdominal operations.

Positioning the patient

The patient's position for laparoscopic surgery depends on whether it is for an upper abdominal, a lower abdominal or a thoracic procedure. The patient is usually positioned so that gravity causes the abdominal organs to fall away from the operation site to facilitate surgical access. For most operations in the upper abdomen, for example cholecystectomy, or gastric or hepatic surgery, the patient is supine in a head-up position, with the surgeon looking in a caudal-to-cranial direction. For operations in the lower abdomen, such as hernioplasty, appendectomy, hysterectomy or colorectal surgery, the patient is in a head-down Trendelenburg position and tilted from side to side as necessary. For operations in the thorax, for example for oesophagus or lung surgery, the patient is placed in a lateral decubitus position, with the side to be operated on uppermost.

The following describes the particular points for typical operations in more detail.

Upper abdominal operations

Cholecystectomy

Since the gall bladder lies on the underside of the liver, the surgeon must approach it from a caudal position, standing at the patient's lower end and looking towards his head. There are two different schools with regard to where the surgeon stands. The "French" school, also known as the "European" school,[9] has the patient positioned supine with the legs slightly abducted and flexed at the hip. The surgeon stands between the legs and views the video screen placed near the patient's right shoulder or on a bridge over the patient's head. This bridge, which is shown in Figure 3.2, makes access to the patient's head very difficult. The first assistant stands to the right, while the second assistant and the scrub nurse stand to the left of the patient (Figure 3.4).

With the "American" method, the patient lies supine or in a slight head-up position, with legs together. The surgeon stands to the left of the patient at about hip level, while the first assistant and the video monitor are on the patient's right. One arm can be abducted to 90 degrees, and the head remains freely accessible (Figure 3.5). There are thus no particular problems associated with this position with regard to the technical aspects of anaesthetic management. Some suggest that the patient be positioned in a left lateral decubitus position for cholecystectomy,[10] since this would facilitate intra-operative endoscopic retrograde cholangiopancreatography (ERCP) should this become necessary.

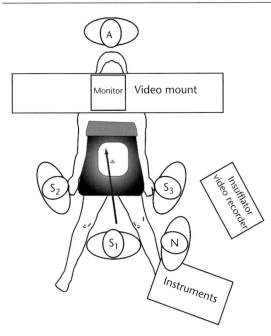

Figure 3.4 Positioning for laparoscopic cholecystectomy according to the European method. The anaesthetist is marked in the diagram with an A, while S_1 represents the surgeon, S_2 and S_3 the surgical assistants, and N the scrub nurse. The video monitor is mounted on a bridge over the patient's head in this diagram.

Gastric and hepatic surgery

For gastric (e.g. fundoplication, ulcer surgery, vagotomy, gastroplasty) or hepatic surgery, the patient is placed in a position similar to that for cholecystectomy. Here, too, the surgeon stands either between the patient's legs or at his side at hip level (Figures 3.4 and 3.5).

Note   Upper abdominal operations:

- Patient supine or in slight head up position, in some cases tilted slightly to the left
- One arm can be free, but both are often positioned alongside the patient

---

Lower abdominal operations

Inguinal hernioplasty

Inguinal hernia repair requires the surgeon to approach the surgical site from the patient's head looking caudal towards the hernia. He stands about even with the patient's shoulder on the side opposite the hernia. Both of the patient's arms are positioned close to his body so that the surgeon has maximal freedom of movement from all sides (Figure 3.6).

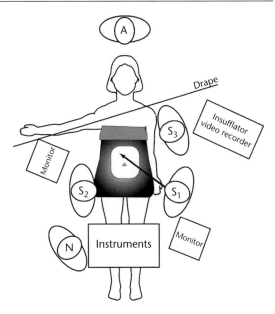

Figure 3.5 Positioning for laparoscopic cholecystectomy according to the American method. The video monitor for the surgeon is mounted to the patient right in this diagram. The assistants follow the operation on the monitor positioned next to the surgeon.

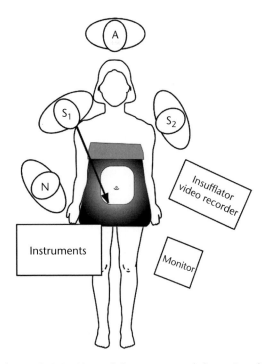

Figure 3.6 Positions of the surgeon and the patient for inguinal hernia repair. The video monitor stands near the patient's feet. Both arms are adducted and the patient's head is draped.

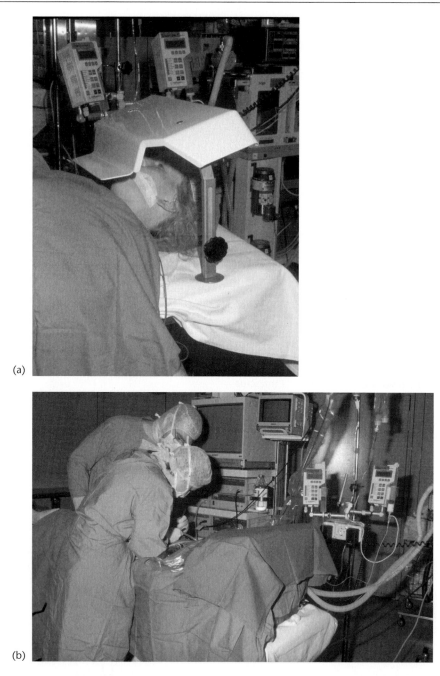

(a)

(b)

Figure 3.7 Shoulder support designed by the German gynaecologist Semm, on which the surgeon can support his or her upper body when operating in the pelvis, lower abdomen or groin. The support protects the patient's head and eyes from mechanical damage, but limits the anaesthetist's access to the arms, the head and the endotracheal tube.

This is highly inconvenient for the anaesthetist, since he cannot access peripheral venous cannulae. If only one side is to be operated on, the arm opposite the surgeon can usually be abducted. With bilateral hernioplasty, it is not possible to abduct an arm from the patient's body, but it can be positioned above the patient's head (Figure 3.1(b)). This position is particularly useful if an arterial catheter is being used. Unfortunately, this position is not possible when a shoulder support, on which the surgeon can lean, is

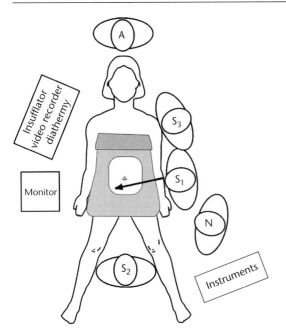

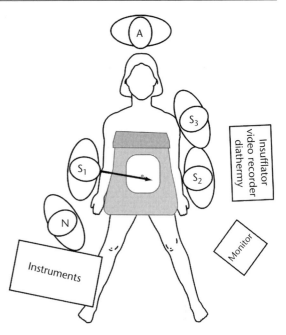

Figure 3.8 Position of the patient and surgeons for append-ectomy and operations on the ascending colon. The patient's right arm can be abducted, allowing access to venous catheter. The head is easily accessible. The anaes-thetist is marked in the diagram with an A, while S_1 repre-sents the surgeon, S_2 and S_3 the surgical assistants, and N the scrub nurse. Surgeon and assistants follow the oper-ation on the video monitor mounted across the patient from their position.

Figure 3.9 For operations on sigmoid and descending colon the surgeon stands to the patient's right with the surgical assistants positioned across from him. Both of the patient's arms are adducted, making access to venous catheters difficult. The head is freely accessible.

installed (Figure 3.7). A further problem in the pos-itioning for herniotomy is that the patient's head is often completely draped, to prevent accidental con-tamination of instruments and surgical personnel. A patient in such a position requires an athletic anaes-thetist (see Figure 3.1).

Appendectomy and colorectal surgery

For appendectomy, as for most colorectal operations, the surgeon's direction of sight is not nearly as paral-lel to the vertical axis of the patient's body as with hernia repair. The surgeon stands on the side of the patient opposite the lesion (Figure 3.8). For oper-ations on the sigmoid and descending colon the sur-geon stands on the patient's right side (Figure 3.9).

Gynaecological laparoscopic surgery

For all gynaecological laparoscopic operations, for example sterilization, ovarian cysts, uterine myomas or laparoscopically assisted vaginal hysterectomy

(LAVH), the patient is in the lithotomy position. The surgeon stands about level with the patient's chest, one assistant stands next to him, and another stands between the patient's legs. It depends on the surgeon as to whether the operation is to be carried out from one side only, or if he wants to change sides during the procedure. One arm can be abducted (usually the left) but sometimes both arms have to be placed next to the patient's body. The anaesthetist should ask beforehand in order to plan venous access.

The patient is routinely tilted head-down to allow the pelvic organs to fall free and facilitate surgical access. This is associated with a number of problems, from securing the patient on the operating table, for provid-ing adequate ventilation and detecting if the endo-tracheal tube has migrated into an endobronchial position (*vide supra*).

Urological surgery

The patient's position for most urological surgery, such as orchidopexy, varicoceles, cryptorchism, etc., is similar to that for hernia repair (*vide supra*). The head is draped, but one arm can be positioned over

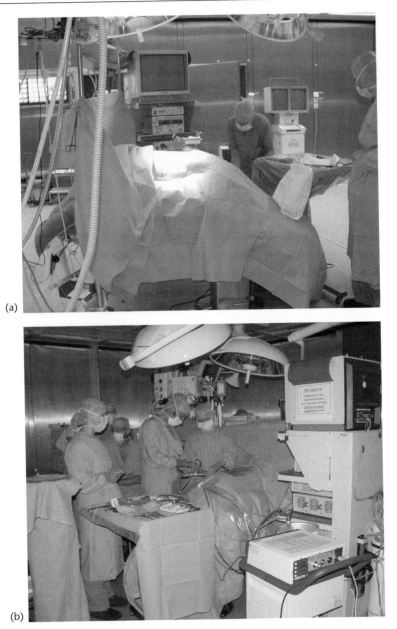

(a)

(b)

Figure 3.10 Patient positioned in a mild jack-knife position for retroperitoneal laparoscopic adrenalectomy. The patient's head is toward the left in (a) and the legs are lowered. The surgeon and his assistant stand on the same side of the patient as seen in (b).

the patient's head. During laparoscopic nephrectomy or transperitoneal adrenalectomy, the patient is in the lateral decubitus position with the affected side up. Retroperitoneal adrenalectomy is performed with the patient prone and the legs slightly lower than the dorsal costal margin (Figure 3.10). Retroperitoneal lymphadenectomy is performed with the patient in a slight Trendelenburg position as for a prostatectomy.

Note   Lower abdominal surgery:

- Patient is usually in a more or less steep, head-down position
- Partial end-expiratory pressure (PEEP) ventilation is recommended
- The tip of the endotracheal tube can migrate with resulting endobronchial intubation

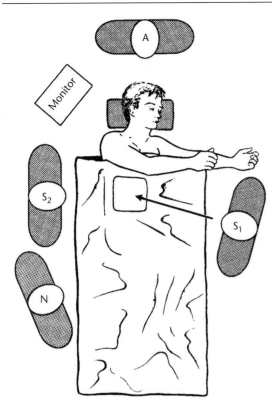

Figure 3.11 Positioning the patient for thoracoscopic surgery. The patient is in a lateral decubitus position with the surgeon standing in front of his chest. The anaesthetist is marked in the diagram with an A, while S_1 represents the surgeon, S_2 the surgical assistants, and N the scrub nurse.

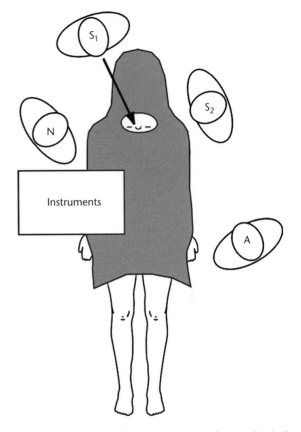

Figure 3.12 Approach to the patient for mediastinal procedures.

Thoracoscopic surgery

Operations on the oesophagus and lungs

Thoracoscopic surgery is usually performed with the patient in a lateral decubitus position. For surgery of the thoracic section of the oesophagus or the right lung, the patient is positioned on his left side. The surgeon stands facing the patient's chest but slightly caudal of the trocar insertion site looking cephalad (Figure 3.11). The lower arm stretches away from the patient's body, while the upper arm is bent at the elbow and brought over the patient's head. Selective ventilation with a double-lumen endotracheal tube is recommended, so that ventilation can be interrupted on the side being operated on. An indwelling arterial catheter is useful for monitoring arterial oxygen tensions and the magnitude of pulmonary shunt perfusion. For more details see Chapter 9.

Thoracoscopic sympathectomy

For this operation, the patient is positioned as for other intrathoracic procedures, except that he is tilted by only about 30 degrees to the contralateral side. The contralateral arm is either abducted or positioned alongside the patient, while the ipsilateral arm is brought over the patient's head and is accessible for the anaesthetist.

Mediastinal surgery

The patient is supine in a slight head-up position, and the surgeon approaches him from cephalad. The patient's head is draped, but at least one arm is usually accessible (Figure 3.12).

Note Thoracoscopic operations:

- Patient usually in lateral decubitus position (exceptions: sympathectomy, coronary artery surgery)
- Use double-lumen endotracheal tube

References

1. Mendonca C, Baguley I, Kuipers AJ, King D, Lam FY. Movement of the endotracheal tube during laparoscopic

hernia repair. *Acta Anaesthesiol Scand* 2000; **44**: 517–519.

2. Lobato EB, Paige GB, Brown MM, Bennett B, Davis JD. Pneumoperitoneum as a risk factor for endobronchial intubation during laparoscopic gynecologic surgery. *Anesth Analg* 1998; **86**: 301–303.

3. Morimura N, Inoue K, Miwa T. Chest roentgenogram demonstrates cephalad movement of the carina during laparoscopic cholecystectomy. *Anesthesiology* 1994; **81**: 1301–1302.

4. Hamm P, Lang C, Fornecker ML, Bruant P, Vuillemin F. Intubation bronchique sélective à répétition au cours d'une cholécystectomie coelioscopique [Recurrent selective bronchial intubation in laparoscopic cholecystectomy]. *Ann Fr Anesth Reanim* 1993; **12**: 67–69.

5. Bronheim D, Abel M, Neustein S. Corneal abrasions following non-ophthalmic surgery: A retrospective review of 35,253 general anesthetics. *Anesthesiology* 1995; **83(Suppl)**: A1071.

6. Mitterschiffthaler G, Theiner A, Posch G, Jäger-Lackner E, Fuith LC. Läsion des Plexus brachialis, verursacht durch fehlerhafte Operationslagerungen [Lesion of the brachial plexus, caused by wrong positioning during surgery]. *Anasth Intensivther Notfallmed* 1987; **22**: 177–180.

7. Romanowski L, Reich H, McGlynn F, Adelson MD, Taylor PJ. Brachial plexus neuropathies after advanced laparoscopic surgery. *Fertil Steril* 1993; **60**: 729–732.

8. Mowschenson PM, Weinstein ME. Why catheterize the bladder for laparoscopic cholecystectomy? *J Laparoendosc Surg* 1992; **2**: 215–217.

9. Perissat J. Laparoscopic cholecystectomy: the European experience. *Am J Surg* 1993; **165**: 444–449.

10. Grieve DA, Merrett ND, Matthews AR, Wilson R. Left lateral laparoscopic cholecystectomy and its relevance to choledocholithiasis. *Aust NZ J Surg* 1993; **63**: 715–718.

Monitoring for minimally invasive operations is essentially the same as for the conventional counterparts with basic monitoring of circulatory and respiratory parameters as well as surveillance of the correct functioning of the auxiliary support apparatus, such as ventilators, drug infusion equipment, etc. However, laparoscopic surgery forces a shift of emphasis to particular aspects of the monitoring spectrum, and mandates the inclusion of some parameters that might not be so crucial for the conventional procedures. Carbon dioxide (CO_2) absorption and alterations of pulmonary function are the two characteristic features that come to mind. The primary aim of monitoring is, of course, to ensure the maximum safety for the patient, but in minimally invasive surgery there is an additional goal of helping to exploit the concept to its fullest extent.

Respiratory monitoring

Monitoring of oxygenation and ventilation is especially important during laparoscopic surgery, because, on the one hand, these functions are directly impaired by the operations themselves, and are additionally challenged by the uptake of CO_2 on the other. Peripheral pulse oximetry and capnometry are usually adequate surrogate measures of arterial oxygen (O_2) and CO_2 tensions, although under some circumstances capnometry may be misleading (see below).

Oxygenation

Pneumoperitoneum and the head-down tilt tend to intensify the occurrence of atelectatic regions in the lung[1] that appear after induction of anaesthesia in the supine patient, and to further increase venous admixture, widening the alveolar–arterial O_2 difference ($AaDO_2$) and increasing the risk of hypoxaemia during laparoscopic procedures. Clinical monitoring of the patient's skin colour is not sufficient, since arterial O_2 desaturation can occur in patients with apparently adequate ventilatory parameters and with no signs of cyanosis. In one study, 16 of 108 patients had arterial O_2 saturation below 90% without visible cyanosis.[2] In addition, the operating theatre is usually darkened during laparoscopic surgery, which makes judging the patient's skin colour even more difficult. Pulse oximetry measures pulsatile changes of light absorption at two wavelengths to calculate the percentage of oxyhaemoglobin in the blood.[3] The method can deliver false readings if other haemoglobins, for example carboxyhaemoglobin (COHb) and methaemoglobin, are present in appreciable concentrations. COHb, which gives false high readings,[4] is frequently increased in smokers, since they can still have COHb concentrations above 5%, hours after the last smoke inhalation. Carbon monoxide is also produced in the abdomen by electrocautery and the use of lasers and is absorbed from there into the blood.[5–7] Methaemoglobinaemia, which causes either incorrectly high or low readings,[8] is less likely to be a problem during laparoscopic surgery, since mentionable amounts usually only appear after infiltration with large amounts of prilocaine, or during infusions of nitroglycerine or sodium nitroprusside in patients with methaemoglobin reductase deficiency. Methylene blue, which is occasionally injected to visualize renal function and ureter patency, can be an iatrogenic source of incorrect pulse oximetry readings and give false low SpO_2 values.[9]

A treacherous cause of arterial O_2 desaturation is the intraoperative migration of the endotracheal tube into an endobronchial position. This is not infrequent during laparoscopic surgery and is facilitated by the relative shift of the carina due to the head-down position and the additional force of the pneumoperitoneum,[10–14] although it can also occur in the reverse Trendelenburg position as well.[15] Table 4.1 summarizes typical causes of intraoperative arterial O_2 desaturation and their treatment.

Ventilation

The defining factor in most laparoscopic operations is the creation of the CO_2 pneumoperitoneum. It was recognized early on that arterial CO_2 tension increases if the absorbed CO_2 is not eliminated by increasing alveolar ventilation.[16] Years of experience and countless studies have shown that the degree of CO_2 adsorption is unpredictable, and it is impossible to calculate beforehand by exactly which amount ventilatory minute volume will have to be increased,[17–19] although attempts in this direction have been made.[20]

Table 4.1 Causes of arterial O_2 desaturation detected by pulse oximetry

Cause	Remarks	Therapy
Increased venous admixture (e.g. atelectasis)	Most common cause	Adapt ventilation (recruitment, PEEP)
Endobronchial intubation	Auscultate	Retract endotracheal tube
Bronchial secretions	Auscultate	Remove by suctioning
Impaired pulmonary perfusion	For example embolism	Specific therapy
Poor peripheral perfusion (centralization, hypothermia, shock, hypovolaemia)	Blood gases to confirm (P_aO_2, pH, lactate)	Treat circulation, active warming
F_IO_2 too low	Rarely sole cause	Increase F_IO_2
Ventilator disconnected	Frequent cause	Reconnect to patient
COHb, Met-Hb	Rare causes	

Met-Hb: methaemoglobin; PEEP: positive end-expiratory pressure.

Hypercapnia and hypocapnia, with their accompanying disturbances of the acid–base status can only be avoided by monitoring partial pressure of CO_2 in arterial blood (P_aCO_2) and adjusting ventilation as necessary. Several monitoring methods are available, each with its advantages and disadvantages. An understanding of the shortcomings of each method, and how it might be affected by the changes during laparoscopic surgery is necessary in order to use each to its fullest advantage.

Capnometry

Capnometry, or measuring the concentration of CO_2 in the expired air, is the easiest, non-invasive method of monitoring ventilation. It is based on the assumption that the end-tidal CO_2 partial pressure ($P_{et}CO_2$) is the same as the CO_2 partial pressure in the alveolar gas mixture (P_ACO_2), and that this in turn approximates the P_aCO_2. The usefulness of $P_{et}CO_2$ for monitoring assumes further that alveolar dead space, and hence the difference between P_aCO_2 and $P_{et}CO_2$ (P_aCO_2 − $P_{et}CO_2$), remains constant during the observation period. This assumption is not consistently valid during anaesthesia and ventilation, since the ventilation–perfusion ratio changes intraoperatively, with a shift in the distribution of the alveoli that are hypoventilated or hyperventilated relative to their perfusion. The hypoventilated areas have no effect on capnometry. The air in the hyperventilated alveoli, however, has a CO_2 tension lower than that in arterial blood. The air from this alveolar dead space "dilutes" the air from the normally ventilated areas, resulting in a $P_{et}CO_2$ that is lower than the P_aCO_2.[21] During normal surgery, this difference is usually of no consequence, but it acquires clinical relevance in laparoscopic operations.

The ventilation–perfusion ratio changes, for example, when pulmonary perfusion is shifted by a fall in blood pressure. Ventilatory distribution changes as a result of increased intra-abdominal pressure or an extreme head-down position. The head-up position converts apical lung segments to West I zones[22] and increases alveolar dead-space ventilation (V_D/V_T). In all of these cases, $P_{et}CO_2$ deviates from the actual P_aCO_2 to an increasing degree, as illustrated in Figure 4.1.[23,24] This deviation is greatest in older patients, especially in those with pre-existing lung disease. Due to the problems mentioned above, capnometry may give incorrect results during prolonged operations, especially in patients with pre-existing pulmonary disease, and it should supplemented with other methods (see below).

When evaluating the changes in $P_{et}CO_2$, the following factors should be taken into account: an increase in $P_{et}CO_2$ is almost always due to an increase in P_aCO_2, which can be caused by hypoventilation, for example, or a rise in body temperature; increased muscle activity; increased CO_2 adsorption or malignant hyperpyrexia. However, a rapid rise in $P_{et}CO_2$, without a concomitant change in P_aCO_2, is routinely observed when pulmonary perfusion improves; for example, when blood pressure increases in response to surgical stimulation. The reason for this is the reduction in the extent of West I areas in the lungs, which reduces alveolar V_D/V_T. A decrease in $P_{et}CO_2$ can indicate hyperventilation. But it can also be caused by a reduction of CO_2 production by the body (anaesthesia effect), or by an increase in alveolar V_D/V_T as a result of regional (e.g. pulmonary embolism, head-up position) or global (e.g. blood pressure decrease) reduction

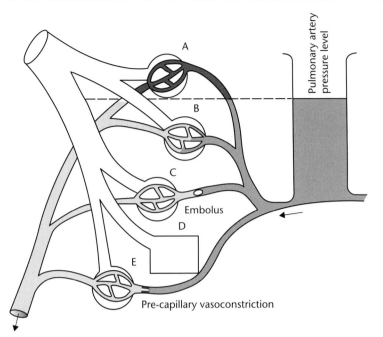

Figure 4.1 Numerous factors influence the reliability of capnometry. Perfusion of the alveoli A, C, D and E is reduced, and the ventilation– perfusion ratio is increased above unity. The result is V_D/V_T with a reduction in $P_{et}CO_2$.

Table 4.2 Interpreting capnometry data

Cause	Clinical consequence
$P_{et}CO_2$ increase	
Hypoventilation	Increase ventilation
Increased CO_2 absorption	Increase ventilation, check for intravasal insufflation
Decrease in V_D/V_T	Observe, and adjust ventilation, if necessary
Malignant hyperpyrexia	Specific therapy
$P_{et}CO_2$ decrease	
Hyperventilation	Reduce ventilation
Gas embolism	Specific therapy (see Chapter 6)
Reduced CO_2 production (effect of anaesthesia)	Adapt ventilation, if necessary
Increased V_D/V_T (positioning, reduced pulmonary perfusion, etc.)	Observe, and adjust ventilation, if necessary

of lung perfusion (Figure 4.1). If one suspects that the capnometry data might be incorrect, blood gases should be measured frequently to clarify the situation. Venous blood samples are adequate for assessing PCO_2. Table 4.2 summarizes the approach to capnometric data.

Transcutaneous CO_2 monitoring

Measuring capillary P_aCO_2 through the intact skin is another non-invasive way to monitor ventilation that is widely used in neonatology and has been shown to

be useful in adults as well.[25–27] The validity of the method rests on two observations, first of all, that the CO_2 tension of capillary blood in hyperaemic skin is virtually identical to that of the arterial blood, and secondly, that CO_2 diffuses rapidly from the capillaries through the epidermis.

In this method, the skin is made hyperaemic by actively heating it to 44°C, and CO_2 is measured in the skin under the heating electrode. Uncorrected transcutaneous CO_2 ($P_{tc}CO_2$) is higher than capillary CO_2 due to the contribution of CO_2 from cutaneous metabolism. A factor is entered manually to correct for this (Figure 4.3). Reduced cutaneous perfusion will produce false high values, because the CO_2 from cutaneous metabolism will accumulate.[28]

In a study in patients undergoing laparoscopic herniotomy and cholecystectomy, we observed a constant difference between measured P_aCO_2 and $P_{tc}CO_2$ ($P_aCO_2 - P_{tc}CO_2$), while $P_aCO_2 - P_{et}CO_2$ tensions increased during the course of the operations (Figure 4.2). Moreover, we found a poor correlation between $P_{et}CO_2$ and the P_aCO_2, which worsened during the operation (Figure 4.3). The correlation between P_aCO_2 and $P_{tc}CO_2$ on the other hand was acceptable (Figure 4.4). This observation has also been confirmed by others.[24]

Transcutaneous CO_2 measurement is a useful supplement to capnometry for monitoring the efficiency of ventilation in patients with pulmonary disease. However, it should not replace capnometry completely, since only

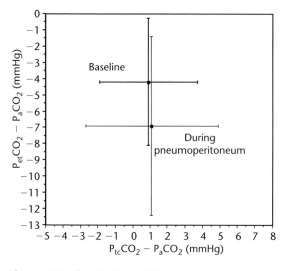

Figure 4.2 The $P_{et}CO_2 - P_aCO_2$ increases during the course of laparoscopic herniotomy, while $P_{tc}CO_2 - P_aCO_2$ remain constant during the same period.

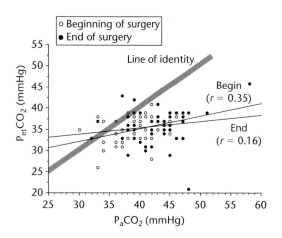

Figure 4.3 The correlation between capnometric and P_aCO_2 is poor at the start of surgery and worsens during laparoscopic cholecystectomy.

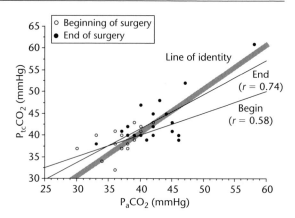

Figure 4.4 $P_{tc}CO_2$ and P_aCO_2 correlate well at the start of surgery, and the correlation improves during laparoscopic cholecystectomy.

Table 4.3 Recommendations for monitoring ventilation during laparoscopic surgery

Operation	Patient status	Recommended monitoring
Short (<2 h)	Young, healthy lungs	Capnometry
	>60 years	Capnometry, occasional venous BGA
	Pulmonary disease (e.g. COLD)	Capnometry, repeated BGA or transcutaneous CO_2 measurement
Long (>2 hours)	All patients	Capnometry, repeated BGA, $P_{tc}CO_2$
Extraperitoneal, retroperitoneal	All patients	Capnometry, repeated BGA, $P_{tc}CO_2$

BGA: blood gas analysis; COLD: chronic obstructive lung disease.

capnometry detects rapid changes of end-tidal CO_2, which might reflect ventilator disconnection, airway obstruction or pulmonary embolism, changes that are not detected by transcutaneous CO_2 monitoring.[29,30] Table 4.3 summarizes the recommended monitoring of ventilation during laparoscopic surgery.

Haemodynamic monitoring

In healthy patients and laparoscopic operations with little risk of circulatory complications, a standard 5-lead electrocardiogram (ECG) and non-invasive blood pressure measurement provide sufficient information; central venous pressure (CVP) monitoring or arterial cannulation is unnecessary. In patients with ischaemic heart disease, automated ST segment analysis of the ECG provides early warning of myocardial ischaemia, which can occur frequently during laparoscopic surgery (see Chapter 2).

However, minimally invasive surgery is frequently indicated in patients with co-morbidity so severe that conventional procedures are contraindicated. Laparoscopic cholecystectomy is a typical example.

These patients will, of course, require much more invasive monitoring, up to and including cardiac output (CO) or ventricular regional wall motion monitoring. For such patients, continuous invasive arterial pressure monitoring contributes substantially to the safety of anaesthetic management, and will facilitate serial blood gas monitoring to assess pulmonary function and perfusion. CVP monitoring might be useful in these patients, if one keeps in mind the problems associated with interpreting CVP changes during pneumoperitoneum as described in Chapter 2. If the patient's condition warrants close control of atrial filling pressures, a pulmonary artery catheter or trans-oesophageal echocardiography (TEE) might be indicated. Patients with impaired ventricular function, but undergoing operations that are known to increase the cardiac workload by increasing the vascular afterload, should have CO, left ventricular filling pressure and systemic vascular resistance monitored to gain the information required for optimal control fluid replacement, and inotrope and vasodilator therapy. With a pulmonary artery catheter, one can measure CO and also right and left ventricular filling pressures. This is a standard method, but it is complicated and associated with serious complications, and should only be employed if strictly indicated. There are a variety of non-invasive method for measuring CO which can provide useful information if their particular limitations and defects are borne in mind. Among these are Doppler sonography and bioimpedance, both of which can be used for CO measurements, but do not allow the measurement of pulmonary artery or left ventricular filling pressures.[31]

Doppler methods measure the velocity of blood flowing in the aorta, from which CO is calculated incorporating the aortic cross section (predicted or measured), heart rate and ejection time. Earlier methods used a transcutaneous approach from the suprasternal notch, which yielded a satisfactory correlation with the results obtained by thermodilution.[32,33] This is not feasible during most laparoscopic operations. Using an oesophageal probe will avoid the problems of access associated with laparoscopic surgery. The initial results were very poor and the correlation between the CO measured by Doppler and that measured by thermodilution varied between -0.02 and $+0.94$.[34] Equipment has improved and studies and reviews show that the correlation between Doppler CO measurement and thermodilution is now much better.[35–37] However, precision is still only fair as measured by the limits of agreement between the methods.[38] Leather and Wouters demonstrated that a redistribution of blood flow induced by lumbar epidural anaesthesia changed the bias of oesophageal

Doppler CO measurement compared to thermodilution from $-0.89 \, l \, min^{-1}$ to $+0.55 \, l \, min^{-1}$. The limits of agreement with thermodilution that were initially between -2.67 and $+0.88 \, l \, min^{-1}$, deteriorated after blood flow redistribution to between -3.21 and $+4.30 \, l \, min^{-1}$, which is inacceptable.[39] The increase in peripheral vascular resistance caused by creating the pneumoperitoneum is likely to cause a redistribution of blood flow as will placing the patient in a steep Trendelenburg or reverse Trendelenburg position. Another factor that might contribute to the high variability of oesophageal Doppler CO monitoring is the fact that it does not include blood flow to the coronaries, the upper extremities and the brain. This error cannot be corrected for with a constant factor, since blood flow to the coronary arteries and the brain are subject to fluctuations which themselves are functions of anaesthesia and surgical stimulation, and do not always represent the same fraction of CO. For example, the typical intraoperative rise in P_aCO_2 will trigger an absolute as well as percentage-wise increase in cerebral blood flow.

Bioimpedance is another well-known, non-invasive method for determining CO that is suitable for continuous monitoring, and which has already been used in studies involving laparoscopic operations.[40,41] With this method, changes in transthoracic impedance are analysed against a high-frequency current. The stroke volume is calculated from the distance between electrodes on the upper and lower thorax aperture, the temporal change in impedance, the baseline impendence and the time. But the distance between the upper and lower electrodes, the constancy of which is most critical, is altered by the creation of the peritoneum and longitudinal data over time are difficult to interpret (see Chapter 2). The bioimpedance technique is also of no use during thoracoscopy, because the changes in baseline impedance caused by creating a pneumothorax are not calculable. Comparative studies show an acceptable total correlation of CO data measured by bioimpedance with those derived from thermodilution, but the values of the individual measurements varied widely ($\pm 1.5 \, l \, min^{-1}$) and exhibited no systematic bias that one could adjust for.[42,43] For these reasons, the bioimpedance technique is hardly suitable for monitoring critically ill patients during laparoscopic–endoscopic operations. Better results might be achieved with the oesophageal placement of the electrodes.[44] A more recent study comparing bioimpedance CO measurements with thermodilution during major abdominal surgery found poor agreement between the two methods and a shift in measurement bias relative to changes in surgical conditions.[45] Pulse contour monitoring and the Fick principle using CO_2 are the two other non-invasive techniques for measuring CO.[35] The former is probably unreliable due to the changes induced by the pneumoperitoneum, and the latter is obviously useless in laparoscopic surgery.

Despite its shortcomings, oesophageal Doppler sonography is, at present, probably the most suitable non-invasive method for monitoring CO in cardiac risk patients. TEE gives information on myocardial contractility, ejection fraction and ventricular filling and complements CO measurements.

Note   Measurement of cardiac function and/or CO is indicated in patients at high cardiac risk.

- **Thermodilution**: invasive but standardized and reliable if properly used
- **Doppler sonograph**: non-invasive and fairly reliable
- **Bioimpedance**: non-invasive but problematic with regard to reliability
- **TEE**: moderately invasive, excellent information on myocardial function and cardiac filling, little information of CO, requires specialized training

---

During laparoscopic surgery, the process of distilling clinical consequences from the haemodynamic monitoring data must include careful differential diagnostic considerations. Changes in blood pressure and/or heart rate, especially increases, may occur in response to surgical stimuli and pain, and thus be an indication of insufficient anaesthesia, but not always. They might also be the first clinical signs of hypercapnia (frequent), hypoxaemia (less frequent), gas embolism (not uncommon), or relative hypovolaemia in a

Table 4.4 Haemodynamic monitoring during laparoscopic surgery

Patient status	Suggested monitoring
Young, no cardiac risks	5-lead ECG, non-invasive blood pressure monitoring
Ischaemic heart disease	5-lead ECG with ST segment analysis, invasive blood pressure monitoring if hypertension a risk
Congestive heart disease compensated	5-lead ECG with ST segment analysis, invasive blood pressure monitoring, CVP
Poorly compensated	Additional cardiac function monitoring (pulmonary artery catheter, oesophageal Doppler, TEE, etc.).

patient with the typical vasoconstriction of pneumoperitoneum. These possible causes must be ruled out before simply deepening the level of anaesthesia. Table 4.4 gives a survey of points to be considered in haemodynamic monitoring.

Neuromuscular monitoring

Neuromuscular monitoring is particularly useful during laparoscopic operations, since adequate relaxation is required for optimal surgical access, while at the same time, one wishes to avoid residual curarization in the postoperative period.[46,47] The latter aspect is especially important in view of the extremely short times required for wound closure after minimally invasive procedures.

Sophisticated monitoring methods are not required, and train-of-four (TOF) stimulation with either tactile or quantitative evaluation (e.g. by accelerography) of the twitch responses and the TOF ratio should suffice. The latter is the quotient obtained by dividing the response to the fourth stimulus by that to the first stimulus. If there are fewer than four responses the TOF ratio is not calculated, and only the number of twitches is noted (TOF number). Residual relaxation can be detected with double-burst stimulation (DBS) consisting of two short series of three stimuli each.[48]

Tactile assessment of the TOF is sufficient for intraoperative management of neuromuscular relaxation. A TOF number of 1–2 indicates an adequate degree of myorelaxation for laparotomy, but there is no universally defined level for laparoscopic procedures. A twitch reduction of approximately 80%, indicated by two to three responses to TOF stimulation, will probably be sufficient to obtain adequate compliance of the abdomen. The presence of singultus will require further relaxation, since the diaphragm is less sensitive to the effect of non-depolarizing neuromuscular blockers than skeletal muscle. Tactile assessment alone is not sufficient for determining eligibility for tracheal extubation. Current guidelines require a TOF quotient of 0.9 or higher.

The ulnar nerve – adductor pollicis muscle unit is normally employed for neuromuscular monitoring. The ulnar nerve is stimulated with closely spaced surface electrodes (ECG electrodes suitable) attached over the course of the nerve at the wrist. However, since the patient's arms are often positioned alongside the body and are thus inaccessible for tactile or accelerographic monitoring, this nerve can only be employed when the response is assessed by electromyography (e.g. Relaxograph®, Datex). One can also stimulate the facial nerve and assess relaxation as the response of the orbicularis oculi or orbicularis oris muscle. The electrodes are placed over the course of the nerve, one approximately over the condyle of the temporal mandibular joint, and the second anterior to the first (Figure 4.5). The current required for supra-maximal stimulation of the ulnar nerve is about 50–70 mA and approximately 30–40 mA for the facial nerve. The orbicularis oculi muscle responds to neuro-muscular blockers in a manner similar to that of the diaphragm.[49] Using these muscles to guide the admin-istration of neuromuscular blockers will guarantee an adequately relaxed patient during the operation, but recovery of the facial muscles may not indicate recov-ery of muscular strength adequate for tracheal extuba-tion.[50,51] Changes of skin or muscle temperature alter the response to relaxometry.[52,53] Response drift can occur during lengthy operations that usually reduces the amplitude of the first twitch compared to base-line.[54] Table 4.5 summarizes the basic principles of neuromuscular monitoring in laparoscopic surgery.

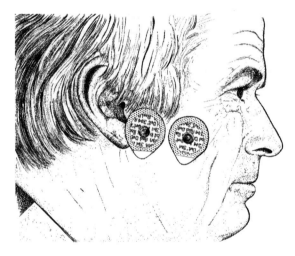

Figure 4.5 Electrode placement for stimulating the facial nerve.

Temperature monitoring

Temperature monitoring is recommended during lengthy laparoscopic operations, since body tempera-ture can decrease sharply, despite the smaller incision and better insulation of the patient compared to con-ventional operations. Care must be taken not to pos-ition the thermistor in the vicinity of the operation site where there is considerable cooling.

References

1. Hedenstierna G, Strandberg Å, Tokics L, Lundqvist H, Brismar B. Correlation of gas exchange impairment to development of atelectasis during anesthesia and muscle paralysis. *Acta Anaesthesiol Scand* 1986; **30**: 183–191.
2. Raeder DB, Warren DL, Morris R, Philip BK, Philip JH. Hypoxemia during ambulatory gynecologic sur-gery as evaluated by the pulse oximeter. *J Clin Monit* 1987; **3**: 244–248.
3. Tremper KK, Barker SJ. Pulse oximetry. *Anesthesiology* 1989; **70**: 98–108.
4. Barker SJ, Tremper KK. The effect of carbon monoxide inhalation on pulse oximetry and transcutaneous PO_2. *Anesthesiology* 1987; **66**: 677–679.
5. Beebe DS, Swica H, Carlson N, Palahniuk RJ, Goodale RL. High levels of carbon monoxide are pro-duced by electro-cautery of tissue during laparoscopic cholecystectomy. *Anesth Analg* 1993; **77**: 338–341.
6. Ott DE. Carboxyhemoglobinemia due to peritoneal smoke absorption from laser tissue combustion at laparoscopy. *J Clin Laser Med Surg* 1998; **16**: 309–315.
7. Esper E, Russell TE, Coy B, Duke BEr, Max MH, Coil JA. Transperitoneal absorption of thermocautery-induced carbon monoxide formation during laparo-scopic cholecystectomy. *Surg Laparosc Endosc* 1994; **4**: 333–335.
8. Eisenkraft JB. Pulse oximeter desaturation due to methemoglobinemia. *Anesthesiology* 1988; **68**: 279–282.
9. Kessler MR, Eide T, Humayun B, Poppers PJ. Spurious pulse oximeter desaturation with methylene blue injection. *Anesthesiology* 1986; **65**: 435–436.

Table 4.5 Clinical application of neuromuscular monitoring for laparoscopic surgery

Phase of operation	Relevant for	Relaxometer	Clinical signs
Intraoperative	Dosing	TOF number 2–3 $T_1 = 10–20\%$	No pressing, no singultus Amply expanded pneumoperitoneum
Emergence	Extubation	DBS without fading TOF ratio $\geqslant 0.9$	Elevate head from table and hold for at least 5 s

TOF: four stimuli at a stimulation frequency of 2 Hz; TOF number: number of detectable responses to TOF stimulation; $T_1\%$: amplitude of first TOF response as percentage of calibrated baseline without relaxation; TOF ratio: amplitude of fourth response divided by that of first response T_4/T_1.

10. Heinonen J, Takki S, Tammisto T. Effect of Trendelenburg tilt and other procedures on the position of endotracheal tubes. *Lancet* 1969; **1**: 850–853.

11. Hamm P, Lang C, Fornecker ML, Bruant P, Vuillemin F. Intubation bronchique sélective à répétition au cours d'une cholécystectomie coelioscopique [Recurrent selective bronchial intubation in laparoscopic cholecystectomy]. *Ann Fr Anesth Reanim* 1993; **12**: 67–69.

12. Morimura N, Inoue K, Miwa T. Chest roentgenogram demonstrates cephalad movement of the carina during laparoscopic cholecystectomy. *Anesthesiology* 1994; **81**: 1301–1302.

13. Lobato EB, Paige GB, Brown MM, Bennett B, Davis JD. Pneumoperitoneum as a risk factor for endobronchial intubation during laparoscopic gynecologic surgery. *Anesth Analg* 1998; **86**: 301–303.

14. Mendonca C, Baguley I, Kuipers AJ, King D, Lam FY. Movement of the endotracheal tube during laparoscopic hernia repair. *Acta Anaesthesiol Scand* 2000; **44**: 517–519.

15. Brimacombe JR, Orland H, Graham D. Endobronchial intubation during upper abdominal laparoscopic surgery in the reverse Trendelenburg position. *Anesth Analg* 1994; **78**: 607.

16. Voigt E. Notwendigkeit der endexpiratorischen CO_2-Kontrolle während laparoskopischer Sterilisation in Allgemeinnarkose mit kontrollierter Beatmung. *Anaesthesist* 1978; **27**: 219–222.

17. Weyland W, Crozier TA, Bräuer A *et al.* Anästhesiologische Besonderheiten der operativen Phase bei laparoskopischen Operationen. *Zentralbl Chir* 1993; **118**: 582–587.

18. Wittgen CM, Naunheim KS, Andrus CH, Kaminski DL. Preoperative pulmonary function evaluation for laparoscopic cholecystectomy. *Arch Surg* 1993; **128**: 880–885.

19. Wurst H, Finsterer U. Pathophysiologische und klinische Aspekte der Laparoskopie. *Anästhesiol Intens Med* 1990; **31**: 187–197.

20. Girardis M, Da Broi U, Antonutto G, Pasetto A. The effect of laparoscopic cholecystectomy on cardiovascular function and gas exchange. *Anesth Analg* 1996; **83**: 134–140.

21. Nunn JF, Hill DW. Respiratory dead space and arterial to end-tidal CO_2 tension difference in anaesthetized man. *J Appl Physiol* 1960; **15**: 383–389.

22. West JB, Dollery CT, Naimark A. Distribution of blood flow in isolated lung: relation to vascular and alveolar pressures. *J Appl Physiol* 1964; **19**: 713–724.

23. Brampton WJ, Watson RJ. Arterial to end-tidal carbon dioxide tension difference during laparoscopy. *Anaesthesia* 1990; **45**: 210–214.

24. Reid CW, Martineau RJ, Miller DR, Hull KA, Baines J, Sullivan PJ. A comparison of transcutaneous, end-tidal and arterial measurements of carbon dioxide during general anaesthesia. *Can J Anaesth* 1992; **39**: 31–36.

25. Goldman MD, Gribbin HR, Martin RJ, Loh L. Transcutaneous pCO_2 in adults. *Anaesthesia* 1982; **37**: 944–946.

26. Kick O, Vanderneersch E, Mulier JP, Vermaut J, Van Aken H. Überwachung des Patienten im Aufwachraum. *Anaesthesist* 1992; **41**: 331–334.

27. Wimberley PD, Grønlund Pedersen K, Thode J, Fogh-Andersen N, Møller Sørensen A, Siggaard-Andersen O. Transcutaneous and capillary pCO_2 and pO_2 measurements in healthy adults. *Clin Chem* 1983; **29**: 1471–1473.

28. Lemke R, Klaus D. Die Bedeutung der nicht-invasiven kontinuierlichen $TcPO_2$- und $TcPCO_2$-Messung bei kreislaufstabilen Patienten und bei Patienten mit Schock. *Intensivmedizin* 1986; **23**: 22–26.

29. Glenski JA, Cucchiara RF, Michenfelder JD. Transesophageal echocardiography and transcutaneous O_2 and CO_2 monitoring for detection of gas embolism. *Anesthesiology* 1986; **64**: 541–545.

30. Bednarz F, Roewer N. Intraoperativer Nachweis von Luftembolien und korpuskulären Embolien mit Hilfe der Pulsoximetrie und Kapnometrie: Vergleichende Untersuchung mit der transösophagealen Echokardiographie [Intraoperative detection of air embolism and corpuscular embolism using pulse oximetry and capnometry. Comparative studies with transesophageal echocardiography]. *Anasth Intensivther Notfallmed* 1989; **24**: 20–26.

31. Prys-Roberts C. Monitoring cardiac output. In: Hutton P, Prys-Roberts C (Eds), *Monitoring in Anaesthesia and Critical Care*. London: W.B. Saunders, 1994; pp. 156–171.

32. Huntsman LL, Steward DK, Barnes SR, Franklin SB, Colocousis JS, Hessel EA. Noninvasive Doppler determination of cardiac output in man. *Circulation* 1983; **67**: 593–602.

33. Chandraratna PA, Nanna M, McKay C *et al.* Determination of cardiac output by transcutaneous continuous-wave ultrasonic Doppler computer. *Am J Cardiol* 1984; **53**: 234–237.

34. Freund PR. Transesophageal Doppler scanning versus thermodilution during general anesthesia: an initial comparison of cardiac output techniques. *Am J Surg* 1987; **153**: 490–494.

35. Berton C, Cholley B. Equipment review: new techniques for cardiac output measurement – oesophageal Doppler, Fick principle using carbon dioxide, and pulse contour analysis. *Crit Care* 2002; **6**: 216–221.

36. Mann C, Boccara G, Pouzeratte Y, Navarro F, Domergue J, Colson P. Monitorage hemodynamique par Doppler oesophagien lors de la cholecystectomie par coelioscopie [Hemodynamic monitoring using esophageal Doppler ultrasonography during laparoscopic cholecystectomy]. *Can J Anaesth* 1999; **46**: 15–20.

37. Royse CF, Royse AG, Blake DW, Grigg LE. Measurement of cardiac output by transoesophageal echocardiography: a comparison of two Doppler methods with thermodilution. *Anaesth Intens Care* 1999; **27**: 586–590.

38. Laupland KB, Bands CJ. Utility of esophageal Doppler as a minimally invasive hemodynamic monitor: a review. *Can J Anaesth* 2002; **49**: 393–401.

39. Leather HA, Wouters PF. Oesophageal Doppler monitoring overestimates cardiac output during lumbar epidural anaesthesia. *Br J Anaesth* 2001; **86**: 794–797.

40. Critchley LAH, Critchley JAJH, Gin T. Haemodynamic changes in patients undergoing laparoscopic cholecystectomy: measurement by transthoracic electrical bioimpedance. *Br J Anaesth* 1993; **70**: 681–683.

41. Rademaker BMP, Odoom JA, deWit LT, Kalkman CJ, ten Brink SA, Ringers J. Haemodynamic effects of pneumoperitoneum for laparoscopic surgery: a comparison of CO_2 with N_2O insufflation. *Eur J Anaesthesiol* 1994; **11**: 301–306.

42. Bernstein DP. Continuous noninvasive real-time monitoring of stroke volume and cardiac output by thoracic electrical bioimpedance. *Crit Care Med* 1986; **14**: 848–890.

43. Shoemaker WC, Appel PL, Kram HB, Nathan RC, Thompson JL. Multicomponent noninvasive physiologic monitoring of circulatory function. *Crit Care Med* 1988; **16**: 482–490.

44. Balestra B, Malacrida R, Leonardi L, Suter P, Marone C. Esophageal electrodes allow precise measurement of cardiac output by bioimpedance. *Crit Care Med* 1992; **20**: 62–67.

45. Critchley LAH, Leung DH, Short TG. Abdominal surgery alters the calibration of bioimpedance cardiac output measurement. *Int J Clin Monit Comp* 1996; **13**: 1–8.

46. Viby-Mogensen J, Jorgensen BC, Ording H. Residual curarisation in the recovery room. *Anesthesiology* 1979; **50**: 539–541.

47. Cammu G, DeVeylder J, Vandenbroucke G, Vandeput D, Foubert L, Deloof T. Postoperative residual curarisation after outpatient surgery. *Eur J Anaesthesiol* 2004; **21 (Suppl)**: A50.

48. Engbaek J, Ostergaard D, Viby-Mogensen J. Double-burst stimulation (DBS): a new pattern of nerve stimulation to identify residual neuromuscular block. *Br J Anaesth* 1989; **62**: 274–278.

49. Donati F, Meistelman C, Plaud B. Vecuronium neuromuscular blockade at the diaphragm, the orbicularis oculi and adductor pollicis muscle. *Anesthesiology* 1990; **73**: 870–875.

50. Sharpe MD, Moote CA, Lam AM, Manninen PH. Comparison of integrated evoked EMG between the hypothenar and facial muscle groups following atracurium and vecuronium administration. *Can J Anaesth* 1990; **38**: 318–323.

51. Rimaniol JM, Dhonneur G, Sperry L, Duvaldestin P. A comparison of the neuromuscular blocking effects of atracurium, mivacurium, and vecuronium on the adductor pollicis and orbicularis oculi muscles in humans. *Anesth Analg* 1996; **83**: 808–813.

52. Thornberry EA, Mazumdar B. The effect of changes in arm temperature on neuromuscular monitoring in the presence of atracurium blockade. *Anaesthesia* 1988; **43**: 447–449.

53. Heier T, Caldwell JE, Sessler DI, Kitts JB, Miller RD. The relationship between adductor pollicis twitch tension and core, skin and muscle temperature during nitrous oxide-isoflurane anesthesia in humans. *Anesthesiology* 1989; **71**: 381–384.

54. Meretolja OA, Brown TCK. Drift of the evoked thenar EMG-signal. *Anesthesiology* 1989; **71**: A825.

Laparoscopy surgery requires a strategic reassessment and adaptation of anaesthetic management in order to derive the greatest possible benefit from the procedures on the one hand, and to anticipate the specific risks and prevent the complications inherent in the technique on the other. When choosing the anaesthetic, the anaesthetist must be fully aware that the main advantage of these minimally invasive surgical procedures is the shortened recovery period and the intended rapid return of the patient to normal daily life. The patient expects early mobilization, a rapid return to oral feeding and prompt discharge from the hospital – frequently within 24 h after an uncomplicated laparoscopic cholecystectomy. This intended fast tracking should not be impeded by postoperative impairment of the patient's recovery by fatigue, lassitude, nausea and vomiting, vertigo or other adverse effects. Even after major operations, such as colectomy, nephrectomy or lymphadenectomy, oral fluids are given on the day of surgery, oral feeding is started on the first postoperative day, and the patient is occasionally discharged from the hospital on the following day.

A further aspect of minimally invasive surgery is the drastic reduction of the time from when, for example, the gall bladder is removed until when the wound is sutured and dressed. Taking the altered time frame into consideration, the anaesthetist can contribute to the smooth handling of the surgical schedule by ensuring short turnover times between the individual patients. In conventional surgery, the anaesthetic could be lightened while the peritoneum was being closed, the various layers of the abdominal wall sutured and the dressing applied, and the patient would be awake immediately afterward. The pharmacokinetics of the anaesthetic were not particularly crucial. This procedure is not possible with laparoscopic surgery, since wound closure only consists of removing the instruments and trocars and stitching up a few holes, and takes only few minutes. This means that a rapid offset and recovery is the *conditio sine qua non* for an anaesthetic for minimally invasive surgery. New hypnotics, volatile anaesthetics, opioids and neuromuscular blockers having the required pharmacokinetic–pharmacodynamic properties have been developed, and advanced methods of

drug delivery and anaesthetic depth monitoring are now available that will allow optimal anaesthetic management of minimally invasive operations with minimal adverse effects and rapid awakening and recovery.

General anaesthesia with controlled ventilation is the method of choice for nearly all minimally invasive procedures with only few possible exceptions. Controlled mechanical ventilation is recommended to counteract the hypercapnia and hypoxia due to impaired lung function, and to meet the simultaneously increased ventilatory requirements. Even where this is not the case, the necessity of neuromuscular relaxation for most laparoscopic operations would make mechanical ventilation mandatory.

Airway

Elevated intra-abdominal pressure (IAP) does not *per se* increase the risk of regurgitating gastric contents, but the risk is higher with the patient in the Trendelenburg position. Endotracheal intubation protects the airway and prevents aspiration pneumonitis in these patients. Some authors see laparoscopic surgery as an indication, or at least not a contraindication, for use of the laryngeal mask airway,[1,2] but their enthusiasm is not shared by all.[3] If one chooses to use a laryngeal airway, some authors recommend using the ProSeal® model instead of the classic model, since they found it provided better ventilation during pneumoperitoneum,[4] and that it was equal to ventilation with a cuffed endotracheal tube.[5] Either would be suited for short diagnostic laparoscopies or for extraperitoneal procedures such as hernia repair.[6] A double lumen endotracheal tube should be used for thoracoscopic operations in order to facilitate collapse of the lung on the side of the operation. This improves surgical access, shortens the operating time and obviates the necessity of intrathoracic gas insufflation with its associated complications.[7]

The optimal anaesthetic for laparoscopic or thoracoscopic operations is one that takes advantage of the excellent pharmacokinetics of drugs such as remifentanil, propofol, desflurane, isoflurane, mivacurium and others with rapid on–off characteristics. This can be a total intravenous technique or a balanced technique with an opioid and a volatile anaesthetic, as long as the components are administered in a way to optimize depth of anaesthesia and recovery. We prefer a total intravenous technique with propofol as the hypnotic and remifentanil, since most meta-analyses have shown that propofol is effective in preventing postoperative nausea and vomiting (PONV), a complication otherwise linked with laparoscopy.[8,9] The newer drugs required for these techniques are more expensive than old faithfuls like fentanyl, thiopental, pancuronium and halothane, but they can be more cost effective by reducing the turnover time between patients and the need for postoperative monitored care, while furthering the goal of early mobilization and hospital discharge. These drugs might not be available in every institution or in every country.

Premedication

We recommend giving patients an oral premedication on the ward to provide anxiolysis before they are brought to the operating theatre, but this is not an absolute necessity and many institutions opt for an intravenous premedication in the holding area or for none at all. When oral premedication is given, a drug should be chosen that does not cause postoperative drowsiness. Short-acting oral benzodiazepines, such as midazolam, lorazepam or temazepam, are good choices. The clinical effects of diazepam, flunitrazepam, barbiturates or similar drugs last too long for most minimally invasive procedures, and will delay awakening and interfere with the recovery period. Whichever drug one chooses, the correct dose and proper time of application are important to ensure getting the maximum benefit from the premedication. Midazolam has a rapid onset of action, but must not be given too soon, since it also has a rapid offset and the sedative and anxiolytic effects might have evaporated before the patient is brought to surgery. Lorazepam, on the other hand, must be given at least an hour before the patient is fetched from the ward, since its effect sets in only slowly. Many institutions choose to give an intravenous premedication with a small dose of midazolam shortly before induction. There are a number of studies which show that this "co-induction" reduces the dose of hypnotic needed to attain the targeted depth of anaesthesia.[10,11] On the other hand, although the propofol dose required for induction is reduced, recovery is prolonged, and this intravenous application does nothing to reduce the patient's anxiety beforehand. Intramuscular premedication used to

be the standard procedure, but the availability of excellent oral drugs and the knowledge that a sip of water with the tablet does not increase the risk of aspiration during induction has rendered the intramuscular route obsolete. Antisialogogues are no longer considered a mandatory component of the premedication, now that the use of ether has been discontinued. When increased salivation might be a problem, such as with a laryngeal mask airway or when ketamine is used, glycopyrrolate or atropine is given intravenously.

Total intravenous anaesthesia

General remarks

In the narrow definition of total intravenous anaesthesia (TIVA), the components of anaesthesia – analgesia, hypnosis and muscle relaxation – are achieved solely with intravenously applied drugs, without using inhalational agents. A totally intravenous technique with a rationally chosen combination of opioid, hypnotic and neuromuscular blocker offers a number of advantages over other types of general anaesthesia. These advantages are associated with the pharmacological properties of the drugs themselves, but are also conferred by being able to avoid the undesired properties of the drugs that can be dispensed with, for example, nitrous oxide (N_2O). The choice of drugs for the TIVA is governed by their pharmacokinetic profiles and by their effects on postoperative recovery.

When comparing pharmacokinetic properties in order to determine which drugs are best suited for an anaesthetic for minimally invasive surgery, one should not be obsessed with terminal elimination half-lives. Much more useful information is given by the

Table 5.1 Premedication agents for minimally invasive surgery

Drug time	Dose (mg)	Administration
Midazolam	7.5–15	20 min before transport to OR
Lorazepam	1–2	60 min before transport to OR
Lormetazepam	1	60 min before transport to OR
Temazepam	20	30 min before transport to OR
Other short-acting, anxiolytic sedatives Diazepam (not recommended)		Sufficiently early to be effective during transport

"context-sensitive half-time". This is a measure of how long it takes for the concentration of a drug to decrease by 50% in the effect site after having been infused for a defined length of time, with the duration of the infusion being the context.[12,13] The context-sensitive half-times of a number of common drugs together with their elimination half-lives determined in bolus injection studies are shown in Figure 5.1. A further parameter that determines how easily the effects of a drug can be titrated to intraoperative demands is $t_{1/2ke0}$. This is a constant that describes the equilibration rate between blood and the effect site and is a measure of hysteresis, the delay between increasing or decreasing plasma concentrations of the drug and a measurable change of its effect.

Choice of opioid

There is one outstanding characteristic of most minimally invasive operations that has a major influence on the rational choice of opioid for the anaesthetic: the surgical stimulus is very intense up to within a few minutes of the end of the operation, and the anaesthetic has to accommodate this fact. Under this constraint, remifentanil is, first and foremost, the opioid of choice for minimally invasive surgery. Sufentanil and alfentanil come in a distant second and third, while fentanyl or morphine are unsuitable, and should be used only when nothing else is available (Table 5.2). The computer simulation shown in Figure 5.1 illustrates that up to an infusion time of about 6 h, sufentanil has a shorter context-sensitive half-time than alfentanil, and thus potentially allows a more rapid awakening, despite its longer terminal elimination half-life.[14] Remifentanil occupies a special position in the palette of opioids, in that its context-sensitive half-time remains virtually unchanged. The time required for effect-site concentrations to decrease by 50% after a constant rate infusion lasting 150 min

is 3.7 min for remifentanil, 34 min for sufentanil, 59 min for alfentanil and an incredible 262 min for fentanyl.[15] The reason for this is that remifentanil is hydrolysed independent of specific organ function by ubiquitous, non-specific esterases in the blood and tissues, including the brain to a virtually inactive metabolite and thus has an unusually high clearance of approximately 3000 ml min^{-1}.[15,16] Due to its large volume of distribution and low clearance, fentanyl is only suitable as a TIVA component for procedures lasting 20–30 min

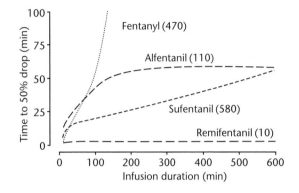

Figure 5.1 Context-sensitive half-times of remifentanil and other fentanyl congeners commonly used in TIVA techniques. The numbers given after each substance is the terminal elimination half-life (in min) after bolus application. This is considerably longer than the context-sensitive half-time – the time required for the effect-site concentration to decrease by 50%, and there is no consistent relationship between the two parameters. This increases dramatically for fentanyl with increasing duration of infusion, but remains nearly constant at a very low level for remifentanil. The diagram illustrates the point made in the text that remifentanil and sufentanil are the opioids most suited for use in a totally intravenous technique for minimally invasive surgery. (Adapted from Egan, *Anesthesiology* 1993; **79**: 881.)

Table 5.2 Pharmacological properties of commonly used opioid

	Remifentanil	Sufentanil	Alfentanil	Fentanyl
Terminal elimination half-life $t_{1/2}$ (min)	10	164–570	110	390–450
Central distribution volume, V_c (l)	7.0	12	2.9	17
Steady-state distribution volume, V_{ss} (l)	25–62	121	23	312
Clearance, Cl (ml min^{-1})	~3000	900	185	700
Protein binding at pH 7.4 (%)	92	92	92	84
pKa	7.1	8.0	6.5	8.4
Non-ionized at pH 7.4 (%)	67	20	89	9
Hepatic extraction ratio	NR	0.7–0.9	0.3–0.5	0.8–1.0

V_c: initial volume of distribution in central compartment; V_{ss}: volume of distribution in quasi-steady state; NR: not reported and not relevant for elimination.

at most.[13] After this time, cumulation causes undue prolongation of respiratory depression and retards recovery. A direct comparison of alfentanil and remifentanil in a total intravenous technique with propofol demonstrated more rapid recovery with remifentanil, as measured by respiratory rate, oxygen (O_2) saturation and number of patients with an Aldrete score of 10 both after 10 and 30 min, even following short procedures lasting only 20 min.[17]

Due to a combination of low degree of ionization and moderate plasma protein binding, remifentanil and alfentanil both have very short onset times. Fentanyl and sufentanil have longer $t_{1/2ke0}$ values and are more difficult to adapt to rapid intraoperative changes in stimulus intensity. During laparoscopic surgery, the elimination of opioids with high hepatic extraction might be impaired due to the reduction in splanchnic and hepatic perfusion.[18–20] This effect can be amplified by volatile anaesthetics, which reduce splanchnic perfusion.

Unlike morphine, the newer opioids have only minor effects on the biliary system, an aspect that is relevant during laparoscopic cholecystectomy. Neither sufentanil nor fentanyl cause a narrowing of the common bile duct.[21] Fentanyl does significantly increase the pressure in the biliary system,[22] but symptomatic choledochoduodenal sphincter spasm is rare with its use.[23] In a direct comparison, alfentanil caused a lower and statistically insignificant pressure increase than fentanyl.[22] The behaviour of remifentanil in this respect is not well known. It has been shown to delay the drainage of radioactive dye into the duodenum,[24] but this delay is shorter than with other studied opioids.

Remifentanil has one characteristic adverse effect, and that is a high incidence of postoperative shivering that is not thermogenetic in nature and not correlated to intraoperative changes in core temperature.[25,26]

Note   Opioids suitable for use as a component of a TIVA or a balanced anaesthetic for minimally invasive surgery are:

- Remifentanil (e.g. Ultiva®)
- Sufentanil (e.g. Sufenta®)
- Alfentanil (e.g. Rapifen®)

Less suitable are:

- Fentanyl, morphine and others

Ketamine should be mentioned when discussing the analgesic component of a total intravenous technique. This unique substance is used in anaesthesia for every kind of surgery in many parts of the world, and it has a number of advantages over opioids. When used for TIVA in combination with propofol, it had a recovery profile similar to that of alfentanil–propofol combination.[27] Dream events were more common on emergence, but were not unpleasant in content. A study comparing of propofol with ketamine or fentanyl for laparoscopic operations found that the only difference was that the patients in the ketamine–propofol group required more pain medication in the immediate postoperative period.[28] However, it seems that the ketamine dose of 1–1.5 mg kg^{-1} used in the study was less than equipotent with the 3–5 µg kg^{-1} dose of fentanyl.

Choice of the hypnotic component

Propofol is essentially the only intravenous hypnotic that is suitable for use in a TIVA for minimally invasive surgery. Methohexital and etomidate have similar elimination kinetics and clearance as propofol, and the recovery time following their use is not relevantly different from that after propofol, but they have little to offer in the way of advantages and a number of drawbacks. Etomidate might be nominally suitable as a component of a TIVA, but it is associated with unpleasant awakening and a higher incidence of PONV than after propofol.[29–31] The well-known inhibition of corticosteroid synthesis by etomidate is probably of no clinical consequence during short-term administration, since it can be overcome if necessary.[32] Awakening takes longer,[31,33] and the incidence of nausea and vomiting was reported to be higher after a TIVA with methohexital than after propofol,[30,34] although other studies could not confirm this finding.[31,33] At any rate, both substances are considerably more expensive than propofol.

The results of a number of studies suggest that propofol has antiemetic properties and also induces a slightly euphoric mood in the patients, a combination of effects that greatly enhances patient satisfaction.[29,35–37] Propofol occasionally causes pain on injection, but this can be attenuated or abolished by applying a tourniquet to the forearm, injecting a small amount (2 ml) of 1% lidocaine into the vein and waiting 10 s, or by waiting until the pre-injected opioid has taken full effect (see below). This pragmatic approach is supported by the results of a recent study.[38] A perhaps more academic concern is that propofol in clinically relevant concentrations ($IC_{50} \sim 9 \mu g\,ml^{-1}$) can inhibit alfentanil and sufentanil metabolism in human liver microsomes.[39] Propofol has also been described to reduce the central volume of distribution of remifentanil by 41% and its clearance by 15%, but this was considered to be without clinical relevance.[40]

Midazolam, which is occasionally used as a component of TIVA for major surgery, is unsuitable in this role for minimally invasive procedures due to its long duration of action.[41] It can be used, however, to reduce the dose of hypnotic necessary for loss of consciousness during induction of anaesthesia[42,43] in a technique known as "co-induction".

Note   Hypnotics suitable for use in a TIVA for minimally invasive surgery:

- Propofol

Perhaps

- Methohexital

For co-induction

- Midazolam

Choice of neuromuscular blocking agent

Adequate muscle relaxation increases the compliance of the abdomen, thus allowing better inflation of the abdomen at a set IAP and thereby facilitating surgical access. Muscle relaxation is therefore a crucial component of expert anaesthetic management. During laparoscopic cholecystectomy or other procedures, deep relaxation makes it easier for larger bits, for example, the gall bladder, to be retrieved through the small incision in the abdominal wall. Muscle relaxation will not always be necessary for extraperitoneal operations, such as hernia repair or nephrectomy. Close co-operation between surgeon and anaesthetist is important in order to adapt the degree of neuromuscular block to the individual stages of the operation.

In laparoscopic surgery, the interval from when the surgeon concludes the intra-abdominal phase of the operation, which requires a good degree of myorelaxation, and final wound closure with dressing is in the order of 5–10 min. Muscle relaxation will have to let up sufficiently during this short period to allow the patient's trachea to be extubated immediately after wound closure. This can be achieved by properly timing the reversal of relaxation and employing higher doses of cholinesterase inhibitors or by using a neuromuscular blocker with a short recovery index, or a combination of the two. Table 5.3 gives a synopsis of the relevant pharmacological data on which a rational choice can be based. The costs of neuromuscular blocking agents vary widely and the newer, short-acting substances are the most expensive. However, understanding the actual cost of a drug requires more than just looking at its shelf price.[44] A carefully performed study has shown that when not only the price of the muscle relaxant, but also the operating room (OR) costs incurred while waiting for the effects to wear off were entered into the calculation, the use of mivacurium led to a saving of approximately £100 per patient over longer acting agents.[45]

We rarely reverse muscle relaxation, since this carries a definite risk of its own, but instead prefer to use short-acting neuromuscular blockers with a rapid recovery index in combination with neuromuscular monitoring. Our choice of agent depends on the expected duration of the operation. With a total expected anaesthesia time of 2 h, we would use cisatracurium, vecuronium or rocuronium with possibly a very slight top-up towards the end if relaxometry indicates a lightening of the block. If the block only had to be intensified to retrieve material at the end of the operation, we would probably only give a small dose of succinylcholine. For shorter operations, we would choose mivacurium or perhaps only succinylcholine for very short diagnostic procedures. For longer operations we would also choose mivacurium, since its recovery index does not increase appreciably with the duration of its administration and one can expect rapid termination of its effect even after an infusion lasting several hours. The effects of mivacurium can be prolonged in patients with insufficient or atypical cholinesterase.[46,47]

Table 5.3 Comparison of pharmacological variables of neuromuscular blockers for use in laparoscopic surgery

	ED$_{95}$ (mg kg^{-1})	Intubating dose (mg kg^{-1})	Onset time (min)	RT$_{25}$ (min)	RT$_{90}$ (min)	Recovery index (min)
Atracurium	0.2	0.4–0.5	2–3	25	70	10–15
Cisatracurium	0.06	0.1–0.15	2–3	25	60	7–9
Mivacurium	0.08	0.2	1.5–2	15	30	6–8
Vecuronium	0.06	0.1	2–3	25	100	10–15
Rocuronium	0.25	0.6	1–1.5	45	90	14–22
Pancuronium	0.07	0.1	3–5	115	240	30–40

ED$_{95}$: dose required to suppress the magnitude of the first twitch (T$_1$) by 95%; RT$_{25}$, RT$_{90}$: times to 25 and 90% recovery of first twitch T$_1$ after the injection of an intubating dose; recovery index: interval between 25 and 75% recovery of T$_1$.

Future pharmaceutical developments may make it possible to specifically reverse the effect of rocuronium rapidly and effectively without the adverse effects seen when cholinesterase inhibitors are administered. Studies have shown that derivatives of cyclodextrine can be synthesized that chelate the rocuronium molecule rendering it inaccessible for the acetylcholine receptors of the neuromuscular junction. The chelated compound is then excreted through the kidneys.[48] One cyclodextrine derivative (ORG 25969) is in pre-clinical testing. When given in a dose of $1\,mg\,kg^{-1}$ this compound shortens the recovery time t_{10-90} from 19 to 2.1 min.[49]

Note Neuromuscular blocking agents suitable for use in minimally invasive surgery:

- Mivacurium
- Rocuronium
- Cisatracurium
- Vecuronium

Basic dosage considerations

Knowing the plasma or effect-site concentrations of the individual components required for hypnosis and surgical tolerance, and considering their additive or synergistic interactions with one other, one can roughly calculate a rationally based dosage schedule for a total intravenous technique based on pharmacokinetic and pharmacodynamic data.

The hypnotic threshold plasma concentration of propofol given alone has been determined to be about $3-5\,\mu g\,ml^{-1}$.[50-52] This is slightly lowered by the addition of an opioid.[51,53,54] The plasma concentration required to suppress reaction to skin incision in 50% of the patients (Cp50i) is reduced significantly by the simultaneous administration of a benzodiazepine or an opioid. Premedication with midazolam, temazepam or lorazepam alone reduces Cp50i by up to 50%.[42,55,56]

Synergistic effects have been demonstrated between propofol and alfentanil or fentanyl by numerous studies.[51,57-60] A fentanyl plasma concentration of $2-4\,ng\,ml^{-1}$, corresponding to an induction dose of 0.2 mg followed by a continuous infusion at a rate of $2-3\,\mu g\,kg^{-1}\,h^{-1}$, reduces the Cp50i of propofol by 80% to $2.7\,\mu g\,ml^{-1}$ (Figure 5.2).[42,51] Equipotent plasma concentrations of sufentanil and alfentanil are $0.4-0.6\,ng\,ml^{-1}$ and $100-300\,ng\,ml^{-1}$, respectively.[61,62] Similar effects have been shown for the combination of alfentanil and propofol.[60] A number of studies have demonstrated the synergistic interactions between propofol and remifentanil with regard to a number of clinical and electrophysiological

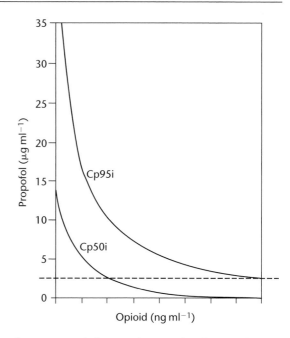

Figure 5.2 Isobologram showing the pharmacodynamic interaction of propofol with an opioid. The curves give the 50 and 95% probability that the patient will tolerate a surgical stimulus at the chosen dosage combination of the two drugs. The dotted line is the hypnotic threshold for propofol; awareness becomes more likely at concentrations under this value.

parameters.[57-59,63] The results of these studies show that a small opioid dose causes a steep reduction in the Cp50i of propofol, but that the interaction curve is hyperbolic, and the relative propofol-sparing effect of the opioid decreases at higher doses.

Since one can achieve the same effect with a propofol-dominated or an opioid-dominated combination of dosages as illustrated by the isobolograms in Figure 5.2, one should choose the combination which gives the shortest recovery time. This can be determined either clinically or theoretically using response surface analysis.[58,64] Just which dose combination this is, depends on the pharmacokinetics of the individual components. Let us just illustrate this concept with two extreme examples. In a combination of propofol with fentanyl, one would give a low dose of fentanyl and titrate the required depth of anaesthesia by increasing the propofol dose. On the other hand, if one decided to combine thiopental with remifentanil, one would give the lowest possible thiopental dose just adequate to prevent awareness and give as much remifentanil as necessary to assure a sufficient depth of anaesthesia. Vuyk and co-workers did a computer simulation that illustrates this point quite nicely.[64]

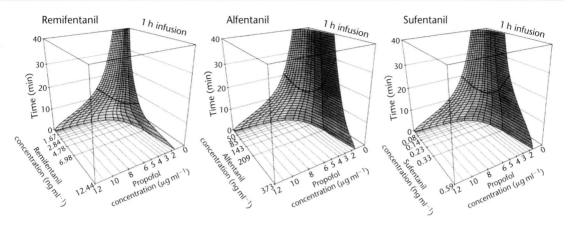

Figure 5.3 Response surface analysis of varying combinations of propofol with remifentanil, alfentanil or sufentanil. The curve on the horizontal plane gives the isobolographic analysis of propofol–opioid dose combinations yielding a 50% probability of no response to surgical stimuli. (Adapted from Ref [64].) The heavy line on the vertical curved plane gives the awakening time after a TIVA lasting 60 min with the various combinations of propofol with the individual opioids.

Figure 5.3, adapted from this study, shows recovery times after a 1-h continuous infusion of propofol and either remifentanil, alfentanil or sufentanil in varying infusion rate combinations, and demonstrates that there is an optimal combination that has the most rapid recovery time. The results also give visible proof of a number of points that have been mentioned so far. The first of these is that awakening is faster after a TIVA with remifentanil than with either alfentanil or sufentanil, and, secondly, that there is virtually no difference between alfentanil and sufentanil with regard to recovery time after a 1-h infusion.

Adding N_2O to the combination of intravenous drugs will reduce the required doses and possibly shorten recovery time.[13,55,56,65] However, as described in more detail in Chapters 2, 6 and 10, N_2O can be hazardous when used during laparoscopic surgery or laser surgery of the upper airways, and one should try to avoid it.

These theoretical considerations should demonstrate that a combination of propofol and remifentanil after oral premedication with a short-acting benzodiazepine, closely approaches the ideal TIVA for all types of minimally invasive surgery with regard to ease of titration to surgical needs, speed of recovery and patient's comfort and satisfaction. Sufentanil, alfentanil or even fentanyl can be used instead of remifentanil in certain, clearly defined situations, or when rapid awakening is not a requirement.

The dosage recommendations based on pharmaco-kinetic–pharmacodynamic data are only to be taken as guidelines for the initial settings. The actual values must be adapted to the intensity of the surgical stimulation and titrated to the patient's needs. Pragmatically determined dosage schedules will be described below.

There is no consensus on the degree of muscle relaxation required for laparoscopic surgery. It might be less than that necessary for laparotomy, where muscle response has to be reduced by 80%, corresponding to one or two twitches following train-of-four (TOF) stimulation. A reduction to two to four TOF responses should be sufficient to provide adequate abdominal compliance. Some patients develop recalcitrant singultus during laparoscopic cholecystectomy that can effectively impede surgical preparation. The diaphragm is much less sensitive to non-depolarizing neuromuscular blocks than skeletal muscle, and singultus can persist despite complete cessation of twitch response to peripheral nerve stimulation. In these cases, the behaviour of the diaphragm will have to guide the administration of the muscle relaxant.

Despite all precautions, relaxation will be sufficiently intense in some patients at the end of the operation as to prevent safe removal of the endotracheal tube. For high-risk patients, the best choice would be to continue ventilation in the post-anaesthetic care unit until the effects of the relaxant have worn off. In all others, reversal of the neuromuscular block is an option, but should not be attempted if the block is too intense, that is twitch strength is decreased by 85% or more, or there are fewer than two responses to TOF stimulation.

Drug application systems for TIVA

For the safe, reliable and economical administration of a TIVA one requires the appropriate equipment.

This includes the syringe pumps, infusion pumps and the correct infusion lines. Peristaltic infusion pumps are used to control the rate of intravenous infusions, and when used for anaesthesia the drugs are added to the infusion solution, usually normal saline or glucose, and infused at the required rate. The one advantage of using such a dilute solution of the drug is that, in a pinch, one can dispense with the pump and regulate the infusion rate by adjusting the drip rate.[66] The main disadvantage is the large fluid volume given to the patient.

Syringe pumps allow a precise application of concentrated solutions of drugs in small volumes. For practical reasons to be mentioned below, the concentration of the drug should not be too high. A wide variety of syringe pumps are available on the market, and listing them would not be feasible. They should have a minimal slack time, achieve the set infusion rate rapidly and be able to keep it constant to within $\pm 2\%$ even at a slow rate, and should be able to accept a variety of different syringe types. Particularly useful are microprocessor-controlled pumps that calculate the infusion rate from patient's weight, drug concentration and required dosage in $mg\,kg^{-1}h^{-1}$ or $\mu g\,kg^{-1}min^{-1}$ entered by the anaesthetist. Some pumps have a pre-programmed, menu-driven drug database that allows one to simply pick and choose the drug and concentration that one needs. All of these sophisticated pumps are more complicated and require more extensive training to use, but once they are mastered they facilitate drug infusions and prevent mistakes resulting from calculation errors.

A constant rate infusion will lead to increasing plasma concentrations over time. Various ways of avoiding an overdose towards the end of the anaesthetic or insufficient depth of anaesthesia at the beginning have been proposed. All of these are based more or less on the bolus, elimination, and transfer (BET) concept.[67] The bolus dose is calculated to saturate the central compartment to a pre-defined initial plasma concentration, while the following infusion compensates for the amount of drug lost from this compartment by elimination or transfer to more peripheral compartments. The rate of elimination remains relatively constant, but the amount of drug transferred into peripheral compartments decreases over time, necessitating a reduction in the infusion rate in order to keep the targeted plasma concentration constant. Examples of simple BET infusion schedules are given below.

Calculating the correct infusion rate required for a constant plasma concentration during the course of a total intravenous technique entails repeatedly solving a number of differential equations. This is not a task for the busy operating theatre, but is just the thing to delegate

to a microprocessor. There are a number of syringe pumps now on the market that are programmed to keep the plasma concentration of the infused drug at a pre-set level by applying a target-controlled infusion (TCI) schedule. The first of these, the Diprifusor® system developed by Kenny and co-workers, controls the infusion of propofol.[68] The software in these pumps incorporates a model based on pharmacokinetic data extracted from studies in thousands of patients and volunteers. Administering an intravenous drug by setting a plasma concentration and not a drug dose takes some getting used to. On the other hand, it is no different than the way one administers inhalational anaesthesia – one dials in the desired concentration and lets the vaporizer or the TCI system give the required volume. Newer pump systems allow several drugs to be applied simultaneously as TCI, and allow one to target plasma concentrations or effect-site concentrations (Figure 5.4).

When administering concentrated solutions of extremely potent drugs, one has to beware of inadvertent bolus applications resulting from occlusion and release of the infusion tubing. To prevent this, only non-compliant tubing should be used to connect the syringe pump to the patient, and the connection should be as close to the venous cannula as possible. If the drug is infused parallel to a running infusion, a check valve should be used to prevent retrograde filling of the infusion system should the venous cannula become occluded. The pump must be equipped with an overpressure alarm, and should actively retract the syringe driver if the alarm is triggered to release pressure in the system. Low-volume, low-compliance systems are available that also incorporate the check valves (Figure 5.5). The drug delivery system must be secured against accidental disconnection that might lead to intraoperative awakening of the patient.

TIVA protocols for laparoscopic surgery

Various opioid–propofol combinations will be described in the following paragraphs. While opioid and propofol doses might differ, other components of the totally intravenous anaesthetic always remain the same. All patients are given an oral premedication as described above. Intubation is facilitated with a neuromuscular blocker chosen according to the criteria described above and dosed according to Table 5.3.

The initially chosen infusion rates of propofol and opioid that are based on the average patient may often not be adequate for the required plane of anaesthesia. The standard procedure in this case is to increase the dose of the analgesic under the assumption that it is

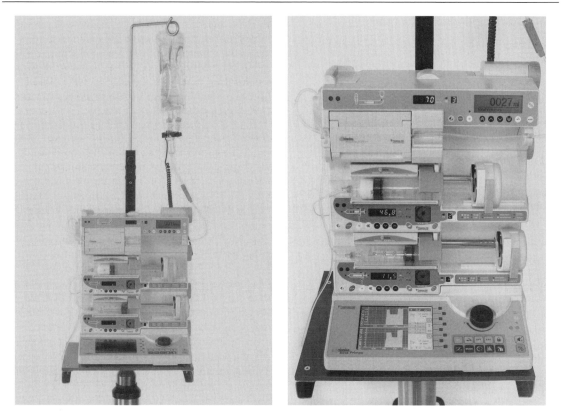

Figure 5.4 An integrated system for administering TIVA. The TCI parameters are set on the control unit, and the calculated plasma and effect-site concentrations of the individual drugs are displayed on the screen. The running infusion is controlled by the peristaltic pump seen at the top of the device.

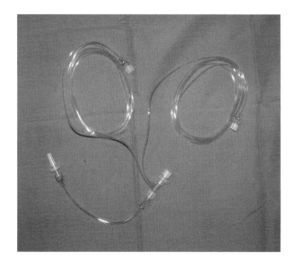

Figure 5.5 Infusion set for use with TIVA. Important features are the low-volume, non-compliant tubing for connecting the syringes to the flowing infusion (upper left and right coils) and the check valves incorporated at relevant points in the system. The short stretch of tubing seen on the lower left is to reduce forces acting on the venous catheter.

pain and not awareness that is causing the signs of too light anaesthesia. If two additional bolus injections of the opioid have no effect, a supplemental dose of the hypnotic is given. During laparoscopic surgery, one must be careful not to misinterpret the blood pressure increase regularly observed during abdominal inflation as an indication that the anaesthetic has to be deepened. This is a trap into which the inexperienced anaesthetist frequently falls. Fortunately enough, the consequence of the anaesthetic overdose is usually only a prolongation of recovery time.

Note   Managing the TIVA:

- Signs of insufficient anaesthetic depth are first treated with additional opioids
- Supplemental doses of the hypnotic are given if the response to the opioid was inadequate

Beware   Blood pressure always increases during inflation of the abdomen as part of the physiological response to increased abdominal pressure. Differentiate as pain response before treating with opioids or hypnotics!

TIVA with propofol–remifentanil

Remifentanil differs in a very practical manner from other frequently used opioids in that it must be given as a constant infusion because of its extremely short half-life. Administering it in individual bolus doses is simply not practical except for very short procedures. If the expected duration of anaesthesia is longer than 10–15 min, administering it as an infusion is necessary. A further consequence of the short elimination half-life is that its analgesic effects wear off rapidly after the infusion is stopped, and postoperative pain can set in early. The problems associated with this will be discussed in the section on postoperative pain therapy.

Remifentanil's rapid onset can cause vagomimetic effects with profound bradycardia, particularly following the initial bolus injection, and atropine or glycopyrrolate should be readily available. This does not usually occur if the initial bolus is given slowly over 60–120 s. Like all intensely acting opioids with rapid onset, remifentanil can induce significant thorax rigidity, which can impair mask ventilation or even render it impossible. This adverse effect is less frequent in patients who have been given a benzodiazepine premedication. The rigidity responds to neuromuscular blockers, and a small dose of succinylcholine (10 mg) can be administered, if ventilation is severely impaired.

Remifentanil is supplied in powder form in vials containing 1 or 5 mg. It has to be dissolved and diluted to the final concentration in 0.9% NaCl or 5% glucose solution before it is used. For use in adult patients we draw the contents of the 5 mg vial into a 50 ml syringe for a final concentration of $100 \mu g \, ml^{-1}$. The average TIVA consumes approximately 1–2 mg of remifentanil per hour. For paediatric anaesthesia, we prefer to dissolve only 1 mg in 50 ml for a final concentration of $20 \mu g \, ml^{-1}$. We use this less concentrated solution to avoid the very low infusion speeds, which not all syringe pumps can reliably apply. If syringe pumps are not available, remifentanil can be diluted in normal saline and administered by infusion pump or through a minidrip set.[66] Five milligrams in 500 ml solution yields a concentration of $10 \, mg \, ml^{-1}$. The

infusion rate (in $ml \, h^{-1}$) of this concentration is easily calculated as the desired dose (in $\mu g \, kg^{-1} min^{-1}$) times body weight (in kg) times 60 (min) divided by 10. For example, a 75 kg patient would require an infusion rate of $90 \, ml \, h^{-1}$ for a dose of $0.2 \, \mu g \, kg^{-1} min^{-1}$. Table 5.4 shows the preparation of these solutions in detail.

Anaesthesia is induced with $0.5–1 \, \mu g \, kg^{-1}$ body weight remifentanil given as a slow intravenous bolus injection, usually by letting the infusion run at a rate of $0.5 \, \mu g \, kg^{-1} min^{-1}$ for 2 min. After the bolus injection, the infusion rate is set at the initial maintenance rate of $0.2 \, \mu g \, kg^{-1} min^{-1}$. As soon as the effect of remifentanil sets in, propofol is given in an induction dose of $1.5–2 \, mg \, kg^{-1}$ body weight and the propofol infusion is started at an initial rate of $6–7 \, mg \, kg^{-1} h^{-1}$. This is reduced after about 15 min to a maintenance rate of $5 \, mg \, kg^{-1} h^{-1}$. As an alternative, propofol can be administered as a TCI. We set the initial target concentration at $4–5 \, \mu g \, ml^{-1}$ and let the pump run until approximately $1.5–2 \, mg \, kg^{-1}$ of propofol have been administered. We then reduce the target concentration to between 2 and $2.5 \, \mu g \, ml^{-1}$. This is, in effect, the intravenous counterpart of the "overpressure" technique used to accelerate induction with inhalational anaesthetics. Our empirical results are supported by the findings of a systematic study, which showed that only 40% of the patients had lost consciousness after 3 min when the target concentration was set at $3 \, \mu g \, ml^{-1}$ as opposed to 90% when the concentration was set at $5 \, \mu g \, ml^{-1}$.[69]

Signs of light anaesthesia are first treated with a bolus injection of $1 \, \mu g \, kg^{-1}$ remifentanil that is repeated after 2 min if there is no response to the first dose. If this is effective in restoring an adequate plane of anaesthesia the infusion rate of remifentanil is increased by $0.2–0.5 \, \mu g \, kg^{-1} min^{-1}$. If the second injection of remifentanil is without effect, a bolus injection of $0.6–0.8 \, mg \, kg^{-1}$ propofol is given, and the infusion rate is increased by $1 \, mg \, kg^{-1} h^{-1}$. Bolus injections are not possible with a TCI system, but we circumvent this problem by increasing the targeted propofol plasma concentration to about $6 \, \mu g \, ml^{-1}$ until approximately 50 mg have been infused and then

Table 5.4 Preparing remifentanil solutions for bolus injection and infusion

Stock solution	5 mg in 5 ml (1 mg ml⁻¹)
Concentration for syringe pump for adults	5 ml stock solution in 50 ml (=100 μg ml⁻¹)
Concentration for bolus injections	1 ml of the syringe solution in 10 ml (=10 μg ml⁻¹)

When using remifentanil from the 1 mg vial, we recommend diluting it in at least 20 ml of liquid (=50 μg ml⁻¹) to reduce the relative amount lost in the system dead space. Concentrations of 10–20 μg ml⁻¹ are recommended for use in children to avoid extremely low infusion rates.

reducing the target concentration to $0.5\,\mu g\,ml^{-1}$ above the previous level (see Table 5.5).

If anaesthesia has been stable for 20 min or more under a constant level of surgical stimulation, we tend to carefully reduce the infusion rates of propofol and remifentanil in order to avoid unnecessarily deep anaesthesia. The median infusion rates required by our patients

Table 5.5 TIVA with propofol and remifentanil for minimally invasive surgery

Dissolve and dilute remifentanil according to Table 5.4	
Induction	
Remifentanil or and	$0.5–1\,\mu g\,kg^{-1}$ slow bolus injection $0.5\,\mu g\,kg^{-1}\,min^{-1}$ for 2 min
Propofol or	$1.5–2\,mg\,kg^{-1}$
Propofol TCI	Target plasma concentration $4–5\,\mu g\,ml^{-1}$
Until	$1.5–2\,\mu g\,kg^{-1}$ have been infused
Then	Target plasma concentration $2.0–2.5\,\mu g\,ml^{-1}$
Maintenance	
Remifentanil	$0.2\,\mu g\,kg^{-1}\,min^{-1}$ initial infusion rate
Propofol	$6–7\,mg\,kg^{-1}\,h^{-1}$ for 15 min $5\,mg\,kg^{-1}\,h^{-1}$ thereafter
or	
Propofol TCI	Target plasma concentration $2.0–2.5\,\mu g\,ml^{-1}$
Intubation	
Endotracheal tube or laryngeal mask airway	
Ventilation	
With O_2–air and minute volume adjusted to eliminate excess carbon dioxide (CO_2)	
If anaesthesia too light	
Remifentanil	$1\,\mu g\,kg^{-1}$ bolus injection, repeated after 2 min, if necessary if opioid effective, increase infusion rate by $0.2–0.5\,\mu g\,kg^{-1}\,min^{-1}$
If opioid ineffective	
Propofol	$0.6–0.8\,mg\,kg^{-1}$ bolus injection and Increase infusion rate by $1\,mg\,kg^{-1}\,h^{-1}$
Propofol TCI	Set target concentration to $6\,\mu g\,ml^{-1}$ until *ca.* 40–60 mg infused Increase target concentration by $0.5\,\mu g\,ml^{-1}$
Anaesthesia stable for 20 min	
Careful stepwise reduction of drug infusion rates Do not reduce propofol infusion rate below $4\,mg\,kg^{-1}\,h^{-1}$	
End	
Stop infusions of remifentanil and propofol about 3 min before last stitch.	
Cave!	
Pain can set in early. Prophylactic analgesics.	

were $0.2\,\mu g\,kg^{-1}\,min^{-1}$ for remifentanil (range 0.05–0.42) and $4.2\,mg\,kg^{-1}\,h^{-1}$ for propofol (range 1.5–7.1). The patients awakened 4–9 min after the drug infusions were stopped. The depth of anaesthesia was monitored by bispectral index (BIS) (see Chapter 4). These empirically determined infusion rates are very similar to those defined by Vuyk on the basis of theoretical calculations aimed at determining the propofol–remifentanil combination with the shortest awakening.[64] These calculations recommend an initial remifentanil dose of $1.5–2\,\mu g\,kg^{-1}$ followed by an infusion rate of $0.37\,\mu g\,kg^{-1}\,min^{-1}$ for 20 min and $0.32\,\mu g\,kg^{-1}\,min^{-1}$ thereafter. Propofol is given as an initial dose of $1.5\,mg\,kg^{-1}$, followed by $8\,mg\,kg^{-1}\,h^{-1}$ for the first 40 min, $6.5\,mg\,kg^{-1}\,h^{-1}$ for the next 150 min and $6\,mg\,kg^{-1}\,h^{-1}$ from then on. The propofol plasma concentration targeted by this infusion regimen is $2.8\,\mu g\,ml^{-1}$, which the authors describe as sufficient to suppress response to surgical stimuli in 95% of the patients when given with remifentanil (Table 5.8). The awakening time after this combination is around 6 min.

TIVA with propofol–sufentanil

We found that when combined with propofol infused at a rate of $6\,mg\,kg^{-1}\,h^{-1}$, a median sufentanil dose of $0.3\,\mu g\,kg^{-1}\,h^{-1}$ was sufficient to provide haemodynamic stability and prevent response to surgical stimuli during laparoscopic cholecystectomy. Anaesthesia is induced with a bolus injection of $0.2–0.3\,\mu g\,kg^{-1}$ sufentanil followed by an infusion with an initial rate of $0.2\,\mu g\,kg^{-1}\,h^{-1}$. We use a sufentanil solution containing $5\,\mu g\,ml^{-1}$ in order to have manageable infusion rates. The onset time is slower with sufentanil than with remifentanil and one must wait 4 or 5 min for an appreciable effect to set it. Propofol is then given as an induction dose of $1–1.5\,mg\,kg^{-1}$, followed by an infusion at a rate of $5–6\,mg\,kg^{-1}\,h^{-1}$, which is then reduced to $4–5\,mg\,kg^{-1}\,h^{-1}$ after 10 min (Table 5.6). This differs slightly from the theoretical dosage recommendations of Vuyk shown in Table 5.8.[64]

As with the remifentanil–propofol combination, light anaesthesia is first treated with an additional dose of the opioid; in this case, a bolus injection of 3–5 µg sufentanil. This is repeated after 5 min if the first injection is without effect. If the additional opioid dose attenuates the patient's response to surgical stimulation, the sufentanil infusion rate is increased by $0.05\,\mu g\,kg^{-1}\,h^{-1}$. If the opioid is not effective, a bolus injection of propofol is administered and the infusion rate is changed as described above. If everything has remained stable for 20 min or more, we reduce the propofol and sufentanil doses in steps, as described above for the remifentanil–propofol combination, starting with the opioid (see Table 5.6).

Table 5.6 TIVA with propofol and sufentanil for minimally invasive surgery

Induction

Sufentanil	0.2–0.3 μg kg^{-1} bolus injection, wait at least 2–3 min
Then	
Propofol	1.5–2 mg kg^{-1} bolus injection
or	
Propofol TCI	Target plasma concentration 4–5 μg ml^{-1}
Until	1.5–2 μg kg^{-1} have been infused
Then	Target plasma concentration 2.0–2.5 μg ml^{-1}

Maintenance

Sufentanil	0.2 μg kg^{-1} h^{-1} initial infusion rate
or	3–5 μg bolus injections as necessary
Propofol	8–10 mg kg^{-1} h^{-1} for 10 min, then 5 mg kg^{-1} h^{-1} thereafter
Propofol TCI	Target concentration 2.0–2.5 μg ml^{-1}

Intubation
Endotracheal tube or laryngeal mask airway

Ventilation
With O_2–air and minute volume adjusted to eliminate excess CO_2

If anaesthesia too light

Sufentanil	3–5 μg kg^{-1} bolus injection, repeated after 5 min, if necessary. If opioid effective, increase infusion rate by 0.05 μg kg^{-1}
If opioid effective, increase	
Propofol	infusion rate by 0.05 μg kg^{-1} h^{-1}. If opioid ineffective 0.6–0.8 mg kg^{-1} bolus injection and Increase infusion rate by mg kg^{-1} h^{-1}
Propofol TCI	Set target concentration to 6 μg ml^{-1} until *ca.* 40–60 mg infused increase target concentration by 0.5 μg ml^{-1}

Anaesthesia stable for 20 min
Careful stepwise reduction of drug infusion rates
Do not reduce propofol below 4 mg kg^{-1} h^{-1}

End
Last sufentanil *ca.* 20–30 min before end of surgery
Stop propofol infusion about 5 min before last stitch and dressing.

Tip: Dilute sufentanil to a concentration of 5 μg ml^{-1} to facilitate handling and to avoid low infusion rates.

Table 5.7 TIVA with propofol and alfentanil for minimally invasive surgery

Induction

Alfentanil	20–30 μg kg^{-1} bolus injection (*ca.* 1.5–2 mg)
then	
Propofol	1–1.5 mg kg^{-1} bolus injection
or	
Propofol TCI	Target plasma concentration 4–5 μg ml^{-1}
Until	1.5–2 μg kg^{-1} have been infused
then	Target plasma concentration 2.0–2.5 μg ml^{-1}

Maintenance

Alfentanil	25–35 μg kg^{-1} h^{-1} initial infusion rate
or	0.5–1.0 mg bolus injections as necessary
Propofol	8–10 mg kg^{-1} h^{-1} for 10 min,
then	5–6 mg kg^{-1} h^{-1} thereafter
Propofol TCI	Target concentration 2.0–2.5 μg ml^{-1}

Intubation
Endotracheal tube or laryngeal mask airway

Ventilation
With O_2–air and minute volume adjusted to eliminate excess CO_2

If anaesthesia too light

Alfentanil	0.5–1 mg bolus injection, repeated after 3 min, if necessary. If opioid effective, increase infusion rate by 5 μg kg^{-1} h^{-1}
If opioid ineffective	
Propofol	0.6–0.8 mg kg^{-1} bolus injection and Increase infusion rate by 1 mg kg^{-1} h^{-1}
Propofol TCI	Set target concentration to 6 μg ml^{-1} until *ca.* 40–60 mg infused Increase target concentration by 0.5 μg ml^{-1}

Anaesthesia stable for 20 min
Careful stepwise reduction of drug infusion rates
Do not reduce propofol below 4 mg kg^{-1} h^{-1}

End
Last alfentanil *ca.* 20–30 min before end of surgery
Stop propofol infusion *ca.* 3 min before last stitch

TIVA with propofol–alfentanil

The combination of propofol and alfentanil is also suitable for minimally invasive surgery lasting up to about 60 min. The time to awakening is essentially the same as after a total intravenous technique with propofol and sufentanil. Alfentanil has the advantage of a more rapid onset of its effects, but it has the disadvantage of being much more expensive than sufentanil in many countries.

Our studies showed that an infusion rate of 25–35 μg kg^{-1} h^{-1}, or approximately 2.5 $\pm$ 1.0 mg h^{-1}, in combination with propofol gave a sufficiently intense analgesia for laparoscopic cholecystectomy. The necessary infusion rate was virtually the same for herniotomy and other laparoscopic operations. Propofol was given as an induction dose of 1–1.5 mg kg^{-1} followed by an infusion of 6 mg kg^{-1} h^{-1} that was reduced to 4–5 mg kg^{-1} h^{-1} after 10 min. Alfentanil can also be

Table 5.8 Infusion rates of remifentanil, sufentanil or alfentanil in combination with propofol calculated to give a 95% probability of no response to surgical stimulation and to have the most rapid recovery times (Vuyk, et al.[64])

	Remifentanil	Sufentanil	Alfentanil
Without propofol			
Target concentration	$8.0\,ng\,ml^{-1}$	$0.2\,ng\,ml^{-1}$	$130\,ng\,ml^{-1}$
Infusion rates			
Bolus	$1.5–2\,\mu g\,kg^{-1}$	$0.25\,\mu g\,kg^{-1}$	$35\,\mu g\,kg^{-1}$
Infusion 1	$22\,\mu g\,kg^{-1}\,min^{-1}$ for 20 min	$0.22\,\mu g\,kg^{-1}\,h^{-1}$	$75\,\mu g\,kg^{-1}\,h^{-1}$ for 30 min
Infusion 2	$19\,\mu g\,kg^{-1}\,min^{-1}$ thereafter	$0.22\,\mu g\,kg^{-1}\,h^{-1}$	$42.5\,\mu g\,kg^{-1}\,h^{-1}$ thereafter
With propofol			
Target concentration	$2.8\,\mu g\,ml^{-1}$	$4.5\,\mu g\,ml^{-1}$	$4.4\,\mu g\,ml^{-1}$
Infusion rates			
Bolus	$1.5\,mg\,kg^{-1}$	$2.8\,mg\,kg^{-1}$	$2.8\,mg\,kg^{-1}$
Infusion 1	$8\,mg\,kg^{-1}\,h^{-1}$ for 40 min	$12\,mg\,kg^{-1}\,h^{-1}$ for 40 min	$12\,mg\,kg^{-1}\,h^{-1}$ for 40 min
Infusion 2	$6.5\,mg\,kg^{-1}\,h^{-1}$ for 150 min	$10\,mg\,kg^{-1}\,h^{-1}$ for 150 min	$10\,mg\,kg^{-1}\,h^{-1}$ for 150 min
Infusion 3	$6\,mg\,kg^{-1}\,h^{-1}$ thereafter	$8\,mg\,kg^{-1}\,h^{-1}$ thereafter	$8\,mg\,kg^{-1}\,h^{-1}$ thereafter

simply given at a set rate of $2\,mg\,h^{-1}$ and supplemented with bolus injections of 0.5 mg if necessary. If two or more additional injections are required in a 10-min period, the infusion rate is increased by $0.5\,mg\,h^{-1}$. Here, as with the other total intravenous technique, the infusion rates can be gradually reduced when the course has been stable for a reasonable length of time (Table 5.7).

Our clinically determined combination of alfentanil and propofol is less propofol-dominated than that calculated by Vuyk[64] (see Table 5.8).

Inhalational anaesthetics and balanced anaesthesia

A monoanaesthetic with a volatile agent has the disadvantage of delayed recovery, perhaps with the exception of desflurane. Time to awakening after a 90 min administration of 1.5 minimal alveolar concentration (MAC) of isoflurane, enflurane or sevoflurane is more than 30 min. This would slow patient turnover, seriously interfere with rational utilization of operating capacity and incurs costs far higher than potential savings from the use of inexpensive volatiles.

Volatile anaesthetics have the further disadvantage that they decrease hypoxic pulmonary vasoconstriction (HPV).[70–72] This vascular reflex reduces the perfusion of non-ventilated alveoli and diminishes the magnitude of pulmonary shunt perfusion (Q_S/Q_T). The extent of non-ventilated lung areas and consequently Q_S/Q_T is increased by controlled ventilation, the head-down position and elevated IAP.[73,74] Interfering with hypoxic vasoconstriction will cause a greater degree of arterial O_2 desaturation at a constant inspiratory O_2 concentration. This effect is enhanced by N_2O.

The increase of systemic vascular resistance during laparoscopic surgery is accompanied by a marked vasoconstriction in the splanchnic vascular bed. The resulting decrease in hepatic portal blood flow might increase the risk of liver damage by anaerobic halothane metabolism. Halothane also increases the risk of cardiac dysrhythmias due to CO_2 absorption and hypercarbia.[75]

It should be obvious that an inhalational monoanaesthetic is not suitable for minimally invasive surgery. One possible exception might be desflurane with its low solubility, although it would be difficult to find convincing arguments for using it alone. The classical method for reducing the alveolar concentration of the volatile agent required for surgical tolerance is to combine it with N_2O. N_2O will be discussed shortly at the end of this section. It is dealt with in Chapter 2 and will figure prominently in Chapter 6. A further way to reduce the required alveolar concentration is to combine the volatile with an opioid. This will be described in the following paragraphs.

Note
- Monoanaesthetic with an inhalational agent is not suited for minimally invasive surgery
- The hypnotic effects of inhalational anaesthetics in low concentrations can be exploited in a balanced anaesthetic

Balanced anaesthesia, the combination of an opioid with a volatile anaesthetic, can be used to advantage in minimally invasive surgery. As with propofol, the addition of an opioid causes a dramatic reduction in the alveolar concentration of the inhalational anaesthetic required for hypnosis as well as suppressing response

Table 5.9 Reduction of isoflurane minimal alveolar concentration by opioids

Opioid	MAC reduction (50% at)	Source
Fentanyl	1.67 ng ml^{-1}	McEwan et al.[76]
Sufentanil	0.145 ng ml^{-1}	Brunner et al.[77]
Alfentanil	28.8 ng ml^{-1}	Westmoreland et al.[80]
Remifentanil	1.37 ng ml^{-1}	Lang et al.[79]

to painful stimulation.[76–83] Whereas an alveolar concentration of 1.5–2 MAC is required to produce a sufficiently deep plane of anaesthesia when used alone, only about 0.5–0.8 MAC is necessary with the simultaneous administration of a relatively small dose of an opioid. For example, about 1 mg of alfentanil reduces the MAC of isoflurane by more than 50%.[80] Equianalgesic doses of other opioids will have the same effect (Table 5.9). Using this combination not only reduces the recovery time but also the adverse effects associated with the use of high concentrations of volatile anaesthetics. Volatile anaesthetics have the one advantage over short-acting hypnotics that they are virtually ubiquitously available and do not require additional equipment, such as syringe pumps, for their exact administration.

The ideal balanced anaesthetic combines a poorly soluble inhalational anaesthetic and an opioid with a short context-sensitive half-time that is not affected by changes in hepatic perfusion. The inhalational agent of choice should be eliminated rapidly with little or no metabolism, should be without relevant side effects and should not interfere with the elimination of other drugs. The first choice would be isoflurane or desflurane followed by sevoflurane and perhaps enflurane. The high lipid solubility of halothane, along with its pronounced metabolism, its sensitization of the myocardium to the dysrhythmogenic effects of catecholamines, and its inhibition of opioid clearance, make it a poor choice.

Note Suitable components of a balanced anaesthetic for minimally invasive surgery:

Inhalational agents
Isoflurane, desflurane, sevoflurane and enflurane
Opioids
Remifentanil, sufentanil and alfentanil

Halothane and fentanyl are unsuitable and are not recommended.

The volatile anaesthetic is administered in an end-tidal concentration that will ensure lack of intraoperative awareness. This is about 0.5–0.7 MAC for all inhalational agents. The opioid is given at the same dosage as described above for TIVA. Signs of a too light plane of anaesthesia are initially treated with additional bolus injections of the opioid.

We compared a balanced anaesthetic with isoflurane and alfentanil to a total intravenous technique with propofol and alfentanil for laparoscopic cholecystectomy. Isoflurane was given at an end-tidal concentration of 0.6% (0.5 MAC), while alfentanil was infused as described above for the TIVA. Median awakening time after the balanced technique was 14 min compared to 12 min after the TIVA (Crozier et al., unpublished data).

Remifentanil is an excellent combination partner for balanced anaesthesia. In one study comparing isoflurane–remifentanil and propofol–remifentanil for arthroscopy lasting about 80 min, the patients with the balanced anaesthetic were awake after an average of 6.7 min, while the mean awakening time following the total intravenous technique was 9.6 min.[84] The need for postoperative supplemental analgesics and the incidence of adverse events were the same in both groups, although the patients requested the first analgesic earlier after the balanced technique. Table 5.10 describes a balanced anaesthetic with isoflurane or desflurane combined with remifentanil or alfentanil. One study compared desflurane–remifentanil with propofol–remifentanil for laparoscopic cholecystectomy.[85] Time to extubation was 5–6 min in both groups, but the patients with the balanced anaesthetic required more supplemental opioid analgesics and had a higher incidence of nausea and vomiting.

Nitrous oxide

The use of N_2O for laparoscopic surgery is problematic for two reasons. One of these is the distension of hollow viscera caused by the diffusion of N_2O into air-filled spaces. The volume of the stomach and intestines was doubled after a 2-h anaesthetic with N_2O;[86] an effect that can interfere with surgical access and impede the course of the operation, if the bowels are not prepared and the stomach not emptied of gas prior to surgery.[87] This might only be an academic worry, since surgeons were unable to tell if N_2O had been used for the anaesthetic during a 75 min laparoscopic cholecystectomy, and were not hampered by bowel distension.[88] However, this might be an issue in operations lasting several hours. It is our experience that surgical access for laparoscopic fundoplication is considerably impaired by distended bowel loops after several hours of N_2O anaesthesia.

Table 5.10 Balanced anaesthesia with isoflurane or desflurane with remifentanil or alfentanil for minimally invasive surgery

Induction	Remifentanil	$0.5–1\ \mu g\ kg^{-1}$ bolus injection and infusion
	or	
	Alfentanil	$20–30\ \mu g\ kg^{-1}$ bolus injection (ca. 1.5–2 mg)
	then	
	Propofol	$1.5–2.0\ mg\ kg^{-1}$ bolus injection
Maintenance	Isoflurane	End-tidal concentration should be around 0.7–0.9% (ca. 0.5 MAC)
	Desflurane	End-tidal concentration should be around 4–5% (higher if using alfentanil)
	Remifentanil	$0.2\ \mu g\ kg^{-1}\ min^{-1}$
	or	
	Alfentanil	$25–35\ \mu g\ kg^{-1}\ h^{-1}$ (ca. 2–3 mg h^{-1})
Intubation	Endotracheal tube or laryngeal mask airway	
Ventilation	With O_2–air and minute volume adjusted to eliminate excess CO_2	

The first measure at signs of too light anaesthesia is to give a supplemental dose of the opioid. If the first dose is not sufficiently effective it is repeated once more after several minutes. If the second dose is also without effect, the inspiratory concentration of the volatile anaesthetic is increased.

End	Last alfentanil ca. 20–30 min before end of surgery
	Slightly reduce ventilation, allow patient to breathe spontaneously (but avoid hypoventilation)
	Stop remifentanil infusion 3 min before last stitch
	Stop isoflurane when instruments are removed; desflurane slightly later

A further reason not to use N_2O in an anaesthetic for laparoscopic surgery is that it can delay the dissolution of gas bubbles in the circulation,[89] even if these contain only CO_2. This increases the risk of clinically relevant pulmonary gas embolism, particularly during intra-abdominal laser surgery.[90]

A final controversy revolves around the question of whether N_2O increases the incidence of PONV.[35,91–93] If it did increase postoperative emesis even slightly, its use would contravene one of the basic intentions of minimally invasive surgery.

Note

- N_2O enhances the circulatory effects of entrained venous gas and reduces the volume of entrained gas required to cause a lethal embolism
- N_2O can easily be dispensed with for anaesthesia

Postoperative nausea and vomiting

PONV is one of the two major factors preventing early discharge after day-care surgery and is also a major reason for re-admission to the hospital. It significantly increases the costs of monitoring, nursing and treatment, and is rivalled only by pain as a cause of patient discomfort.[94] Prevention of PONV is an important contribution to the rational management of patients undergoing minimally invasive surgery.

Laparoscopy was once thought to be a risk factor for PONV, but this has not been confirmed in controlled studies. Large studies on thousands of patients have distilled four factors that predict the likelihood of PONV. These are female gender, non-smoker, a history of travel sickness or PONV and postoperative opioid administration.[95] Female patients suffer from PONV three times more frequently than males.[95,96] Non-smokers are at increased risk of PONV,[96] as are patients with a history of PONV or travel sickness.[95–97] The first three factors are beyond the control of the anaesthetist, but he or she can still influence the risk of PONV to a certain degree by carefully planning the management of the anaesthetic and postoperative pain relief. Opioids given for postoperative pain control are the fourth major risk factor for PONV,[95,96] and their use can be minimized by rational planning of analgesic regimens (see Chapter 7). Volatile anaesthetics increase the risk of PONV,[98] and simply avoiding their use reduces the incidence by 18%.[99] Eliminating N_2O from the anaesthetic regimen probably decreases the incidence of PONV.[9,100] Reversing the effects of the neuromuscular blockers with neostigmine is a further factor that increases PONV.[101]

Effective measures for the treatment and prophylaxis of PONV have been determined by countless clinical studies. 5-HT$_3$ receptor antagonists are the drugs of first choice for treating PONV, followed by antihistamines, such as dimenhydrinate or cyclizine, and droperidol. Metoclopramide has been shown to be ineffective.[102] Scopolamine is a popular substance, but its efficacy in the treatment of PONV is limited, and its high incidence of adverse effects, such as visual disturbances, dry mouth, dizziness and agitation, will limit its usefulness.[103] Dexamethasone has been demonstrated to be effective in the prevention, but not in the treatment of PONV.[104]

The overall probability of PONV is 10% in patients without risk factors. The presence of one, two, three or four risk factors is associated with an incidence of PONV of 20, 40, 60 and 80%, respectively.[105,106] Current recommendations for PONV prophylaxis incorporate this observation into a graded, multimodal approach.[107,108] Patients at moderate risk for PONV (one risk factor) should be given a TIVA without N_2O and a prophylactic dose of an antiemetic, preferably 4 mg dexamethasone. In addition to these measures, patients at high risk (two or more risk factor) should be given a prophylactic dose of a second antiemetic. Patients with failed prophylaxis should not be given a second dose of the prophylactic agent, but one acting at a different site.

Regional and local anaesthesia

Regional or local anaesthesia has the advantage that the patient is awake and can be rapidly mobilized as soon as the motor blockade recedes. Some authors see a further advantage in the fact that the patient can automatically adapt his alveolar ventilation to eliminate absorbed CO_2. But there are only very few laparoscopic or endoscopic procedures that could be carried out under regional or local anaesthesia. The choice is severely limited by the physiological consequences of the operation, the pain localization and, above all, the patient's possible reluctance to accept the technique. Regional anaesthesia is most useful for short procedures with low-pressure pneumoperitoneum, with at most a slightly head-down position and without expected surgical complications (e.g. adhesions). Among these are laparoscopic tubal ligation, diagnostic procedures, gamete transfer, cryptorchism, etc. Laparoscopic tubal ligation is frequently performed in spinal or local anaesthesia.[109,110] N_2O is recommended as insufflation gas instead of CO_2 for laparoscopy with local anaesthesia, since it causes less peritoneal irritation and is better tolerated by the patient.[109] Extraperitoneal hernia repair is a further indication for epidural anaesthesia,[111–113] however, conversion to general anaesthesia can become necessary if the peritoneum is perforated.

Although regional anaesthesia is not generally recommended for upper abdominal surgery, since part of the afferent innervation runs through the vagus and phrenic nerves, and complete sensory blockade is not always assured, it has been performed successfully. In one institution, epidural anaesthesia is the method of choice for laparoscopic cholecystectomy in patients with severe obstructive lung disease,[114] while Edelman and colleagues described a laparoscopic cholecystectomy performed under epidural anaesthesia during pregnancy.[115]

Regional anaesthesia is not feasible as the sole anaesthetic for thoracoscopic operations in any case. For laparoscopic procedures, the level of anaesthesia has to reach Th4 to completely block all peritoneal afferents, but segments Th1 to Th4 should be spared to avoid blocking the thoracic sympathetic accelerant nerves. This is hardly possible, since the extent of sympathetic block usually exceeds that of analgesia, and there will be a risk of severe bradycardia during pneumoperitoneum.

Increased abdominal pressure impeding breathing, a head-down position and other associated factors cause severe distress in some patients that can interfere with surgery or even render it impossible to complete. The increased respiratory efforts required to eliminate excess CO_2 can cause considerable movement in the surgical field making delicate work increasingly difficult. Gas-free abdominal wall lift techniques that do not require increased IAP might avoid these problems.

It remains to be seen if regional anaesthesia is a suitable method for extraperitoneal procedures, such as hernia repair. The extremely high CO_2 uptake from the tissues will impose a heavy demand on the ventilatory capacity that the patient might not be willing to tolerate or even be physically able to cope with. Gas-free techniques might offer an acceptable alternative.

Fluid management during laparoscopic surgery

The elevated IAP of pneumoperitoneum establishes a pressure gradient between the intra-abdominal and intrathoracic segments of the inferior vena cava that interferes with venous return to the heart and thus induces circulatory changes resembling those seen in hypovolaemia. Hypotension is absent only because pneumoperitoneum increases peripheral vascular resistance. This is usually clinically irrelevant for short procedures or for surgery in the Trendelenburg position. Occasionally, however, this relative hypovolaemia can contribute to significant intraoperative hypotension. This is particularly the case in operations, such as retroperitoneal laparoscopic adrenalectomy, in which the patient's legs are lowered and there is no pneumoperitoneum to stimulate cardiovascular responses. Bandages or elastic stockings can be useful in preventing venous pooling in the legs, but these measures are not always sufficient. In these cases, cardiac filling must be restored by infusing a sufficient fluid volume to compensate for that sequestered in dependent body areas. Crystalloids are the fluids of choice, since they can be removed from the circulation again with greater ease. Signs of over-infusion, with right and left ventricular overload may occur when the patient is returned to the horizontal supine position, and the fluid pooled in the legs is shifted to the thorax. Rapidly acting diuretics, such as furosemide, can be given to accelerate excretion of the excess fluid from the circulation.

References

1. Swann DG, Spens H, Edwards SA, Chestnut RJ. Anaesthesia for gynaecological laparoscopy – a comparison between the laryngeal mask airway and tracheal intubation. *Anaesthesia* 1993; **48**: 431–434.
2. Maltby JR, Beriault MT, Watson NC. Use of the laryngeal mask is not contraindicated for laparoscopic cholecystectomy. *Anaesthesia* 2001; **56**: 800–802.
3. Rabey PG, Murphy PJ, Langton JA, Barker P, Rowbotham DJ. Effect of the laryngeal mask airway on lower oesophageal sphincter pressure in patients during general anaesthesia. *Br J Anaesth* 1992; **69**: 346–348.
4. Lu PP, Brimacombe J, Yang C, Shyr M. ProSeal versus the classic laryngeal mask airway for positive pressure ventilation during laparoscopic cholecystectomy. *Br J Anaesth* 2002; **88**: 824–827.
5. Maltby JR, Beriault MT, Watson NC, Liepert D, Fick GH. The LMA-ProSeal is an effective alternative to tracheal intubation for laparoscopic cholecystectomy. *Can J Anaesth* 2002; **49**: 857–862.
6. Edelman DS, Misiakos EP, Moses K. Extraperitoneal laparoscopic hernia repair with local anesthesia. *Surg Endosc* 2001; **15**: 976–980.
7. Harris RJ, Benveniste G, Pfitzner J. Cardiovascular collapse caused by carbon dioxide insufflation during one-lung anaesthesia for thoracoscopic dorsal sympathectomy. *Anaesth Intens Care* 2002; **30**: 86–89.
8. Sneyd JR, Carr A, Byrom WD, Bilski AJ. A meta-analysis of nausea and vomiting following maintenance of anaesthesia with propofol or inhalational agents. *Eur J Anaesthesiol* 1998; **15**: 433–445.
9. Tramer M, Moore A, McQuay H. Meta-analytic comparison of prophylactic antiemetic efficacy for postoperative nausea and vomiting: propofol anaesthesia vs omitting nitrous oxide vs total i.v. anaesthesia with propofol. *Br J Anaesth* 1997; **78**: 256–259.
10. Djaiani G, Ribes-Pastor MP. Propofol auto-co-induction as an alternative to midazolam co-induction for ambulatory surgery. *Anaesthesia* 1999; **54**: 63–67.
11. Tighe KE, Warner JA. The effect of co-induction with midazolam upon recovery from propofol infusion anaesthesia. *Anaesthesia* 1997; **52**: 1000–1004.
12. Hughes MA, Glass PSA, Jacobs JR. Context-sensitive half-time in multicompartment pharmacokinetic models for intravenous anesthetic drugs. *Anesthesiology* 1992; **76**: 334–341.
13. Shafer SL, Varvel JR. Pharmacokinetics, pharmacodynamics, and rational opioid selection. *Anesthesiology* 1991; **74**: 53–63.
14. Youngs EJ, Shafer SL. Pharmacokinetics parameters relevant to recovery from opioids. *Anesthesiology* 1994; **81**: 833–842.
15. Westmoreland CL, Hoke JF, Sebel PS, Hug Jr CC, Muir KT. Pharmacokinetics of remifentanil (GI87084B) and its major metabolite (GI90291) in patients undergoing elective inpatient surgery. *Anesthesiology* 1993; **79**: 893–903.
16. Egan TD, Lemmens HJ, Fiset P *et al.* The pharmacokinetics of the new short-acting opioid remifentanil (GI87084B) in healthy adult male volunteers. *Anesthesiology* 1993; **79**: 881–892.
17. Wuesten R, Van Aken H, Glass PS, Buerkle H. Assessment of depth of anesthesia and postoperative respiratory recovery after remifentanil- versus alfentanil-based total intravenous anesthesia in patients undergoing ear–nose–throat surgery. *Anesthesiology* 2001; **94**: 211–217.
18. Ishizaki Y, Bandai Y, Shimomura K, Abe H, Ohtomo Y, Idezuki Y. Changes in splanchnic blood flow and cardiovascular effects following peritoneal insufflation of carbon dioxide. *Surg Endosc* 1993; **7**: 420–423.
19. Hashikura Y, Kawasaki S, Munakata Y, Hashimoto S, Hayashi K, Makuuchi M. Effects of peritoneal insufflation on hepatic and renal blood flow. *Surg Endosc* 1994; **8**: 759–761.
20. Tunon MJ, Gonzalez P, Jorquera F, Llorente A, Gonzalo Orden M, Gonzalez Gallego J. Liver blood flow changes during laparoscopic surgery in pigs. A study of hepatic indocyanine green removal. *Surg Endosc* 1999; **13**: 668–672.
21. Vieira ZE, Zsigmond EK, Duarate B, Renigers SA, Hirota K. Evaluation of fentanyl and sufentanil on the diameter of the common bile duct by ultrasonography in man: a double blind placebo controlled study. *Int J Clin Pharmacol Ther* 1994; **32**: 274–277.
22. Hynynen MJ, Turunen MT, Korttila KT. Effects of alfentanil and fentanyl on common bile duct pressure. *Anesth Analg* 1986; **65**: 370–372.
23. Jones RM, Detmer M, Hill AB, Bjoraker DG, Pandit U. Incidence of choledochoduodenal sphincter spasm during fentanyl-supplemented anesthesia. *Anesth Analg* 1981; **60**: 638–640.
24. Fragen RJ, Vilich F, Spies SM, Erwin WD. The effect of remifentanil on biliary tract drainage into the duodenum. *Anesth Analg* 1999; **89**: 1561–1564.
25. Crozier TA, Kietzmann D, Dobereiner B. Mood change after anaesthesia with remifentanil or alfentanil. *Eur J Anaesthesiol* 2004; **21**: 20–24.
26. Sessler DI, Israel D, Pozos RS, Pozos M, Rubinstein EH. Spontaneous post-anesthetic tremor does not resemble thermoregulatory shivering. *Anesthesiology* 1988; **68**: 843–850.
27. Crozier TA, Sumpf E. Der Einfluß einer totalen intravenösen Anästhesie mit S-(+)-Ketamin/Propofol

auf hämodynamische, endokrine und metabolische Streßreaktionen im Vergleich zu Alfentanil/Propofol bei Laparotomien. *Anaesthesist* 1996; **45**: 1015–1023.

28. Vallejo MC, Romeo RC, Davis DJ, Ramanathan S. Propofol–ketamine versus propofol–fentanyl for out-patient laparoscopy: comparison of postoperative nausea, emesis, analgesia, and recovery. *J Clin Anesth* 2002; **14**: 426–431.

29. Fruergaard K, Jenstrup M, Schierbeck J, Wiberg-Jorgensen F. Total intravenous anaesthesia with propofol or etomidate. *Eur J Anaesthesiol* 1991; **8**: 385–391.

30. de Grood PM, Harbers JB, van Egmond J, Crul JF. Anaesthesia for laparoscopy. A comparison of five techniques including propofol, etomidate, thiopentone and isoflurane. *Anaesthesia* 1987; **42**: 815–823.

31. Crozier TA, Müller JE, Quittkat D, Sydow M, Wuttke W, Kettler D. Totale intravenöse Anaesthesie mit Methohexital–Alfentanil oder Propofol–Alfentanil bei Unterbauchlaparotomien: Klinische Aspekte und Einfluß auf die Stressreaktion [Total intravenous anesthesia with methohexital–alfentanil or propofol–alfentanil for lower abdominal surgery: Clinical aspects and effect on the stress response]. *Anaesthesist* 1994; **43**: 594–604.

32. Crozier TA, Schlaeger M, Wuttke W, Kettler D. TIVA mit Etomidat-Fentanyl versus Midazolam-Fentanyl. Der perioperative Streß der Koronarchirurgie überwindet die Kortisolsynthesehemmung nach einer totalen intravenösen Anästhesie mit Etomidate-Fentanyl [TIVA with etomidate–fentanyl versus midazolam–fentanyl. The perioperative stress of coronary artery surgery overrides the inhibition of cortisol synthesis after a total intravenous anaesthetic with etomidate–fentanyl]. *Anaesthesist* 1994; **43**: 605–613.

33. Blobner M, Schneck HJ, Felber AR, Goegler S, Feussner H, Jelen-Esselborn S. Vergleichende Untersuchungen der Aufwachphase: Laparoskopische Cholezystektomie nach Isofluran-, Methohexital- und Propofolanästhesie [Comparative study of the recovery phase. Laparoscopic cholecystectomy following isoflurane, methohexital and propofol anesthesia]. *Anaesthesist* 1994; **43**: 573–581.

34. Doze VA, Westphal LM, White PF. Comparison of propofol with methohexital for outpatient anesthesia. *Anesth Analg* 1986; **65**: 1189–1195.

35. Raftery S, Sherry E. Total intravenous anaesthesia with propofol and alfentanil protects against postoperative nausea and vomiting. *Can J Anaesth* 1992; **39**: 37–40.

36. Möllhoff T, Burgard G, Prien T. Übelkeit und Erbrechen nach gynäkologischen Laparoskopien [Nausea and vomiting after gynaecological laparoscopy]. *Anästhesiol Intens Med Notfallmed Schmerzther* 1995; **30**: 23–27.

37. Klockgether-Radke A, Piorek V, Crozier TA, Kettler D. Nausea and vomiting after laparoscopic surgery. A comparison of propofol and thiopentone/halothane anaesthesia. *Eur J Anaesthesiol* 1996; **13**: 3–9.

38. Schaub E, Kern C, Landau R. Pain on injection: a double-blind comparison of propofol 1% with iv lidocaine pre-treatment versus Propofol-Lipuro 1%. *Eur J Anaesthesiol* 2004; **21(Suppl 32)**: A535.

39. Janicki PK, James MF, Erskine WA. Propofol inhibits enzymatic degradation of alfentanil and sufentanil by isolated liver microsomes in vitro. *Br J Anaesth* 1992; **68**: 311–312.

40. Bouillon T, Bruhn J, Radu-Radulescu L, Bertaccini E, Park S, Shafer S. Non-steady state analysis of the pharmacokinetic interaction between propofol and remifentanil. *Anesthesiology* 2002; **97**: 1350–1362.

41. Vuyk J, Hennis PJ, Burm AG, de Voogt JW, Spierdijk J. Comparison of midazolam and propofol in combination with alfentanil for total intravenous anesthesia. *Anesth Analg* 1990; **71**: 645–650.

42. Short TG, Plummer JL, Chui PT. Hypnotic and anaesthetic interactions between midazolam, propofol and alfentanil. *Br J Anaesth* 1992; **69**: 162–167.

43. Vinik HR. Intravenous anaesthetic drug interactions: practical applications. *Eur J Anaesthesiol* 1995; **12(Suppl 12)**: 13–19.

44. Crozier TA, Kettler D. Cost effectiveness of general anaesthesia: inhalation vs i.v. *Br J Anaesth* 1999; **83**: 547–549.

45. Puura AI, Rorarius MG, Manninen P, Hopput S, Baer GA. The costs of intense neuromuscular block for anesthesia during endolaryngeal procedures due to waiting time. *Anesth Analg* 1999; **88**: 1335–1339.

46. Fox MH, Hunt PCW. Prolonged neuromuscular block associated with mivacurium. *Br J Anaesth* 1995; **74**: 237–238.

47. Maddineni VR, Mirakhur RK. Prolonged neuromuscular block following mivacurium. *Anesthesiology* 1993; **78**: 1181–1184.

48. Vermeyen KM, Sparr HJ, Beaufort AM *et al.* Reversal of rocuronium induced neuromuscular block by Org 25969: pharmacokinetics. *Eur J Anaesthesiol* 2004; **21(Suppl 32)**: A576.

49. Sorgenfrei I, Larsen PB, Norrild K *et al.* Rapid reversal of rocuronium by the cyclodextrine ORG 25969: a two centre dose finding and safety study. *Eur J Anaesthesiol* 2004; **21(Suppl 32)**: A571.

50. Schüttler J, Stoeckel H, Schwilden H. Pharmacokinetic and pharmacodynamic modeling of propofol (Diprivan) in volunteers and surgical patients. *Postgr Med J* 1985; **61(Suppl 3)**: 53–55.

51. Smith C, McEwan AI, Jhaveri R *et al.* The interaction of fentanyl on the Cp50 of propofol for loss of consciousness and skin incision. *Anesthesiology* 1994; **81**: 820–828.

52. Vuyk J, Engbers FHM, Lemmens HJM *et al.* Pharmacodynamics of propofol in female patients. *Anesthesiology* 1992; **77**: 3–9.

53. Moffat AC, Murray AW, Fitch W. Opioid supplementation during propofol anaesthesia. *Anaesthesia* 1989; **44**: 644–647.

54. Vuyk J, Engbers FH, Burm AG *et al.* Pharmacodynamic interaction between propofol and alfentanil when given for induction of anesthesia. *Anesthesiology* 1996; **84**: 288–299.

55. Turtle MJ, Cullen P, Prys-Roberts C, Coates D, Monk CR, Faroqui MH. Dose requirements of propofol during nitrous oxide anaesthesia in man. II. Patients premedicated with lorazepam. *Br J Anaesth* 1987; **59**: 283–287.

56. Davidson JAH, Macleod AD, Howie JC, White M, Kenny GNC. Effective concentration 50 for propofol with and without 67% nitrous oxide. *Acta Anaesthesiol Scand* 1993; **37**: 458–464.

57. Bouillon TW, Bruhn J, Radulescu L *et al.* Pharmacodynamic interaction between propofol and remifentanil regarding hypnosis, tolerance of laryngoscopy, bispectral index, and electroencephalographic approximate entropy. *Anesthesiology* 2004; **100**: 1353–1372.

58. Kern SE, Xie G, White JL, Egan TD. A response surface analysis of propofol–remifentanil pharmacodynamic interaction in volunteers. *Anesthesiology* 2004; **100**: 1373–1381.

59. Milne SE, Kenny GN, Schraag S. Propofol sparing effect of remifentanil using closed-loop anaesthesia. *Br J Anaesth* 2003; **90**: 623–629.

60. Vuyk J, Lim T, Engbers FH, Burm AG, Vletter AA, Bovill JG. The pharmacodynamic interaction of propofol and alfentanil during lower abdominal surgery in women. *Anesthesiology* 1995; **83**: 8–22.

61. White PF, Coe V, Shafer A, Sung ML. Comparison of alfentanil with fentanyl for outpatient anesthesia. *Anesthesiology* 1986; **64**: 99–106.

62. O'Connor M, Sear JW. Sufentanil to supplement nitrous oxide in oxygen during balanced anaesthesia. *Anaesthesia* 1988; **43**: 749–752.

63. Mertens MJ, Olofsen E, Engbers FH, Burm AG, Bovill JG, Vuyk J. Propofol reduces perioperative remifentanil requirements in a synergistic manner: response surface modeling of perioperative remifentanil–propofol interactions. *Anesthesiology* 2003; **99**: 347–359.

64. Vuyk J, Mertens MJ, Olofsen E, Burm AG, Bovill JG. Propofol anesthesia and rational opioid selection: determination of optimal EC50–EC95 propofol–opioid concentrations that assure adequate anesthesia and a rapid return of consciousness. *Anesthesiology* 1997; **87**: 1549–1562.

65. Shafer A, Doze DA, Shafer SL, White PF. Pharmacokinetics and pharmacodynamics of propofol infusions during general anesthesia. *Anesthesiology* 1988; **69**: 348–356.

66. Fragen RJ, Fitzgerald PC. Is an infusion pump necessary to safely administer remifentanil? *Anesth Analg* 2000; **90**: 713–716.

67. Schwilden H. A general method for calculating the dosage scheme in linear pharmacokinetics. *Eur J Clin Pharmacol* 1981; **20**: 379–386.

68. White M, Kenny GN. Intravenous propofol anaesthesia using a computerised infusion system. *Anaesthesia* 1990; **45**: 204–209.

69. Chaudhri S, White M, Kenny GN. Induction of anaesthesia with propofol using a target-controlled infusion system. *Anaesthesia* 1992; **47**: 551–553.

70. Sykes MK, Loh L, Seed RF, Kafer ER, Chakrabarti NK. The effect of inhalational anaesthetics on hypoxic pulmonary vasoconstriction and pulmonary vascular resistance in the perfused lungs of the dog and cat. *Br J Anaesth* 1972; **44**: 776–788.

71. Mathers J, Benumof JL, Wahrenbrock EA. General anesthetics and regional hypoxic pulmonary vasoconstriction. *Anesthesiology* 1977; **46**: 111–114.

72. Bjertnæs LJ. Hypoxia-induced vasoconstriction in isolated perfused lungs exposed to injectable or inhalation anesthetics. *Acta Anaesthesiol Scand* 1977; **21**: 133–147.

73. Hedenstierna G. Gas exchange during anaesthesia. *Br J Anaesth* 1990; **64**: 507–514.

74. Hedenstierna G, Strandberg Å, Tokics L, Lundqvist H, Brismar B. Correlation of gas exchange impairment to development of atelectasis during anesthesia and muscle paralysis. *Acta Anaesthesiol Scand* 1986; **30**: 183–191.

75. Scott DB, Julian DG. Observations on cardiac arrhythmias during laparoscopy. *Br Med J* 1972; **12**: 411–413.

76. McEwan AI, Smith C, Dyar O, Goodman D, Glass PSA. Isoflurane MAC reduction by fentanyl. *Anesthesiology* 1993; **78**: 864–869.

77. Brunner MD, Braithwaite P, Jhaveri R *et al.* MAC reduction of isoflurane by sufentanil. *Br J Anaesth* 1994; **72**: 42–46.

78. Lake CL, DiFazio CA, Moscicki JC, Engle JS. Reduction of halothane MAC: comparison of morphine and alfentanil. *Anesth Analg* 1985; **64**: 807–810.

79. Lang E, Kapila A, Shlugman D, Hoke JF, Sebel PS, Glass PS. Reduction of isoflurane minimal alveolar concentration by remifentanil. *Anesthesiology* 1996; **85**: 721–728.

80. Westmoreland CL, Sebel PS, Gropper A. Fentanyl or alfentanil decreases the minimum alveolar anesthetic concentration of isoflurane in surgical patients. *Anesth Analg* 1994; **78**: 23–28.

81. Sebel PS, Glass PSA, Fletcher JE, Murphy MR, Gallagher C, Quill T. Reduction of MAC of desflurane with fentanyl. *Anesthesiology* 1992; **76**: 52–59.

82. Hall RI, Murphy MR, Hug CC. The enflurane-sparing effect of sufentanil in dogs. *Anesthesiology* 1987; **67**: 518–525.

83. Hall RI, Szlam F, Hug CCJ. The enflurane-sparing effect of alfentanil in dogs. *Anesth Analg* 1987; **66**: 1287–1291.

84. Wilhelm W, Huppert A, Brun K, Gruness V, Larsen R. Remifentanil mit Propofol oder Isofluran. Ein Vergleich des Aufwachverhaltens bei arthroskopischen Eingriffen. [Remifentanil with propofol or isoflurane. A comparison of the recovery times after arthroscopic surgery]. *Anaesthesist* 1997; **46**: 335–338.

85. Grundmann U, Silomon M, Bach F *et al.* Recovery profile and side effects of remifentanil-based anaesthesia with desflurane or propofol for laparoscopic cholecystectomy. *Acta Anaesthesiol Scand* 2001; **45**: 320–326.

86. Eger EI, II, Saidman LJ. Hazards of nitrous oxide anesthesia in bowel obstruction and pneumothorax. *Anesthesiology* 1965; **26**: 61–66.

87. Krogh B, Jørn Jensen P, Henneberg SW, Hole P, Kronborg O. Nitrous oxide does not influence operating conditions or postoperative course in colonic surgery. *Br J Anaesth* 1994; **72**: 55–57.

88. Taylor E, Feinstein R, White PF, Soper N. Anesthesia for laparoscopic cholecystectomy: is nitrous oxide contraindicated? *Anesthesiology* 1992; **76**: 541–543.

89. Steffey EP, Johnson BH, Eger EI. Nitrous oxide intensifies the pulmonary arterial pressure response

to venous injection of carbon dioxide in the dog. *Anesthesiology* 1980; **52**: 52–55.

90. Greville AC, Clements EAF, Erwin DC, McMillan DL, Wellwood JM. Pulmonary air embolism during laparoscopic laser cholecystectomy. *Anaesthesia* 1991; **46**: 113–114.

91. Felts JA, Poler SM, Spitznagel EL. Nitrous oxide, nausea, and vomiting after outpatient gynecologic surgery. *J Clin Anaesth* 1990; **2**: 168–171.

92. Hovorka J, Korttila K, Erkola O. Nitrous oxide does increase nausea and vomiting following gynaecological laparoscopy. *Can J Anaesth* 1989; **36**: 145–148.

93. Sukhani R, Lurie J, Jabamoni R. Propofol for ambulatory gynecologic laparoscopy: does omission of nitrous oxide alter postoperative emetic sequelae and recovery? *Anesth Analg* 1994; **78**: 831–835.

94. Macario A, Weinger M, Carney S, Kim A. Which clinical anesthesia outcomes are important to avoid? The perspective of patients. *Anesth Analg* 1999; **89**: 652–658.

95. Apfel CC, Läärä E, Koivuranta M, Greim CA, Roewer N. A simplified risk score for predicting postoperative nausea and vomiting. *Anesthesiology* 1999; **91**: 693–700.

96. Cohen MM, Duncan PG, DeBoer DP, Tweed WA. The postoperative interview: assessing risk factors for nausea and vomiting. *Anesth Analg* 1994; **78**: 7–16.

97. Koivuranta M, Läärä E, Snare L, Alahuhta S. A survey of postoperative nausea and vomiting. *Anaesthesia* 1997; **52**: 443–449.

98. Apfel CC, Kranke P, Katz MH *et al.* Volatile anaesthetics may be the main cause for early but not delayed postoperative nausea and vomiting: a randomized controlled trial of factorial design. *Br J Anaesth* 2002; **88**: 659–668.

99. Apfel CC, Korttila K, Abdalla M, Biedler A, Pocock S, Roewer N. An international multicenter protocol to assess the single and combined benefits of antiemetic strategies in a controlled clinical trial of a 2 × 2 × 2 × 2 × 2 factorial design (IMPACT). *Control Clin Trial* 2003; **24**: 736–751.

100. Divatia JV, Vaidya JS, Badwe RA, Hawaldar RW. Omission of nitrous oxide during anesthesia reduces the incidence of postoperative nausea and vomiting. A meta-analysis. *Anesthesiology* 1996; **85**: 1055–1062.

101. Tramer M, Fuchs-Buder T. Omitting antagonism of neuromuscular block: effect on postoperative nausea and vomiting and risk of residual paralysis. A systematic review. *Br J Anaesth* 1999; **82**: 379–386.

102. Henzi I, Walder B, Tramer M. Metoclopramide in the prevention of postoperative nausea and vomiting: a quantitative systematic review of randomized, placebo-controlled studies. *Br J Anaesth* 1999; **83**: 761–771.

103. Kranke P, Morin AM, Roewer N, Wulf H, Eberhardt LHJ. The efficacy and safety of transdermal scopolamine for the prevention of postoperative nausea and vomiting: a quantitative systematic review. *Anesth Analg* 2002; **95**: 133–143.

104. Liu K, Hsu CC, Chia YY. The effect of dose of dexamethasone for antiemesis after major gynecological surgery. *Anesth Analg* 1999; **89**: 1316–1318.

105. Apfel CC, Kranke P, Eberhardt LHJ, Roos IA, Roewer N. A comparison of predicting models for postoperative nausea and vomiting. *Br J Anaesth* 2002; **88**: 234–240.

106. Pierre S, Benais H, Pouymayou J. Apfel's simplified score may favourably predict the risk of postoperative nausea and vomiting. *Can J Anaesth* 2002; **49**: 237–242.

107. Habib AS, Gan TJ. Evidence-based management of postoperative nausea and vomiting: a review. *Can J Anaesth* 2004; **51**: 326–341.

108. Apfel CC, Roewer N. Postoperative Übelkeit und Erbrechen [Postoperative nausea and vomiting]. *Anaesthesist* 2004; **53**: 377–391.

109. Penfield AJ. Laparoscopic sterilization under local anesthesia. *Obstet Gynecol* 1977; **49**: 725–727.

110. Burke RK. Spinal anesthesia for laparoscopy. A review of 1063 cases. *J Reprod Med* 1978; **21**: 59–62.

111. Ferzli GS, Dysarz FA. Extraperitoneal endoscopic inguinal herniorrhaphy performed without carbon dioxide insufflation. *J Laparoendosc Surg* 1994; **4**: 301–304.

112. Hirschberg T, Olthoff D, Borner P. Vergleichende Untersuchungen zur Durchfuhrung der totalen extraperitonealen Hernioplastik in kombinierter Spinal-Epidural-Anästhesie versus balancierter Allgemeinanästhesie [Comparative studies of total extraperitoneal hernioplasty in combined spinal epidural anesthesia versus balanced general anesthesia]. *Anaesthesiol Reanim* 2002; **27**: 144–151.

113. Salihoglu Z, Demiroluk S, Yavuz N. Minimally invasive preperitoneal inguinal hernia repair with epidural anaesthesia. *Anaesth Intens Care* 2002; **30**: 813–814.

114. Gramatica Jr L, Brasesco OE, Mercado Luna A *et al.* Laparoscopic cholecystectomy performed under regional anesthesia in patients with chronic obstructive pulmonary disease. *Surg Endosc* 2002; **16**: 472–475.

115. Edelman DS. Alternative laparoscopic technique for cholecystectomy during pregnancy. *Surg Endosc* 1994; **8**: 794–796.

COMPLICATIONS AND CONTRAINDICATIONS OF LAPAROSCOPIC SURGERY

6

Laparoscopic operations carry a distinct risk of complications despite their minimal invasiveness, as shown in Table 6.1. In one study, the incidence of typical anaesthesiological complications, such as hypo- or hypertension, tachycardia, hypercapnia, dysrhythmia, hypoxaemia or hypothermia, in the course of laparoscopic cholecystectomy was 19.8% compared to 14.8% with open cholecystectomy, but 3.7% with short gynaecological laparoscopic procedures.[1] The most frequent complication during laparoscopic cholecystectomy was hypotension, which was seen in 13% of the patients. Arterial hypertension is a regular occurrence and most reviews do not even count it as a complication. Hypothermia, nausea and vomiting, hypoxaemia and pain head the list of the postoperative adverse events (Table 6.2). Subcutaneous emphysema, the incidence of which depends on the type of operation, is a typical surgical complication of laparoscopic operations that can have considerable anaesthetic implications in the postoperative period. The most important complications will be described and discussed in the following chapters.

Gas embolism

Intravascular gas embolism is one of the most serious complication of laparoscopic surgery. Depending on the gas used for insufflation, the speed of entrainment, the volume of gas entering the blood stream and the anaesthetic, the clinical impact of this complication ranges from a virtually inapparent course to death on the table. The incidence and the severity of gas embolism also depends on the type of endoscopic operation performed. Besides being aware of the factors that lead to embolization, the anaesthetist must also be well acquainted with those that aggravate the clinical effects of a gas embolism once it has occurred.

Gas embolism occurs frequently during hysteroscopy, and small amounts of gas can be detected in the right heart with a precordial Doppler stethoscope in up to 50% of all patients,[2] while larger amounts that can be auscultated with a normal stethoscope are found in 10–15% of the patients.[3] Pressurized air was originally used to dilate the uterus but the unacceptably high incidence of fatal gas embolism triggered a search for a safer insufflation gas.[2–5] The most important development towards preventing fatal gas embolisms was the introduction of carbon dioxide (CO_2) as insufflation gas (see Chapter 2). Other gases, such as oxygen (O_2) or helium (He), have been studied for use as insufflation gas, but they offer no advantage over CO_2 with regard to

---

Table 6.1 Complications of laparoscopic operations with relevance to anaesthesia

Cardiovascular
Hypotension, hypertension, tachycardia, bradycardia, dysrhythmias

Pulmonary
Hypercapnia, hypoxaemia, atelectasis, barotrauma

Related to gas insufflation
Subcutaneous emphysema, gas embolism, pneumothorax, pneumomediastinum, extreme CO_2 absorption

Surgical
Haemorrhage, damage to hollow viscera, damage to nerves

Mechanical
Damage to nerves or eyes (positioning and draping), dislodgement of endotracheal tube with endobronchial intubation

Miscellaneous
Hypothermia, nausea and vomiting, hyperkalemia, renal failure

---

Table 6.2 Incidence of adverse postoperative events after laparoscopic cholecystectomy (LC), open cholecystectomy (OC) or gynaecological laparoscopy (GL)[1]

Event	LC	OC	GL
All (%)	52.5	58.8	20.0
Hypothermia (%, skin temperature <35°C)	31.4	11.8	Not studied
PONV (%)	12.9	16.4	5.7
Hypoxaemia (%, SO_2 <90% when breathing room air)	10.9	25.9	1.3
Severe pain (%)	4.0	12.9	4.4

PONV: postoperative nausea and vomiting; SO_2: oxygen saturation.

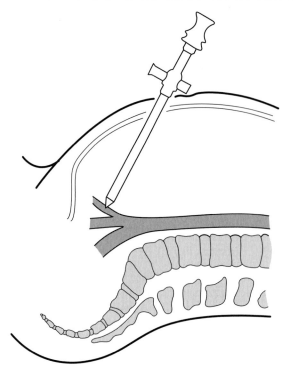

Figure 6.1 Diagram of vascular injury during initial blind introduction of the trocar.

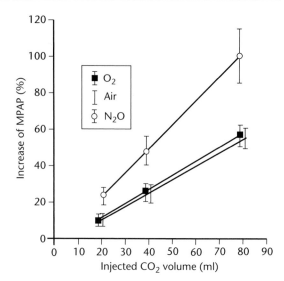

Figure 6.2 Increase of MPAP following intravenous injection of CO_2 while breathing room air, 100% O_2, or $N_2O:O_2$ 79:21. (Data from Ref [21].)

gas embolism. Quite the contrary, due to their physico-chemical properties they carry the same risk of fatal embolism as air.[6]

Clinically apparent gas embolism occurs much less frequently during laparoscopy than during hyster-oscopy,[4,7–13] although the incidence of gas bubbles detected in the right heart by echocardiography during laparoscopic cholecystectomy was almost 70%.[14] Animal studies have shown that the incidence of gas embolism is nearly 100% during laparoscopic dissection of the liver.[15] The reason for the lower incidence of clinically relevant embolic events despite the high prevalence of intracardiac gas bubbles is possibly due to the lower insufflation pressure and the vascular anatomy. Gas cannot pass directly from the abdominal cavity through the uninjured peritoneum into the blood stream, and significant intravascular entrainment of gas occurs during laparoscopic cholecystectomy only when the insufflation needle is incorrectly positioned or when veins are injured that for some reason cannot collapse. This happens frequently during the early stages of insufflation, since the Veress needle is introduced blindly and the tip can be inserted into a vein despite all precautions (Figure 6.1).[10] Small peritoneal veins can be torn by the trocar during insertion and remain open until they are compressed by an increase in intra-abdominal pressure (IAP). This would explain

the high incidence of detectable gas bubbles following the beginning of insufflation.[14] Intravascular gas insufflation occurring intraoperatively can result from the insufflation trocar becoming dislodged from an originally correct position.[16] Gas can also pool in the venous system and cause symptomatic systemic embolization after some delay.[17] Gas embolism has also been described during the use of gas-cooled laser probes or fluid dissectors on well-vascularized organs, such as the liver.[12,18–20]

The only initial effect of a small amount of gas on the circulation is an increase of pulmonary artery pressure, the magnitude of which depends primarily on the type of insufflated gas. Injecting 20 ml of air intravenously increases the mean pulmonary artery pressure (MPAP) in a spontaneous breathing dog by an average of 87%, while the MPAP increase after injecting the same volume of CO_2 is only 10%.[21] A larger volume of gas reduces blood flow in the lung by obstructing pulmonary arteries and blocking right ventricular outflow.

Nitrous oxide (N_2O) intensifies the circulatory effects of a gas embolism, causing smaller intravascular bubbles to acquire clinical relevance. Injecting 20 ml of air into a dog breathing a N_2O–O_2 mixture raises pulmonary artery pressure not by 87% as when breathing room air, but by 148%.[21] N_2O reduces the median lethal volume (LD_{50}) of an intravenous injection of gas by approximately 60–80%.[22] It also magnifies the circulatory effects of intravascular CO_2 bubbles and intensifies the resulting MPAP increase (Figure 6.2).[21]

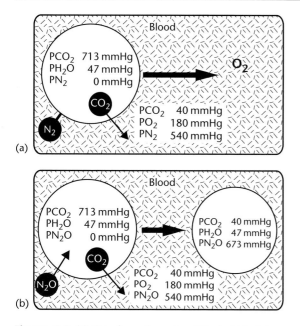

(a)

(b)

Figure 6.3 (a) Transformation of a CO_2 bubble into a N_2O bubble in blood saturated with N_2O. The partial pressures are given without regard to the hydrostatic pressure of the surrounding blood. (b) During ventilation with $O_2:N_2$ mixture the CO_2 bubbles dissolve rapidly, since N_2 has a low diffusion coefficient and enters the bubbles more slowly than CO_2 diffuses out. PCO_2, PH_2O, PN_2, PN_2O and PO_2 are partial pressures of CO_2, H_2O, N_2, N_2O and O_2, respectively.

The elevated pressure also returns to normal more slowly in the presence of N_2O.

Why do entrained CO_2 bubbles that dissolve very rapidly in blood under normal circumstances, cause such severe circulatory problems when N_2O is in the inspiratory gas mixture? One has to imagine that in this case the blood is saturated with poorly soluble but highly diffusible N_2O. N_2O diffuses into the CO_2 bubbles at approximately the same rate as CO_2 diffuses outward. O_2 also diffuses into the bubbles but significantly more slowly, since its diffusion coefficient is about 30 times less than that of N_2O. In quasi equilibrium, somewhat smaller bubbles will remain, filled with N_2O and some CO_2 (Figure 6.3). These slowly resolving N_2O bubbles remain in the pulmonary circulation and are responsible for the clinical symptoms.

Detection and symptoms of gas embolism

The symptoms of gas embolism (Table 6.3) result from the acute obstruction of the pulmonary circulation, and affect both the arterial and venous systems.[23] A sufficiently large embolism increases central venous pressure (CVP) and causes signs of venous congestion.

Table 6.3 Symptoms of gas embolism

- Fall of end-tidal CO_2 (increased dead-space ventilation)
- Dysrhythmias (bradycardia, ventricular ectopic beats, tachycardia, asystole)
- Hypotension (decreased left ventricular filling)
- Fall in arterial O_2 saturation
- Increased CVP and venous congestion
- ECG signs of acute right heart strain
- Auscultatory phenomena (tympanic second heart sound, mill-wheel murmur)

Tricuspid regurgitation can be observed even with otherwise inapparent gas embolism.[24] An acute increase in right ventricular pressure induces typical changes in the electrocardiography (ECG), such as tall R-waves in V_1, peaked P-waves best seen in the inferior leads, right axis deviation, atrial dysrhythmias and right bundle branch block. Left ventricular filling pressure falls and with it systemic arterial pressure.

The reduction of pulmonary perfusion increases the extent of the West I zones in the lungs. These are the areas in which the ventilation–perfusion relationship is shifted towards dead-space ventilation. The resulting fall of the capnometric end-tidal CO_2 concentration is one of the most sensitive indicators of an embolism. The widespread misconception that the CO_2 bubbles trapped in the pulmonary circulation would be exhaled and thereby increase the end-tidal CO_2 concentration is not supported by clinical observations and has been disproved in animal studies.[25]

Acute right ventricular dilation in combination with inadequate myocardial perfusion predisposes to cardial dysrhythmias. Bradycardia followed by tachydysrhythmia is frequently the initial manifestation of an embolism, but an immediate onset with tachycardia and ventricular ectopic beats is also observed. Polymorphic ectopic beats which rapidly progress to asystole are the consequence if the obstruction of the pulmonary circulation persists.

Transoesophageal echocardiography (TEE) is the most sensitive method for detecting intracardial gas[25,26] followed by Doppler ultrasonography. Gas bubbles can be detected in the inferior vena cava and the right heart before they become apparent as acoustical Doppler phenomena or as a fall in end-tidal CO_2 partial pressure ($P_{et}CO_2$).[24] One study showed that auscultation with a precordial or oesophagus stethoscope has a sensitivity similar to that of capnometry or pulmonary artery pressure monitoring.[25]

The auscultatory phenomena of venous gas embolism depend on the amount of gas trapped in the right heart. Small gas bubbles can only be detected by pre-cordial Doppler ultrasonography as brief swishing sounds. A slightly greater amount of gas in the right ventricle gives a tympanic character to the pulmonic component of the second heart sound due to rising pulmonary artery pressure, and with increasing gas volume the typical splashing, churning sound reminiscent of a washing machine, and known as a mill-wheel murmur, can be heard. A Doppler stethoscope should be used as an early warning system for operations with a high risk of embolism, since this allows prompt countermeasures to be taken to stop further gas entrainment and to prevent the accumulation of relevant amounts of gas. Capnometric evidence of embolism has a greater clinical relevance than ultrasonographic phenomena, since it reflects an actual reduction of pulmonary perfusion.

There is a certain risk of paradoxical embolization into the systemic circulation through arteriovenous shunts in the lung or through a patent foramen ovale (present in 30% of all adults), particularly when pulmonary artery pressure is increased.[27] This can occlude cerebral or coronary arteries causing permanent neurological damage or myocardial infarction.[28–30]

Secondary pulmonary failure can occur even after successful management of the initial event.[31–33] The pathogenesis of this is not completely resolved but inflammatory and coagulatory reaction cascades, activated by the endothelial adhesion of leucocytes and thrombocytes in the affected vascular bed, are thought to be involved.[34–36]

Therapy of gas embolism

The therapy of symptomatic pulmonary gas embolism requires a concerted approach with the goal of alleviating the clinical symptoms and stabilizing vital functions. At the same time, one has to prevent the further entrainment of gas, and the expansion of gas already in the circulation.

On the slightest suspicion of a clinically relevant embolism, or the occurrence of unexpected, severe circulatory symptoms, insufflation must be stopped immediately and the patients' lungs ventilated with 100% O_2. The patient is brought into a steep head-down, left lateral decubitus position (Durant position) under the assumption that this will facilitate the escape of gas from the pulmonary artery and the right ventricular outflow tract.[37] However, this position is not unanimously considered to offer any advantage over the horizontal supine position.[38]

Circulatory complications are then treated following the guidelines for cardiopulmonary resuscitation: closed chest cardiac compression, catecholamines for asystole, and defibrillation for ventricular fibrillation or ventricular tachycardia. Inotropes are administered to support the right ventricle. Vasopressors should be used to treat severe hypotension and to maintain a minimal coronary perfusion.

Some recommend introducing a central venous catheter into the right ventricle and aspirating the trapped gas. One study showed that intracardiac gas aspiration was no more effective in the management of gas embolism than proper positioning,[39] while others found it to be effective when a multiorifice catheter was used, but even then only if the gas had entered the heart via the superior vena cava.[40,41] If the patient has an indwelling central venous catheter, one can attempt to aspirate gas, but one should not interrupt other measures in order to insert a catheter.

After the event the patient should be allowed to awaken rapidly under intensive care monitoring in order to assess the neurological status. One should look for symptoms arising from a paradoxical embolization. Hyperbaric O_2 therapy may be beneficial in cerebral gas embolism.[28,42] Further close monitoring is indicated to detect a delayed occurrence of pulmonary complications.

CO_2 embolism usually resolves rapidly, and the patients normally recover without permanent sequelae; however, this is not always the case.[10,13,17] Acute right ventricular decompensation can drastically worsen the prognosis in patients with congestive heart failure and pre-existing elevated pulmonary artery pressure, while coronary artery occlusion can precipitate fatal myocardial infarction.

Note

- Stop gas insufflation immediately!
- Increase inspiratory O_2 concentration to 100% O_2 and hyperventilate
- Position patient head-down, left lateral decubitus (Durant position)
- Attempt intracardiac gas aspiration if central venous catheter is present (but do not waste time trying to insert a catheter)
- Give inotropes to support right ventricle
- Treat severe hypotension with vasopressors
- Closed chest cardiac compression for asystole

Prevention of gas embolism

It is primarily the surgeon's responsibility to prevent gas embolism, since this complication is usually caused by an incorrect position of the insufflating needle or trocar. It is the responsibility of the anaesthetist to undertake everything possible to remove the risk of clinically relevant embolisms, and to minimize the clinical effects of a pulmonary gas embolism by early detection and effective, competent treatment. This includes avoiding the use of N_2O, which seriously aggravates the clinical course of gas embolism.[21]

Subcutaneous emphysema

Subcutaneous emphysema, gas in the soft tissues of the subcutis, is a fairly common complication of laparoscopic surgery. There is a smooth swelling of the skin, and crepitations; which are felt on palpation. Gas can also collect in the mediastinum or pericardium, where it reveals its presence by the typical Hamman sign, a precordial crunching, crackling sound that is synchronous with the heart beat. Patients with extensive subcutaneous emphysema eliminate the excess CO_2 absorbed from the tissues by breathing deeply at a high respiratory rate. This hyperpnoea occasionally gives them a quite disturbing feeling of breathlessness, which can be alleviated to a certain extent by the careful administration of opiates.

Subcutaneous emphysema can arise from incorrect positioning or secondary dislodgement of the insufflation needle or trocar (Figure 6.4). It can also occur in the course of an endoscopic operation when the peritoneum is breached (such as in transperitoneal hernia repair or retroperitoneal operations) or whenever artificial cavities are formed by gas insufflation (such as during preperitoneal hernia repair, nephrectomy or mediastinal operations). Subcutaneous emphysema occurs with such regularity during some operations, that it should not be considered a complication, but a typical event.

The subcutaneous emphysema arising during intraperitoneal, laparoscopic operations involves the abdomen and the flanks and occasionally extends to the chest and mediastinum. In isolated cases, it can extend to the neck and face, and in some patients the eyes are swollen shut (Figure 6.5). Figure 6.6 shows a chest X-ray of a patient with fairly extensive subcutaneous emphysema. One can see the gas inclusion in subcutaneous tissue, in the structure of the pectoral muscle and in the fine line along the right border of the mediastinum. The direct and indirect pathways by which the gas spreads from the peritoneum are shown in Figure 6.7. Following hernia repair and retroperitoneal operations, the emphysema can extend to the abdomen, the flanks, scrotum and thighs. Gas can also travel through the retroperitoneal space into the mediastinum and from there into the neck and face. The anatomical structures along which it spreads are shown in Figure 6.8.

A potentially dangerous situation can arise if the emphysema affects the soft tissues of the pharynx. The swelling can be so extensive that the airway is only kept patent by the endotracheal tube and extubation would lead to acute airway obstruction and suffocation.[43] Faced with extensive cervicofacial subcutaneous emphysema, the anaesthetist should always inspect the pharynx and hypopharynx for swelling. An air leak should be heard in adults and older children after the cuff of the endotracheal tube is deflated. If

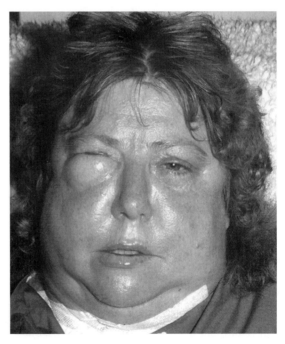

Figure 6.5 Patient with subcutaneous emphysema extending to the neck and face. If the pharynx is affected to the same degree there is a risk of airway occlusion when the endotracheal tube is removed.

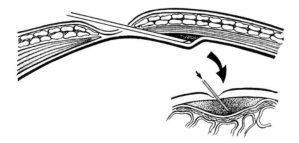

Figure 6.4 Gas is insufflated subcutaneously from a malpositioned trocar.

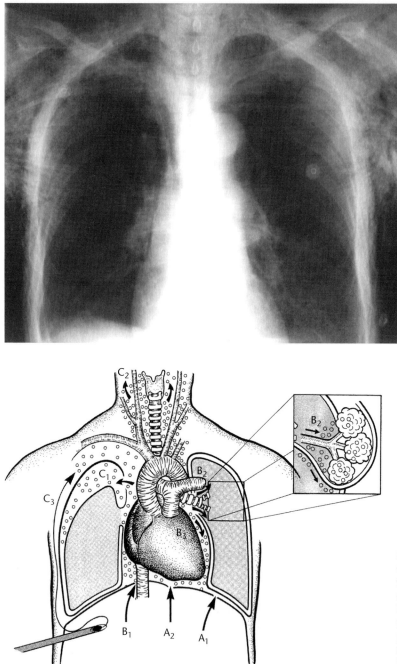

Figure 6.6 Chest X-ray of a patient with subcutaneous emphysema. Gas can be seen as darker layers in the soft tissue of the patient's right side. A pennate structure is visible on the upper chest extending towards the arms that is caused by gas in the intramuscular septa in the pectoral muscle.

Figure 6.7 Diagram of the pathways by which the gas spreads. A_1: foramen of Bochdalek; A_2: foramen of Morgagni; B_1: paraoesophageal hiatus; B_2: along the bronchi; B_3: pneumopericardium; C_1: mediastinal pleural conduits; C_2: cervical soft tissue; C_3: subcutaneously from trocar insertion site.

pharyngeal swelling prevents a free view of the glottis, and if no air flow around the endotracheal tube is detectable after deflation of the cuff, the endotracheal tube should be left in place until the swelling subsides. This usually takes about 2–5 h.

Subcutaneous emphysema alone can be a risk factor for the patient, since CO_2 absorption can rise to over 700 ml min^{-1} in patients with extensive emphysema. This is an increase of total CO_2 uptake of more than 300% over the rate in patients without emphysema. These patients require ventilatory minute volumes 30 l min^{-1} and more to maintain normocapnia. Hypercapnia has to be tolerated in some patients, since inspiratory pressures reach 50 mmHg and ventilation cannot be increased further without risk of barotrauma.[44]

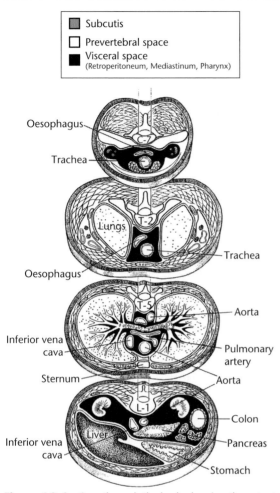

Subcutis

Prevertebral space

Visceral space
(Retroperitoneum, Mediastinum, Pharynx)

Oesophagus

Trachea

Lungs   T-2

Trachea

Oesophagus

T-5

Aorta

Inferior vena cava

Pulmonary artery

Sternum

Aorta

L-1

Colon

Inferior vena cava

Liver

Pancreas

Stomach

Figure 6.8 Sections through the body showing the extent of the retroperitoneal space.

Newer studies show that postoperative absorption of CO_2 from the emphysema is so slow that spontaneous respiration is adequate to eliminate it.[44] However, there is the risk that ventilatory reserve might be exhausted in patients with severe restrictive or obstructive lung disease, or respiratory muscle disorders. If such high-risk patients develop subcutaneous emphysema, the endotracheal tube should be left in place as a precautionary measure. The patients are allowed to breathe spontaneously, perhaps with pressure support, and the course of end-tidal CO_2 and respiratory mechanics are monitored to determine the necessity for mechanical ventilation. If the endotracheal tube has already been removed, respiration (frequency, capnometry, blood gases) must be monitored closely. The decision for reintubation and assisted ventilation (synchronized intermittent mandatory ventilation, SIMV) with pressure support, continuous positive airway pressure (CPAP) should be made liberally and early if there are signs of respiratory insufficiency or impending exhaustion. It is difficult to define a reliable limit beyond which invasive respiratory support is necessary and warranted. Maximal breathing capacity is a parameter that can help in the preoperative assessment of how likely postoperative respiratory support will be required. However, it is based on a very short measuring period, is very dependent on patient cooperation, and gives no information on how long the ventilatory effort can be sustained before the respiratory muscles are exhausted.

Pneumothorax, pneumomediastinum

Pneumothorax is not a rare occurrence following laparoscopic operations.[45–47] Gas passes from the peritoneum directly into the pleural space either through preformed channels, or it spreads from the mediastinum along the bronchi and bronchioles until it breaks through a weak spot into the thorax (Figure 6.7). Barotrauma due to excessive airway pressure with alveolar rupture and consequent pneumothorax is another possibility.

The intraoperative manifestations of a pneumothorax can be an increase in inspiratory pressure, a decrease of peripheral O_2 saturation, or even a drop in arterial pressure and a simultaneous rise of CVP with tension pneumothorax. Differentiating pneumothorax from gas embolism is crucial.[48] Breath sounds are absent or diminished on one side in pneumothorax but not in gas embolism. Postoperatively, the patients complain of dyspnoea and have asymmetrical chest excursions.

Asymptomatic pneumothorax requires no treatment, since the CO_2 is rapidly absorbed. End-expiratory pressure can be initiated or increased to counteract the compression of the lung parenchyma.[47] Pneumothorax with severe clinical symptoms calls for immediate action. The insufflated gas should be vented and if the symptoms persist, intrathoracic pressure should be relieved by drainage, perhaps with insertion of a pleural catheter. If this is adequate to relieve the symptoms, the laparoscopic operation can be continued, if not, the operation should be converted to an open procedure.

Cardiac dysrhythmias

The incidence of cardiac dysrhythmia during laparoscopic operations given in the literature ranges from 5% to 47%.[49–51] This can be a simple bradycardia or tachycardia, but life-threatening dysrhythmias such as polymorphic ventricular ectopic beats, ventricular fibrillation or primary asystole can occur. There are certain associations between the type of dyshyrthmia and its triggering factors, and each requires its own preventive measures. Bradydysrhythmia leading to asystole is the most common type of arrhythmia.[49] The underlying cause is an intense vagal stimulus such as peritoneal distension during initial insufflation or traction on the viscera. Bradydysrhythmia is also an early symptom of gas embolism.

Tachydysrhythmia and ventricular ectopic beats are normally a sign of sympathetic nervous system activation, which can be due to hypercapnia or hypoxaemia. They usually occur later in the course of the operation than vagally induced dysrhythmias. The impact of CO_2 on the incidence of dysrhythmias is illustrated by the findings that the incidence was reduced from 17% to 4% when N_2O replaced CO_2 as insufflation gas.[50] The incidence of dysrhythmias is also influenced by the choice of anaesthetic. This is illustrated nicely by the results of a study which showed that ectopic beats occurred at an $P_{et}CO_2$ of 35 mmHg under halothane, but with enflurane they did not appear until $P_{et}CO_2$ had increased to 50 mmHg.[51]

Prevention and therapy of dysrhythmias during laparoscopic operations depends on avoiding or correcting triggering factors. Pharmacological interventions follow standard therapy guidelines.

Haemorrhage

Intraoperative haemorrhage is a potentially serious complication. Massive bleeding from the cystic artery is frequently the reason for converting a laparoscopic cholecystectomy to an open procedure.[52,53] This type of arterial bleeding is obvious and rapidly detected. Less common, but more serious, are injuries to great abdominal vessels that may be inflicted with the Veress needle or the trocars at the beginning of the operation.[54] The topography of iliac vessels, aorta and vena cava favour this type of injury. Tissue can move to cover the perforation and the haemorrhage can spread imperceptibly in the retroperitoneum (Figure 6.9). The surgeon will not see any signs of bleeding, but the anaesthetist will be alerted to the problem by the developing haemodynamic instability. The surgeon should be informed if the patient exhibits signs of unexpected hypovolaemia, and should subject the abdominal cavity to a careful inspection.

Epigastric arteries can be injured during insertion of the trocar. The vessels are frequently compressed by the trocar, so that bleeding, which can be brisk, does not set in until the trocar is removed. This complication can be detected by inspecting the puncture sites before the laparoscope is removed completely.

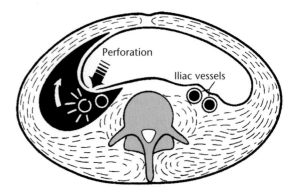

Figure 6.9 Retroperitoneal haemorrhage. The large retroperitoneal vessels (aorta, vena cava, iliac vessels) can be injured during the introduction of the Veress needle or the trocars and can cause serious bleeding. The haemorrhage can spread in the retroperitoneum without being noticed by the surgeon. The anaesthetist is often the first to detect the occult bleeding when it begins to cause circulatory symptoms.

Injury to internal organs

The intestines, stomach and urinary bladder can be injured during insertion of the Veress needle. Lifting the abdominal wall while introducing the needle will lower the risk (Figure 6.10). This complication is more likely if there are adhesions between the hollow viscera and the parietal peritoneum. A puncture of this type is unlikely to cause specific anaesthesiological problems.

Bipolar electrocoagulation is used for intraoperative haemostasis and for tissue dissection. Unipolar electrodes can cause thermal damage to intra-abdominal organs including intestinal lesions with perforations that only become apparent postoperatively.[55,56]

Perioperative peripheral neuropathy

Perioperative peripheral neuropathy is a problem of any type of surgery under anaesthesia. Precautionary measures are thought to prevent the occurrence, and this has been supported by a recent advisory even though the authors could not identify conclusive evidence of a causal relationship in every case.[57] The positions commonly used during laparoscopic operations have an inherent risk of nerve damage, particularly of the brachial plexus and sciatic nerve or peripheral nerves in the arms and legs (Table 6.4).[58-61] The steep Trendelenburg and lithotomy positions as well as abduction of the arms predispose to peripheral

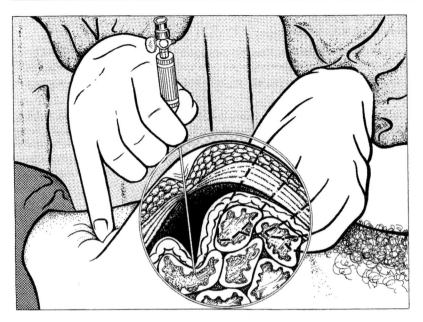

Figure 6.10 Hollow viscera can be injured by the blindly inserted Veress needle. The risk can be reduced by lifting the abdominal wall.

Table 6.4 Perioperative neuropathies typical of laparoscopic surgery

Nerve	Cause	Prevention
Brachial plexus	Pressure or tension on the plexus	Position the shoulder pads carefully, reduce abduction of the arm
Radial nerve	Pressure on the upper arm	Position arm alongside patient
Sciatic nerve	Stretching by hyperflexion	Reduce flexion of the legs in the lithotomy position
Peroneal nerve	Pressure on head of fibula	Carefully pad the knees (lithotomy position)
Obturator nerve	Surgical damage	

neuropathy. Abduction during lithotomy is worse than flexion since it puts more traction on the obturator nerve.[62]

The brachial plexus has long been known to be especially vulnerable in the steep head-down position.[63–65] Pressure from the shoulder pads that prevent the patient from sliding from the table can damage the brachial plexus. A medial position of the pads can directly injure the long thoracic nerve and parts of the plexus causing acute serratus anterior paralysis with the typical symptoms of "hod carrier's palsy" ("Steinträgerlähmung"), while pads positioned too far laterally injure a different set of nerves by compressing the plexus between the clavicle and the upper ribs causing "rucksack palsy". Fastening the patient by the wrists causes plexus damage both by costoclavicular compression and as well by traction on upper portions of the plexus.

The radial nerve can be damaged by pressure on the medial upper arm, for example from the surgeon leaning towards the patient's head for a better view of the true pelvis. The use of a video camera will remove the need of the surgeon to lean in this direction, and positioning the arms at the patient's side will avoid this type of injury altogether. Sciatic and femoral neuropathy occurs primarily in the lithotomy position. Delayed appearance of neuropathy or paralysis of the obturator nerve has been described as a complication of pelvic lymphadenectomy.[66,67]

Miscellaneous complications

Cephalad displacement of the diaphragm and intrathoracic organs under the influence of gravity and increased IAP causes a shift of the tip of the endotracheal tube relative to the trachea. This can cause a one-sided intubation with all the associated consequences.[68–74] This complication can be detected by auscultation of the lungs after the patient has been positioned and the abdomen inflated, and treated by correcting the position of the endotracheal tube. Access to the patient is nearly impossible in a number of minimally invasive procedures (see Chapter 3), and the anaesthetist should be aware of the situations, in which endobronchial intubation can occur, and know which signs should be observed with particular diligence. An unexplained fall in peripheral O_2 saturation, increase of inspiratory pressure or reduction of pulmonary compliance should be taken as signs of endobronchial intubation until proven otherwise.

Hypothermia occurs fairly frequently despite the small wound and the fact that the patient is almost completely draped and places a considerable burden on the cardiovascular system.[75,76] The main cause of hypothermia is thought to be the gas insufflation, since the temperature drop correlates with the insufflated gas volume ($-0.3°$ per 50 l gas[77]) and to a certain extent with the temperature of the insufflated gas.[78,79] Warming the insufflation gas does not prevent the drop in core temperature, but humidifying it does.[80,81] The use of heating mats and convective warming can help prevent cooling. Using suitable instruments and careful technique helps to avoid gas loss, thus reducing the volume of insufflated gas and the magnitude of heat loss.

Nausea and vomiting following laparoscopic surgery were found to be frequent in a number of studies,[82–84] but these data are not confirmed by other studies.[1] The incidence of nausea and vomiting is usually lower after a totally intravenous anaesthetic with propofol and an opiate than after inhalational anaesthesia or a balanced technique with a volatile anaesthetic,[83,85] although contradictory data have been published.[82]

Basal atelectases and pneumonia are seen in 1–2% of the patients following laparoscopic cholecystectomy. This is approximately the same incidence as seen following the open procedure.[86]

Completely covering the face during the operation predisposes the patient to mechanical damage to the eyes. The danger is enhanced if the surgeon leans on the head. An arm support will obstruct direct access to the patient's head and face, but will prevent pressure damage to the eyes (see Chapter 3). The eyes should be taped shut with non-irritating adhesive tape or protected with disposable goggles. The use of salve is not recommended since it does not offer any better protection and can cause corneal oedema and conjunctivitis.[87]

There are isolated reports that pneumoperitoneum can cause hyperkalaemia, which have been confirmed in animal studies.[88,89] It is not clear whether this occurs independently or is simply an epiphenomenon associated with the hypercapnia and respiratory acidosis frequently observed during pneumoperitoneum. It may be associated with the observation that the increase in IAP causes a reduction of diuresis and creatinine clearance that can progress to frank renal failure in isolated cases.[90–92]

The reduction of blood flow in the legs and pelvic vessels caused by the pneumoperitoneum and reverse Trendelenburg position predisposes to deep vein thrombosis.[93] Data are only available from small patient collectives,[94] but hypercoagulability is seen even after these minimally invasive operations.[95] Preventive measures such as low-dose heparin, compression stockings, or intraoperative intermittent pneumatic compression is indicated in these patients.[96]

There is a theoretical risk of intra-abdominal explosions when N_2O is used for insufflation. The dreadful name of this complication sounds as implausible as the ballistic organ syndrome,[97] but it actually has been reported. Although not combustible itself, N_2O supports combustion of methane or hydrogen, which are produced in the intestinal lumen.[98] These gases are normally not present in the peritoneum in relevant amounts, since they do not diffuse rapidly enough through the intact intestine.[99] However, their concentrations could increase significantly if the wall of the intestine were to be breached. Reports of the actual occurrence of intra-abdominal explosions seem to confirm this possibility.[100,101]

Complication spectrum of individual operations

Individual laparoscopic operations are associated with specific risks and complications (Table 6.5). Laparoscopic hernioplasty and other operations that invade the extraperitoneal space (nephrectomy, retroperitoneal adrenalectomy, retroperitoneal lymphadenectomy) have an increased risk of massive CO_2 absorption with excessive hypercapnia. The minute ventilation required to maintain normocapnia can exceed 30 l min^{-1}, and permissive hypercapnia should be considered in patients with pre-existing lung pathology.

During laparoscopic operations performed in a steep Trendelenburg position (e.g. hernioplasty, gynaecological operations, operations on rectum and sigmoid colon) the tip of the endotracheal tube can migrate to an endobronchial position and cause hypoxaemia. The lungs should be auscultated frequently to detect this, and the endotracheal tube should be retracted, if it should occur.

Table 6.5 Complications and risks of individual laparoscopic operations relevant to anaesthesia

Operation	Complications and risks
Cholecystectomy	Bleeding from the cystic artery, bile leakage
Hernioplasty	Massive CO_2 absorption, hypercapnia, facial and pharyngeal subcutaneous emphysema, endotracheal tube migration to endobronchial position causing hypoxaemia
Retroperitoneal procedures (lymphadenectomy, adrenalectomy, etc.)	Massive CO_2 absorption, hypercapnia
Gynaecological operations, rectum, sigmoid colon operations	Endotracheal tube can migrate to endobronchial position causing hypoxaemia
Adrenalectomy for hyperaldosteronism (Conn syndrome)	Hypertensive reaction to surgical stimulation, postural hypotension after positioning with legs lowered
Fundoplication	Pneumothorax, tension pneumothorax, pneumomediastinum, facial and pharyngeal subcutaneous empysema
Surgery of liver and spleen	Haemorrhage from organ or supplying vessels. Gas embolism when gas-cooled laser is used for hepatic surgery

Table 6.6 Adverse events that can necessitate terminating the laparoscopic operation

Complication	How to proceed
Gas embolism with severe circulatory symptoms	Stop insufflation, check for gas entry site, reinsert trocars, careful resumption of insufflation, convert or terminate if symptoms recur
Tension pneumothorax	Stop insufflation, ventilate with positive end-expiratory pressure, drain pleura if necessary. If the symptoms recur with insufflation convert to open procedure or continue with suction on pleural drainage
Excessive CO_2 absorption	Stop insufflation, convert to other method

Laparoscopic adrenalectomy for Conn syndrome is complicated by the arterial hypertension and relative volume depletion in these patients. Hypotension occurs due to venous pooling in the dependent legs, and adequate fluid substitution with crystalloid solutions is required. The patients have a relative fluid overload when they are returned to a level supine position and this fluid must be removed from the circulation postoperatively. Surgical stimulation can cause an exaggerated blood pressure response that frequently does not respond to deepening the anaesthetic. Beta-adrenergic blockers and nitroglycerine are effective in controlling this hypertension.

Pneumothorax and pneumomediastinum can occur during laparoscopic fundoplication. An open communication between the peritoneum and the pleural cavity compresses the lungs, but this can be compensated for by increasing end-expiratory pressure and decreasing intra-abdominal inflation pressure. Tension pneumothorax occurs when gas enters the thorax from the peritoneum by a valve mechanism. It can be severe enough to require draining. Pneumomediastinum is usually innocuous itself, but gas can pass through the mediastinum and cause facial and hypopharyngeal subcutaneous emphysema. This is also a typical complication of extraperitoneal gas insufflation during laparoscopic hernioplasty.

Surgery of the liver and spleen can cause appreciable blood loss, and haemorrhage can be so brisk as to interfere with the operation. Lasers are used for coagulation during liver surgery. Some of these are gas cooled and can cause severe gas embolism.

Criteria for aborting the laparoscopic procedure

There are a number of complications that will force the conversion to an open procedure or even require premature termination of laparoscopic operations (Table 6.6). Most of these are surgical complications and only peripherally involve the anaesthetist. Among these are haemorrhage, extensive adhesions, lack of orientation in the operation site, and damage to anatomical structures.[52,67,102–105]

The most important non-surgical complications are gas embolism, tension pneumothorax and extremely high degree of CO_2 absorption. In every case, gas insufflation has to be stopped immediately and IAP vented. This is frequently sufficient to allay the symptoms. In cases of gas embolism, insufflation can usually be carefully recommenced when the circulation is stabilized, the gas entry site has been identified and dealt with, and the trocars have been repositioned. In cases of tension pneumothorax, the most important initial measure is to relieve intrathoracic pressure. If the symptoms recede rapidly, insufflation can be re-instituted carefully. If the symptoms reappear the laparoscopic procedure has to be terminated or, if this is not possible or feasible, it can be continued after a chest tube has been placed to prevent intrathoracic pressure build-up.

Insufflation should be stopped if CO_2 absorption significantly exceeds the ventilatory capacity of the lungs to deal with it. The gas is usually absorbed from an extensive subcutaneous emphysema that normally cannot be drained. Our studies have shown that absorption decreases rapidly once insufflation has been terminated.[44] However, since it cannot be excluded that absorption will increase again once insufflation is recommenced, it is probably best to convert to an open technique, if possible, or, if not, to use a markedly reduced inflation pressure.

Contraindications

The list of contraindications for laparoscopic surgery is in continuous flux (Table 6.7). Not too long ago morbid obesity was considered an absolute contra-indication for laparoscopic procedures, since the

cardiopulmonary changes induced by the pneumoperitoneum were thought to carry too high a risk. Now they are the method of choice, even, or especially, for the extremely obese patient. It is generally recognized that while the intraoperative course might indeed be quite tempestuous, the postoperative recovery period is usually much shorter and passes with fewer complications than after conventional open procedures. Therefore, when determining if one should perform a laparoscopic operation on a patient, one must consider not only the risk of the laparoscopic operation, but also compare it to the risks associated with the conventional technique – even high risks are acceptable if the risks of the alternatives are greater. The postoperative course must be taken into consideration as well. A typical illustration of this is the divergent behaviour of intraoperative complications and postoperative advantages of laparoscopic cholecystectomy. The pneumoperitoneum and extreme reverse Trendelenburg position of the laparoscopic procedure cause considerable intraoperative cardiovascular problems, but the better postoperative pulmonary function, more rapid recovery and earlier mobilization compared with the open operation more than makes up for this.

Patients with severe cardiovascular or pulmonary diseases are commonly described in the literature as absolutely unsuited for elective laparoscopic operations. Pneumoperitoneum does increase circulatory afterload, reduce preload, and interfere with ventilation of the lungs to an extent which may exceed the adaptive capacity of these patients. But co-existing diseases of this severity are probably contraindications for any kind of elective surgery. However, one should not simply regard them as a contraindication to every vitally indicated operation, but should first

Table 6.7 Anaesthesiological contraindications for laparoscopic surgery

Condition	Assessment
Congestive heart disease (NYHA II–IV)	No contraindication for vitally indicated laparoscopic cholecystectomy or other intra-abdominal operations. Probably contraindication for laparoscopic hernia repair
Ischaemic heart disease	No contraindication for laparoscopic cholecystectomy or other intra-abdominal operations with adequate monitoring
Obstructive and restrictive pulmonary diseases	No contraindication for laparoscopic cholecystectomy or other intra-abdominal operations with low risk of excessive CO_2 absorption. Relative contraindication for laparoscopic hernia repair or other extraperitoneal operations
Morbid obesity	No contraindication for most intra-abdominal operations. Caution required for procedures in Trendelenburg position.
Pregnancy	No contraindication
Patent foramen ovale	Risk of paradoxical embolization. Relative contraindication for laparoscopic operations
Right-to-left shunt	High risk of paradoxical embolization. Contraindication for laparoscopic operations

NYHA: New York Health Association.

consider the perioperative complications and risks associated with the surgical alternatives. Studies have also shown that high-risk (American Society of Anesthesiology, (ASA) II–III) patients with predominantly congestive heart failure tolerate the circulatory load induced by the pneumoperitoneum astonishingly well[106,107] and thus should be able to undergo laparoscopic surgery with careful monitoring and management. Even patients with heart transplants tolerate laparoscopic surgery well.[108] The decision will be more difficult in patients with manifest congestive heart failure who need emergency surgery, but even in these cases there probably is no absolute contraindication for the laparoscopic technique.

An example for the opposite case is hernia repair. The conventional Lichtenstein operation for tension-free mesh repair of inguinal hernias is minimally invasive and can be performed under local anaesthesia while the laparoscopic procedure requires general anaesthesia. However, the laparoscopic approach is considered by many to offer so many advantages over the conventional operation that they outweigh the associated intraoperative risks.[109] Other studies find the exact opposite: patients in the laparoscopic operation group were discharged and returned to work earlier, but complication rates and the incidence of recurrence were higher.[110] All things considered, severe concomitant cardiopulmonary disease should be regarded as a contraindication for laparoscopic hernia repair.

Significant impairment of pulmonary function is a contraindication for all laparoscopic operations that have the risk of extensive CO_2 absorption. In these patients, ventilation can probably not be increased to the degree required to eliminate the excess CO_2 and to prevent intraoperative hypercapnia and respiratory acidosis with their associated complications. Among these are nearly all extraperitoneal procedures such as retroperitoneal lymphadenectomy, and extraperitoneal hernioplasty. The decision is more difficult in the case of hiatus hernia repair or nephrectomy, since the postoperative respiratory impairment and the incidence of pulmonary complications after conventional surgery is significant. Laparoscopic cholecystectomy is the method of choice for patients with significant respiratory disease, since functional residual capacity is less impaired and the duration of hypoxaemia is much shorter than after the open procedure.

Pregnancy is often listed as a contraindication for laparoscopic surgery. This is probably based on subconscious wariness and perhaps also on the fear of litigation should the child eventually has any sort of developmental difficulties. Nearly all reports in the literature show that laparoscopic surgery is completely uneventful during surgery if care is taken not to injure the uterus or its blood supply.[111–117] Fetal death has been reported when gas is insufflated into the uterus. Pneumoperitoneum and hypercapnia reduce uterine blood flow.[118,119] Inflation pressure should be kept to a minimum and hypercapnia should be avoided by adapting ventilation to changes in end-tidal CO_2. Although surgery is generally not advisable during pregnancy, should it become necessary all available data suggest that for most operations the laparoscopic approach has no more risk for mother and foetus than the conventional method. The choice is therefore up to the surgeon and the mother.

Morbidly obese patients have a tendency to develop hypoxaemia when breathing spontaneously in a supine position. Arterial O_2 desaturation is even observed during mechanical ventilation with 100% O_2.[120–122] The degree of hypoxaemia is increased by the pneumoperitoneum and the Trendelenburg position, but is somewhat, albeit not reliably reduced if the patient is in a head-up position as for upper abdominal procedures.[123,124] On the other hand, obese patients have a very high risk of postoperative pulmonary complications after conventional surgery, particularly upper abdominal operations.[125] This is reduced after laparoscopic surgery.[126] In view of these changes, the laparoscopic approach is definitely indicated in the morbidly obese patient for upper abdominal operations. The indication for lower abdominal and pelvic surgery is not that easy to decide and depends on the operation itself and the perioperative risks associated with the conventional technique.

Patients with a patent foramen ovale are at risk of arterial embolization with gas bubbles or debris (see above). Some authors therefore suggest avoiding laparoscopic surgery in these patients, and this caution is supported by reports of paradoxical embolism.[127] On the other hand, considering that a substantial percentage of the population actually has a patent foramen ovale, the incidence of this complication in laparoscopic surgery is rare. However, patients with an intracardiac right-to-left shunt are at a much higher risk for paradoxical embolism and should therefore be considered ineligible for laparoscopic surgery.

References

1. Rose DK, Cohen MM, Soutter DI. Laparoscopic cholecystectomy: the anaesthetist's point of view. *Can J Anaesth* 1992; **39**: 809–815.
2. Crozier TA, Luger A, Dravecz M *et al.* Gasembolie und Kreislaufstillstand bei Hysteroskopien: Fallberichte von drei Patientinnen [Gas embolism with cardiac arrest during hysteroscopy. A case report on 3 patients].

Anasthesiol Intensivmed Notfallmed Schmerzther 1991; **26**: 412–415.

3. Brundin J, Thomasson K. Cardiac gas embolism during carbon dioxide hysteroscopy: risk and management. *Eur J Obstet Gynecol Reprod Biol* 1989; **33**: 241–245.

4. Gomar C, Fernandez C, Villalonga A, Nalda MA. Carbon dioxide embolism during laparoscopy and hysteroscopy. *Ann F Anesth Reanim* 1985; **4**: 380–381.

5. Obenhaus T, Maurer W. CO2-Embolie bei Hysteroskopie [CO2 embolism during hysteroscopy]. *Anaesthesist* 1990; **39**: 243–246.

6. Wolf JS, Carrier S, Stoller ML. Gas Embolism: Helium is more lethal than carbon dioxide. *J Laparoendosc Surg* 1994; **4**: 173–177.

7. Yacoub OF, Cardona I, Coveler LA, Dodson MG. Carbon dioxide embolism during laparoscopy. *Anesthesiology* 1982; **57**: 533–535.

8. Ostman PL, Pantle-Fisher FH, Faure EA, Glosten B. Circulatory collapse during laparoscopy. *J Clin Anesth* 1990; **2**: 129–132.

9. Morison DH, Riggs JRA. Cardiovascular collapse in laparoscopy. *Can Med Assoc J* 1974; **111**: 433–437.

10. Lantz PE, Smith JD. Fatal carbon dioxide embolism complicating attempted laparoscopic cholecystectomy – case report and literature review. *J Forensic Sci* 1994; **39**: 1468–1480.

11. Kadar N. Early recourse to laparoscopy in the management of suspected ectopic pregnancy. Accuracy and morbidity. *J Reprod Med* 1990; **35**: 1153–1156.

12. Greville AC, Clements EAF, Erwin DC, McMillan DL, Wellwood JM. Pulmonary air embolism during laparoscopic laser cholecystectomy. *Anaesthesia* 1991; **46**: 113–114.

13. Beck DH, McQuillan PJ. Fatal carbon dioxide embolism and severe haemorrhage during laparoscopic salpingectomy. *Br J Anaesth* 1994; **72**: 243–245.

14. Derouin M, Couture P, Boudreault D, Girard D, Gravel D. Detection of gas embolism by transesophageal echocardiography during laparoscopic cholecystectomy. *Anesth Analg* 1996; **82**: 119–124.

15. Schmandra TC, Mierdl S, Bauer H, Gutt C, Hanisch E. Transoesophageal echocardiography shows high risk of gas embolism during laparoscopic hepatic resection under carbon dioxide pneumoperitoneum. *Br J Surg* 2002; **89**: 870–876.

16. Hall D, Goldstein A, Tynan E, Braunstein L. Profound hypercarbia late in the course of laparoscopic cholecystectomy: detection by continuous capnometry. *Anesthesiology* 1993; **79**: 173–174.

17. Root B, Levy MN, Pollack S, Lubert M, Pathak K. Gas embolism death after laparoscopy delayed by "trapping" in portal circulation. *Anesth Analg* 1978; **57**: 232–237.

18. Smith JAS. Possible venous air embolism with a new water jet dissector. *Br J Anaesth* 1993; **70**: 466–467.

19. Mastragelopulos N, Sarkar MR, Kaissling G, Bähr R, Daub D. Argongas-Embolie während laparoskopischer Cholecystektomie mit dem Argon-Beam-One-Coagulator [Argon gas embolism in laparoscopic cholecystectomy with the Argon Beam One coagulator]. *Chirurgie* 1992; **63**: 1053–1054.

20. Baggish MS, Daniell JF. Catastrophic injury secondary to the use of coaxial gas-cooled fibers and artificial sapphire tips for intrauterine surgery. *Lasers Surg Med* 1989; **9**: 581–584.

21. Steffey EP, Johnson BH, Eger EI. Nitrous oxide intensifies the pulmonary arterial pressure response to venous injection of carbon dioxide in the dog. *Anesthesiology* 1980; **52**: 52–55.

22. Munson ES, Merrick HC. Effect of nitrous oxide on venous air embolism. *Anesthesiology* 1966; **27**: 783–787.

23. Muth CM, Shank ES. Gas embolism. *N Engl J Med* 2000; **342**: 476–482.

24. Fahy BG, Hasnain JU, Flowers JL, Plotkin JS, Odonkor P, Ferguson MK. Transesophageal echocardiographic detection of gas embolism and cardiac valvular dysfunction during laparoscopic nephrectomy. *Anesth Analg* 1999; **88**: 500–504.

25. Couture P, Boudreault D, Derouin M *et al*. Venous carbon dioxide embolism in pigs: An evaluation of end-tidal carbon dioixde, transesophageal echocardiography, pulmonary artery pressure, and precordial auscultation as monitoring modalities. *Anesth Analg* 1994; **79**: 867–873.

26. Bednarz F, Roewer N. Intraoperativer Nachweis von Luftembolien und korpuskulären Embolien mit Hilfe der Pulsoximetrie und Kapnometrie: Vergleichende Untersuchung mit der transösophagealen Echokardiographie [Intraoperative detection of air embolism and corpuscular embolism using pulse oximetry and capnometry. Comparative studies with transesophageal echocardiography]. *Anasth Intensivther Notfallmed* 1989; **24**: 20–26.

27. Schwerzmann M, Seiler C, Lipp E *et al*. Relation between directly detected patent foramen ovale and ischemic brain lesions in sport divers. *Ann Intern Med* 2001; **134**: 21–24.

28. McGrath BJ, Zimmerman JE, Williams JF, Parmet J. Carbon dioxide embolism treated with hyperbaric oxygen. *Can J Anaesth* 1989; **36**: 586–589.

29. Knauth M, Ries S, Pohimann S *et al*. Cohort study of multiple brain lesions in sport divers: role of a patent foramen ovale. *Br Med J* 1997; **314**: 701–705.

30. Agostoni P, Gasparini G, Destro G. Acute myocardial infarction probably caused by paradoxical embolus in a pregnant woman. *Heart* 2004; **90**: e12.

31. Still JA, Lederman DS, Renn WH. Pulmonary edema following air embolism. *Anesthesiology* 1974; **40**: 194–196.

32. Chandler WF, Dimshell DG, Taren JA. Acute pulmonary edema following venous air embolism during a neurosurgical procedure. *J Neurosurg* 1974; **40**: 400–404.

33. Desai S, Roaf E, Liu P. Acute pulmonary edema during laparoscopy. *Anesth Analg* 1982; **61**: 699–700.

34. Nossum V, Hjelde A, Brubakk AO. Small amounts of venous gas embolism cause delayed impairment of endothelial function and increase polymorphonuclear neutrophil infiltration. *Eur J Appl Physiol* 2002; **86**: 209–214.

35. Clark MC, Flick MR. Permeability edema caused by venous air embolism. *Am Rev Resp Dis* 1984; **129**: 633–635.

36. Flick MR, Porel A, staub NC. Leukocytes are required for increased lung microvascular permeability after microembolization in sheep. *Circ Res* 1981; **48**: 344–351.

37. Durant TM, Oppenheimer MJ, Lynch PR, Ascanio G, Webber D. Body position in relation to venous air embolism: A roentgenologic study. *Am J Med Sci* 1954; **227**: 269–281.

38. Mehlhorn U, Burke EJ, Butler BD *et al*. Body position does not affect the hemodynamic response to venous air embolism in dogs. *Anesth Analg* 1994; **79**: 734–739.

39. Alvaran SB, Toung JK, Graff TE, Benson DW. Venous air embolism: comparative merits of external cardiac massage, intracardiac aspiration, and left lateral decubitus position. *Anesth Analg* 1978; **57**: 166–170.

40. Artru AA. Placement of a multiorificed catheter in the inferior portion of the right atrium; percentage of gas retrieved and success rate of resuscitation after venous air embolism in prone dogs positioned with the abdomen hanging freely. *Anesth Analg* 1994; **79**: 740–744.

41. Colley PS, Artru AA. Bunegin-Albin catheter improves air retrieval and resuscitation from lethal venous air embolism in upright dogs. *Anesth Analg* 1989; **68**: 298–301.

42. Benson J, Adkinson C, Collier R. Hyperbaric oxygen therapy of iatrogenic cerebral arterial gas embolism. *Undersea Hyperb Med* 2003; **30**: 117–126.

43. Chien GL, Soifer BE. Pharyngeal emphysema with airway obstruction as a consequence of laparoscopic inguinal herniorrhaphy. *Anesth Analg* 1995; **80**: 201–203.

44. Sumpf E, Crozier TA, Ahrens D, Brauer A, Neufang T, Braun U. Carbon dioxide absorption during extraperitoneal and transperitoneal endoscopic hernioplasty. *Anesth Analg* 2000; **91**: 589–595.

45. Chui PT, Gin T, Chung SC. Subcutaneous emphysema, pneumomediastinum and pneumothorax complicating laparoscopic vagotomy. Report of two cases. *Anaesthesia* 1993; **48**: 978–981.

46. Mangar D, Kirchhoff GT, Leal JJ, Laborde R, Fu E. Pneumothorax during laparoscopic Nissen fundoplication. *Can J Anaesth* 1994; **41**: 854–856.

47. Joris JL, Chiche JD, Lamy ML. Pneumothorax during laparoscopic fundoplication: diagnosis and treatment with positive end-expiratory pressure. *Anesth Analg* 1995; **81**: 993–1000.

48. Carrero Cardenal EJ. Differentiating massive carbon dioxide embolism from tension pneumothorax during laparoscopic cholecystectomy. *Eur J Anaesthesiol* 2002; **19**: 459–460.

49. Myles PS. Bradyarrhythmias and laparoscopy: a prospective study of heart rate changes with laparoscopy. *Aust NZ J Obstet Gynaecol* 1991; **31**: 171–173.

50. Scott DB, Julian DG. Observations on cardiac arrhythmias during laparoscopy. *Br Med J* 1972; **12**: 411–413.

51. Harris MN, Plantevin OM, Crowther A. Cardiac arrhythmias during anaesthesia for laparoscopy. *Br J Anaesth* 1984; **56**: 1213–1217.

52. Perissat J. Laparoscopic cholecystectomy: the European experience. *Am J Surg* 1993; **165**: 444–449.

53. Smith JF, Boysen D, Tschirhart J, Williams T, Vasilenko P. Comparison of laparoscopic cholecystectomy versus elective open cholecystectomy. *J Laparoendosc Surg* 1992; **2**: 311–317.

54. Apelgren KN, Scheeres DE. Aortic injury. A catastrophic complication of laparoscopic cholecystectomy. *Surg Endosc* 1994; **8**: 689–691.

55. Burmucic R. Späte Symptomatik einer Darmverbrennung nach laparoskopischer Tubensterilisation. [Late manifestation of a burn of intestine caused by laparoscopic tubal sterilization]. *Wien Med Wochenschr* 1979; **129**: 157–158.

56. Peterson HB, Ory HW, Greenspan JR, Tyler Jr CW. Deaths associated with laparoscopic sterilization by unipolar electrocoagulating devices, 1978 and 1979. *Am J Obstet Gynecol* 1981; **139**: 141–143.

57. Task Force on Prevention of Perioperative Peripheral Neuropathies. Practice advisory for the prevention of perioperative peripheral neuropathies: a report by the American Society of Anesthesiologists Task Force on Prevention of Perioperative Peripheral Neuropathies. *Anesthesiology* 2000; **92**: 1168–1182.

58. Nicholson MJ, McAlpine FS. Neural injuries associated with surgical positions and operations. In: Martin JT (Ed.), *Positioning in Anesthesia and Surgery*. Philadelphia: W.B. Saunders, 1978; pp. 193–224.

59. Stöhr M. Nervenläsionen in Narkose. In: *Iatrogene Nervenläsionen*. Stuttgart: Georg Thieme Verlag, 1980; pp. 146–159.

60. Lachman E, Rosenberg P, Gino G, Levine S, Goldberg S, Borstein M. Axonal damage to the left musculocutaneous nerve of the left biceps muscle during laparoscopic surgery. *J Am Assoc Gynecol Laparosc* 2001; **8**: 453–455.

61. Ullrich W, Biermann E, Kienzle F, Krier C. Lagerungsschäden in Anästhesie und operativer Medizin (Teil 1) [Damage due to patient positioning in anesthesia and surgical medicine (Part 1)]. *Anasthesiol Intensivmed Notfallmed Schmerzther* 1997; **32**: 4–20.

62. Litwiller JP, Wells Jr RE, Halliwill JR, Carmichael SW, Warner MA. Effect of lithotomy positions on strain of the obturator and lateral femoral cutaneous nerves. *Clin Anat* 2004; **17**: 45–49.

63. Pommerenke WT, Ristern WA. The scalenus anticus syndrome as a complication after gynecologic operations. *Am J Obstet Gynecol* 1944; **47**: 395–399.

64. Clausen EG. Postoperative ("anesthetic") paralysis of the brachial plexus. A review of the literature and report of nine cases. *Surgery* 1942; **12**: 933–942.

65. Mitterschiffthaler G, Theiner A, Posch G, Jäger-Lackner E, Fuith LC. Läsion des Plexus brachialis, verursacht durch fehlerhafte Operationslagerungen [Lesion of the brachial plexus, caused by wrong positioning during surgery]. *Anasth Intensivther Notfallmed* 1987; **22**: 177–180.

66. Fishman JR, Moran ME, Carey RW. Obturator neuropathy after laparoscopic pelvic lymphadenectomy. *Urology* 1993; **42**: 198–200.

67. Kavoussi LR, Sosa E, Chandhoke P *et al*. Complications of laparoscopic pelvic lymph node dissection. *J Urol* 1993; **149**: 322–325.

68. Brimacombe JR, Orland H, Graham D. Endobronchial intubation during upper abdominal laparoscopic surgery

in the reverse Trendelenburg position. *Anesth Analg* 1994; **78**: 607.

69. Hamm P, Lang C, Fornecker ML, Bruant P, Vuillemin F. Intubation bronchique sélective à répétition au cours d'une cholécystectomie coelioscopique [Recurrent selective bronchial intubation in laparoscopic cholecystectomy]. *Ann Fr Anesth Reanim* 1993; **12**: 67–69.

70. Heinonen J, Takki S, Tammisto T. Effect of Trendelenburg tilt and other procedures on the position of endotracheal tubes. *Lancet* 1969; **1**: 850–853.

71. Morimura N, Inoue K, Miwa T. Chest roentgenogram demonstrates cephalad movement of the carina during laparoscopic cholecystectomy. *Anesthesiology* 1994; **81**: 1301–1302.

72. Wilcox S, Vanddam LD. Alas, poor Trendelenburg and his position! A critique of its uses and its effectiveness. *Anesth Analg* 1988; **67**: 574–578.

73. Lobato EB, Paige GB, Brown MM, Bennett B, Davis JD. Pneumoperitoneum as a risk factor for endobronchial intubation during laparoscopic gynecologic surgery. *Anesth Analg* 1998; **86**: 301–303.

74. Mendonca C, Baguley I, Kuipers AJ, King D, Lam FY. Movement of the endotracheal tube during laparoscopic hernia repair. *Acta Anaesthesiol Scand* 2000; **44**: 517–519.

75. Frank SM, Higgins MS, Breslow MJ *et al.* The catecholamine, cortisol, and hemodynamic responses to mild perioperative hypothermia. *Anesthesiology* 1995; **82**: 83–93.

76. Frank SM, Beattie C, Christopherson R *et al.* Unintentional hypothermia is associated with postoperative myocardial ischemia. The Perioperative Ischemia Randomized Anesthesia Trial Study Group. *Anesthesiology* 1993; **78**: 468–476.

77. Ott DE. Laparoscopic hypothermia. *J Laparoendosc Surg* 1991; **1**: 127–131.

78. Ott DE. Correction of laparoscopic insufflation hypothermia. *J Laparoendosc Surg* 1991; **1**: 183–186.

79. Bäcklund M, Kellokumpu I, Scheinin T, von Smitten K, Lindgren L. Warm CO_2 insufflation for laparoscopic surgery. *Eur J Anaesthesiol* 1996; **13**: 159.

80. Bessell JR, Ludbrook G, Millard SH, Baxter PS, Ubhi SS, Maddern GJ. Humidified gas prevents hypothermia induced by laparoscopic insufflation: a randomized controlled study in a pig model. *Surg Endosc* 1999; **13**: 101–105.

81. Nelskyla K, Yli-Hankala A, Sjoberg J, Korhonen I, Korttila K. Warming of insufflation gas during laparoscopic hysterectomy: effect on body temperature and the autonomic nervous system. *Acta Anaesthesiol Scand* 1999; **43**: 974–978.

82. Blobner M, Schneck HJ, Felber AR, Goegler S, Feussner H, Jelen-Esselborn S. Vergleichende Untersuchungen der Aufwachphase: Laparoskopische Cholezystektomie nach Isofluran-, Methohexital- und Propofolanästhesie [Comparative study of the recovery phase. Laparoscopic cholecystectomy following isoflurane, methohexital and propofol anesthesia]. *Anaesthesist* 1994; **43**: 573–581.

83. Klockgether-Radke A, Piorek V, Crozier TA, Kettler D. Nausea and vomiting after laparoscopic surgery. A comparison of propofol and thiopentone/halothane anaesthesia. *Eur J Anaesthesiol* 1996; **13**: 3–9.

84. Hovorka J, Korttila K, Erkola O. Nitrous oxide does increase nausea and vomiting following gynaecological laparoscopy. *Can J Anaesth* 1989; **36**: 145–148.

85. Raftery S, Sherry E. Total intravenous anaesthesia with propofol and alfentanil protects against postoperative nausea and vomiting. *Can J Anaesth* 1992; **39**: 37–40.

86. Williams Jr LF, Chapman WC, Bonau RA, McGee Jr EC, Boyd RW, Jacobs JK. Comparison of laparoscopic cholecystectomy with open cholecystectomy in a single center. *Am J Surg* 1993; **165**: 459–465.

87. Bronheim D, Abel M, Neustein S. Corneal abrasions following non-ophthalmic surgery: A retrospective review of 35,253 general anesthetics. *Anesthesiology* 1995; **83(Suppl)**: A1071.

88. Pearson MRB, Sander ML. Hyperkalaemia associated with prolonged insufflation of carbon dioxide into the peritoneal cavity. *Br J Anaesth* 1994; **72**: 602–604.

89. Hassan H, Gjessing J, Tomlin PJ. Hypercapnia, hyperkalaemia. *Anaesthesia* 1979; **34**: 897–899.

90. Hashikura Y, Kawasaki S, Munakata Y, Hashimoto S, Hayashi K, Makuuchi M. Effects of peritoneal insufflation on hepatic and renal blood flow. *Surg Endosc* 1994; **8**: 759–761.

91. Kubota K, Kajiura N, Teruya M *et al.* Alterations in respiratory function and hemodynamics during laparoscopic cholecystectomy under pneumoperitoneum. *Surg Endosc* 1993; **7**: 500–504.

92. Richards WO, Scovill W, Shin B, Reed W. Acute renal failure associated with increased intra-abdominal pressure. *Ann Surg* 1983; **197**: 183–187.

93. Beebe DS, McNevin MP, Crain JM *et al.* Evidence of venous stasis after abdominal insufflation for laparoscopic cholecystectomy. *Surg Gynecol Obstet* 1993; **176**: 443–447.

94. Mayol J, Vincent Hamelin E, Sarmiento JM *et al.* Pulmonary embolism following laparoscopic cholecystectomy: report of two cases and review of the literature. *Surg Endosc* 1994; **8**: 214–217.

95. Caprini JA, Arcelus JI, Laubach M *et al.* Postoperative hypercoagulability and deep-vein thrombosis after laparoscopic cholecystectomy. *Surg Endosc* 1995; **9**: 304–309.

96. Millard JA, Hill BB, Cook PS, Fenoglio ME, Stahlgren LH. Intermittent sequential pneumatic compression in prevention of venous stasis associated with pneumoperitoneum during laparoscopic cholecystectomy. *Arch Surg* 1993; **128**: 914–918.

97. Barry M. The ballistic organ syndrome. In: Vandermeer J, Roberts M (Eds), *The Thackery T Lambshead Pocket Guide to Eccentric and Discredited Diseases*, 83rd edition. San Francisco: Night Shade Books, 2003.

98. Neuman GG, Sidebotham G, Negolanu E *et al.* Laparoscopy explosion hazards with nitrous oxide. *Anesthesiology* 1993; **78**: 875–879.

99. Hunter JG, Staheli J, Oddsdottir M, Trus T. Nitrous oxide pneumoperitoneum revisited. Is there a risk of combustion? *Surg Endosc* 1995; **9**: 501–504.

100. Drummond GB, Scott DB. Laparoscopy explosion hazards with nitrous oxide. *Br Med J* 1976; **1**: 586.

101. El-Kady AA, Abd-El-Razek M. Intraperitoneal explosion during female sterilization by laparoscopic electrocoagulation. *Int J Gynaecol Obstet* 1976; **14**: 487–488.

102. Lee VS, Chari RS, Cucchiaro G, Meyers WC. Complications of laparoscopic cholecystectomy. *Am J Surg* 1993; **165**: 527–532.

103. Siewert JR, Feussner H, Scherer MA, Brune IB. Fehler und Gefahren der laparoskopischen Cholecystektomie [Errors and danger in laparoscopic cholecystectomy]. *Chirurg* 1993; **64**: 221–229.

104. Wolfe BM, Gardiner BN, Leary BF, Frey CF. Endoscopic cholecystectomy. An analysis of complications. *Arch Surg* 1991; **126**: 1192–1196.

105. Tabboush ZS. When hypotension during laparoscopic cholecystectomy indicates termination of the laparoscopy. *Anesth Analg* 1994; **79**: 195–196.

106. Safran D, Sgambati S, Orlando III R. Laparoscopy in high-risk cardiac patients. *Surg Gynec Obstet* 1993; **176**: 548–554.

107. Zollinger A, Krayer S, Singer T *et al.* Haemodynamic effects of pneumoperitoneum in elderly patients with an increased cardiac risk. *Eur J Anaesth* 1997; **14**: 266–275.

108. Joshi GP, Hein HA, Ramsay MA, Foreman ML. Hemodynamic response to anesthesia and pneumoperitoneum in orthotopic cardiac transplant recipients. *Anesthesiology* 1996; **85**: 929–933.

109. Memon MA, Cooper NJ, Memon B, Memon MI, Abrams KR. Meta-analysis of randomized clinical trials comparing open and laparoscopic inguinal hernia repair. *Br J Surg* 2003; **90**: 1479–1492.

110. Neumayer L, Giobbie-Hurder A, Jonasson O *et al.* Open mesh versus laparoscopic mesh repair of inguinal hernia. *N Engl J Med* 2004; **350**: 1819–1827.

111. Elerding SC. Laparoscopic cholecystectomy in pregnancy. *Am J Surg* 1993; **165**: 625–627.

112. Schorr RT. Laparoscopic cholecystectomy and pregnancy. *J Laparoendosc Surg* 1993; **3**: 291–293.

113. Rizzo AG. Laparoscopic surgery in pregnancy: long-term follow-up. *J Laparoendosc Adv Surg Tech A* 2003; **13**: 11–15.

114. Oelsner G, Stockheim D, Soriano D *et al.* Pregnancy outcome after laparoscopy or laparotomy in pregnancy. *J Am Assoc Gynecol Laparosc* 2003; **10**: 200–204.

115. Al-Fozan H, Tulandi T. Safety and risks of laparoscopy in pregnancy. *Curr Opin Obstet Gynecol* 2002; **14**: 375–379.

116. Reedy MB, Kallen B, Kuehl TJ. Laparoscopy during pregnancy: a study of five fetal outcome parameters with use of the Swedish Health Registry. *Am J Obstet Gynecol* 1997; **177**: 673–679.

117. Curet MJ, Allen D, Josloff RK *et al.* Laparoscopy during pregnancy. *Arch Surg* 1996; **131**: 546–550.

118. Walker AM, Oakes GK, Ehrenkranz R, McLaughlin M, Chez RA. Effects of hypercapnia on uterine and umbilical circulations in conscious pregnant sheep. *J Appl Physiol* 1976; **41**: 727–733.

119. Southerland LC, Cruz AM, Duke T, Ferguson JG, Crone LA. Intraabdominal CO_2-insufflation in the pregnant ewe: uterine blood flow, intraamniotic pressure and cardiopulmonary effects. *Can J Anaesth* 1995; **42(Suppl)**: A21A.

120. Santesson J. Oxygen transport and venous admixture in the extremely obese. Influence of anaesthesia and artificial ventilation with and without positive endexpiratory pressure. *Acta Anaesthesiol Scand* 1976; **20**: 387–392.

121. Hedenstierna G, Santesson J, Norlander O. Airway closure and distribution of inspired gas in the extremely obese, breathing spontaneously and during anaesthesia with intermittent positive pressure ventilation. *Acta Anaesthesiol Scand* 1976; **20**: 334–342.

122. Peters J, Steinhoff H. Anaesthesieprobleme bei extremer Fettsucht [Anaesthesiological problems in extreme adipositas]. *Anaesthesist* 1983; **32**: 324–327.

123. Vaughan RW, Bauer S, Wise L. Effect of position (semirecumbent versus supine) on postoperative oxygenation in markedly obese patients. *Anesth Analg* 1976; **55**: 37–40.

124. Casati A, Comotti L, Tommasino C *et al.* Effects of pneumoperitoneum and reverse Trendelenburg position on cardiopulmonary function in morbidly obese patients receiving laparoscopic gastric banding. *Eur J Anaesthesiol* 2000; **17**: 300–305.

125. Eichenberger A, Proietti S, Wicky S *et al.* Morbid obesity and postoperative pulmonary atelectasis: an underestimated problem. *Anesth Analg* 2002; **95**: 1788–1792.

126. Nguyen NT, Lee SL, Goldman C *et al.* Comparison of pulmonary function and postoperative pain after laparoscopic versus open gastric bypass: a randomized trial. *J Am Coll Surg* 2001; **192**: 469–476.

127. Uchida S, Yamamoto M, Masaoka Y, Mikouchi H, Nishizaki Y. A case of acute pulmonary embolism and acute myocardial infarction with suspected paradoxical embolism after laparoscopic surgery. *Heart Vessels* 1999; **14**: 197–200.

Patterns and mechanism of post-laparoscopy pain

The majority of laparoscopic operations are performed as short-stay or even day-care surgery. Although pain is less severe and of shorter duration than following open procedures (Table 7.1), it can still be sufficiently intense to prevent early discharge. The pain after laparoscopic surgery has a spatial distribution and character that is so unique that it is often referred to as the "post-laparoscopic pain syndrome".[1,2] Pain arises from the trocar insertion sites, the intra-abdominal trauma and also from the rapid distension of the peritoneum with traumatic traction on blood vessels and nerves, irritation of the phrenic nerve and release of inflammatory mediators (see reviews in Refs [3,4]). The pain presents as parietal pain in the insertion sites, visceral pain from the intra-abdominal wound and the irritated peritoneum, and pain referred to the shoulder tip, a characteristic feature, or to the back. Post-laparoscopic pain is most frequently located in the upper abdomen, independent of the intra-abdominal localization of the operation site.

Pain tops the list of complaints following laparoscopic surgery, with up to 96% of the patients complaining of postoperative pain (Table 7.1). It is most intense immediately after the operation, but decreases rapidly. In one study, the patients quantified the initial intensity as 60 on a 100 point visual analogue scale (VAS),[5] but it had decreased under therapy to approximately 30 VAS points within 2 h. This is equivalent to a verbal pain score of 2–2.5 on a six-point scale (see Table 7.2). Women consistently reported more intense pain than

men.[6] In a survey of patients in our institution, the median pain score was 8 VAS points (range 0–64) immediately after laparoscopic cholecystectomy under total intravenous anaesthesia with propofol–alfentanil and diclofenac as prophylactic analgesic. The pain had decreased to 0 VAS points (range 0–26) at the end of the 10-h postoperative observation period (unpublished data). In all published studies, pain decreased to below 15 VAS points by the third postoperative day (Figure 7.1). Joris and co-workers described the discordant temporal behaviour of the various types of pain following laparoscopic cholecystectomy.[7] Visceral pain was predominant during the first 24 h, but this abated and was superseded in significance by shoulder pain on the following day.

Pain localized in the tip of the shoulder, usually on the right side, and the back are typical for laparoscopy. This is accompanied by visceral upper abdominal pain,

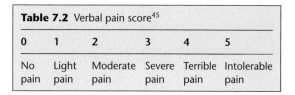

Table 7.2 Verbal pain score[45]

0	1	2	3	4	5
No pain	Light pain	Moderate pain	Severe pain	Terrible pain	Intolerable pain

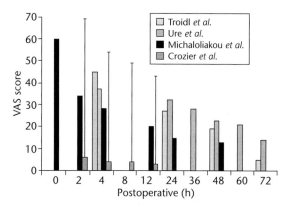

Figure 7.1 Time course of pain intensity after laparoscopic surgery. Mean VAS scores reported in different studies are shown. The differences between the various studies reflect the choice of anaesthetic, postoperative pain therapy and differing assessment times.

Table 7.1 Incidence of moderate to severe postoperative pain after laparoscopic surgery

Author	Operation	Incidence (%)
Crozier[a]	Cholecystectomy	76
Ure[6]	Cholecystectomy	95
Götz[44]	Appendectomy	87
Pier[8]	Cholecystectomy	95
Michaloliakou[5]	Cholecystectomy	96

[a]unpublished date.

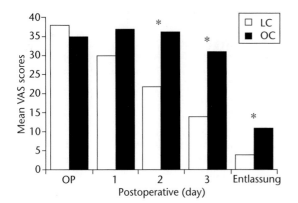

Figure 7.2 Time course of pain intensity after laparoscopic and open cholecystectomy (LC and OC, respectively). Mean values of VAS scores are shown (VAS scores) (*$P < 0.01$).[6]

Table 7.3 Studies on pain intensity and analgesic requirements after cholecystectomies and appendectomies performed either with the laparoscopic or the conventional open technique

Author	Pain intensity	Analgesic requirements
Laparoscopic cholecystectomy (LA)		
Attwood[46]	LC < OC	nd
Barkun[47]	LC ≈ OC	LC < OC
Kunz[48]	LC < OC	LC ≈ OC
Putensen-Himmer[49]	LC ≈ OC	LC < OC
Rademaker[50]	LC ≈ OC	LC ≈ OC
Ure[6]	LC < OC	LC < OC
Laparoscopic appendectomy (LC)		
Attwood[51]	LA < OA	nd
Lejus[52]	LA ≈ OA	LA ≈ OA
McAnena[53]	nd	LA < OA
Ure[54]	LA ≈ OA	LA ≈ OA

OC: open cholecystectomy; OA: open appendectomy; L < O: laparoscopic procedure superior to open procedure; ≈: no difference detectable between the two techniques; nd: no data.

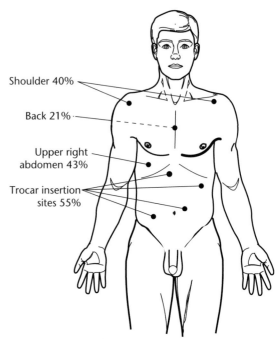

Figure 7.3 Localization of post-laparoscopy pain.

the intensity of which can exceed that of the surgical wound. In a prospective study, about half of the patients reported pain in the trocar insertion sites, usually in the navel, 43% had pain in the upper right abdomen, 40% described pain in the shoulders and about 20% complained of pain in the back. The incidence of shoulder and upper abdominal pain can, however, amount to over 80% (Figure 7.3) and is largely independent of the type of laparoscopic operation. The incidence is similar after cholecystectomy, appendectomy and gynaecological operations.[8–10] The intensity of this pain reaches its maximum on the first or second postoperative day. The severest pain is localized in the upper right abdomen, followed by the trocar insertion

sites, and the intraperitoneal wound (46% and 36% of patients, respectively; see Figure 7.4). Although most patients have back and shoulder pain, only few (2% and 4%, respectively) describe this as severe.

The pathogenesis of the characteristic post-laparoscopic pain syndrome has not been entirely explained. Its localization in the shoulder and upper abdominal areas suggest subdiaphragmatic, peritoneal irritation. There is evidence that the insufflation gas is responsible for the irritation, since insufflation with carbon dioxide produces more severe intraoperative and immediate postoperative pain in awake patients than, for example, nitrous oxide.[11] Only 8% of the patients operated with a gasless abdominal wall lift device complained of postoperative shoulder pain compared with 46% with pneumoperitoneum.[12]

A subphrenic gas bubble, detectable in over 90% of patients and persisting at least 48 h after deflation of the pneumoperitoneum, is thought to contribute to the typical upper abdominal and shoulder pain.[1,2,13,14] Active aspiration of the residual gas at the end of the operation reduces postoperative pain.[14] One popular hypothesis is that the retained carbon dioxide causes a local acidosis in the peritoneal lining which induces pain. In a prospective, randomized study, however, no difference was found between insufflation with carbon dioxide as opposed to argon with regard to the development of post-laparoscopic pain syndrome,[1]

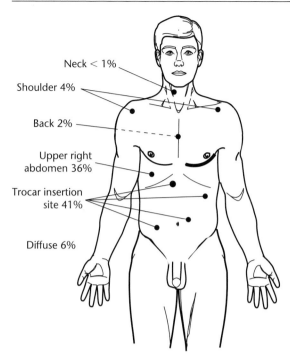

Neck < 1%

Shoulder 4%

Back 2%

Upper right
abdomen 36%

Trocar insertion
site 41%

Diffuse 6%

Figure 7.4 Localization of the severest post-laparoscopy pain.[6]

but on the other hand, no difference was found in intra-abdominal pH values.

Pain relief

The majority of patients require an analgesic after laparoscopic surgery.[5,6] Opioids are effective in reducing post-laparoscopic pain, but the adverse effects, such as nausea, vomiting and sedation, associated with their use can delay patient mobilization and discharge from the post-anaesthetic care unit and from the hospital. Other approaches have therefore been evaluated to provide adequate pain relief in patients undergoing laparoscopic surgery. Among these are instillation of local anaesthetics into the abdominal cavity, topical application of local anaesthetics directly under the diaphragm, infiltration of the incision sites and the prophylactic administration of non-opioid analgesics.

The typical localization of post-laparoscopy pain in the right upper abdomen, regardless of the site of the intra-abdominal wound, and the projection of pain to the associated head zone in the shoulder, fostered the assumption that peritoneal irritation was the initiating event, and prompted treatment with intraperitoneal local anaesthetics. A number of studies have been reported, but their results are conflicting. The most positive effects were seen following diagnostic

laparoscopy or laparoscopic pelvic surgery. Narchi and colleagues report that 80 ml of either 0.5% lidocaine or 0.125% bupivacaine instilled into the abdomen reduced analgesic requirements and the severity of shoulder pain but not abdominal pain.[15] Similar results were reported by Loughney[16] and Helvacioglu.[17] Some authors reported that intraperitoneal instillation of local anaesthetics was ineffective after laparoscopic cholecystectomy,[7,18,19] but they did not report if the patients had been tilted head-down to bathe the upper peritoneum. Schulte-Steinberg and co-workers found no effect of 20 ml bupivacaine 0.25% i.p. but a significant reduction of global postoperative pain by the interpleural injection of 30 ml bupivacaine 0.25%.[20] On the other hand, Labaille and co-workers demonstrated that intraperitoneal ropivacaine (20 ml of a 0.25% solution) significantly reduced visceral pain and morphine consumption.[21] Chundrigar and colleagues also reported significant pain relief following laparoscopic cholecystectomy when 20 ml bupivacaine 0.25% were applied directly to the gall bladder bed.[22]

Non-steroidal anti-inflammatory drugs (NSAID) have been used in the treatment of post-laparoscopy pain under the assumption that peritoneal inflammation and prostaglandin synthesis are major determinants of pain. Numerous studies have been published comparing a wide variety of substances against placebo as well as against one another. Most studies demonstrated that NSAID were effective in reducing post-laparoscopy pain[23–26] but some studies were unable to demonstrate more effect of the NSAID over placebo. In most of these, pain levels were lower in the treatment group, but the calculated P values were greater than 0.05, indicating that the sample size might have been too small,[27,28] or that the study design was faulty. The study drug was frequently given too late to have developed its full effect by the time postoperative pain was assessed. Newer cyclo-oxygenase 2 (Cox-2) inhibitors have been shown to be effective in reducing post-laparoscopy pain,[26] but their relative efficacy is questioned.[29] The topical application of NSAID might even be effective, since the use of a piroxicam patch was shown to alleviate the shoulder pain of laparoscopic surgery.[30]

Although NSAID provide at least a certain degree of pain relief following laparoscopic procedures, some authors warn against their use, since as potent inhibitors of prostacyclin synthesis they can reduce renal blood flow, which is already compromised by the increased abdominal pressure, and ultimately precipitate renal failure.[31] Ketorolac is reported to be particularly dangerous in this respect.[32] In fact, ketorolac has been taken off the market in some countries because of the incidence and severity of its adverse effects.

Impairment of renal function is much less likely with the use of acetaminophen (paracetamol) or metamizol (dipyrone). Acetaminophen has been shown to significantly reduce opioid requirements after laparoscopic sterilization.[33] One gram of intravenous acetaminophen was shown to have an analgesic effect equal to that of 10 mg morphine.[34] Metamizol was taken off the market in a number of countries, because of an assumed link to blood disorders, such as agranulocytosis. It has since been relicenced in most of Europe, South America and other countries. Its efficacy for the treatment of acute postoperative pain is well documented.[35] Both of these substances are thought to modulate pain perception by acting on Cox-3 species in the central nervous system,[36,37] and not to affect the constitutive prostagladin synthesis responsible for maintaining renal perfusion and gastric mucosal protection. These substances also interact with spinal and supraspinal serotonergic mechanisms to produce their antinociceptive effects.[38,39] Studies have shown that these Cox-3 inhibitors and classic NSAID act synergistically in reducing acute postoperative pain.[40,41]

Intravenous opioids are, of course, effective in the treatment of post-laparoscopy pain and are the mainstay of rescue analgesia for break-through postoperative pain. Oral oxycodone 10 mg given 1 h before surgery was shown to effectively reduce postoperative pain and analgesic requirements.[42] Intrathecal morphine reduced postoperative morphine consumption following laparoscopic colorectal surgery.[43]

It was shown that the postoperative pain following laparoscopic–endoscopic operations could be treated effectively with non-steroid antiphlogistics, especially if these were administered in time – that is, optimally before the operation.[5,24] This also reflects the results of a randomized, controlled study in our institution (Crozier, unpublished data).

We studied postoperative analgesic requirements following laparoscopic cholecystectomy. The patients were given rectal diclofenac (100 mg) after induction of anaesthesia, and were allowed to self-administer an opioid (piritramide) with a patient-controlled analgesia pump in the postoperative period. The average piritramide dose during the first 10 postoperative hours was 22 mg (equivalent to 15 mg morphine).

The pain caused by laparoscopy and laparoscopic surgery is less severe than that after laparotomy, but can still be quite distressing. The multifactorial genesis of post-laparoscopic pain requires a multimodal approach for effective pain relief.[5] NSAID and other non-opioid analgesics reduce the intensity of postoperative pain, but are usually inadequate as the sole analgesic, and

none of them are very effective for treating referred pain the shoulder and back. The intraperitoneal instillation of local anaesthetics can also be employed for pain reduction in the immediate postoperative period, but prolonged use would require the placement of a subdiaphragmatic catheter. Infiltrating the trocar insertion sites with local anaesthetic affords effective pain relief for a few hours.

Based on these insights, the most efficient pain therapy would consist of the preoperative, prophylactic administration of a non-opioid analgesic, perhaps a combination of an NSAID with a centrally acting Cox-3 inhibitor, the preoperative infiltration of the skin incision sites with a local anaesthetic, the instillation of a local anaesthetic into the upper abdomen prior to abdominal closure and the postoperative supplementary administration of an opioid as rescue medication.

Note   Protocol for postoperative pain relief after laparoscopic surgery:

- Preoperative administration of a non-opioid analgesic (e.g. NSAID, acetaminophen)
- Pre-incisional infiltration of trocar insertion sites with local anaesthetic (e.g. bupivacaine 0.25%)
- Intraperitoneal instillation of local anaesthetic solution before removing trocars (e.g. 40 ml bupivacaine 0.25%, lidocaine 0.5% or ropivacaine 0.25%)
- Rescue medication with small doses of an opioid (e.g. morphine)
- Treat postoperative shivering with clonidine or meperidine[55]

References

1. Pier A, Benedic M, Mann B, Buck V. Das postlaparoskopische Schmerzsyndrom. Ergebnisse einer prospektiven, randomisierten Studie [Postlaparoscopic pain syndrome. Results of a prospective, randomized study]. *Chirurg* 1994; **65**: 200–208.
2. Riedel HH, Semm K. Das postpelviskopische-(laparoskopische) Schmerzsyndrom [The post-laparoscopic pain syndrome]. *Geburtsh Frauenheilk* 1980; **40**: 635–643.
3. Schoeffler P, Diemunsch P, Fourgeaud L. Coelisoscopie ambulatoire. *Cah Anesthesiol* 1993; **41**: 385–391.
4. Alexander JI. Pain after laparoscopy. *Br J Anaesth* 1997; **79**: 369–378.
5. Michaloliakou C, Chung F, Sharma S. Preoperative multimodal analgesia facilitates recovery after ambulatory laparoscopic cholecystectomy. *Anesth Analg* 1996; **82**: 44–51.
6. Ure BM, Troidl H, Spangenberger W, Dietrich A, Lefering R, Neugebauer E. Pain after laparoscopic

cholecystectomy. Intensity and localization of pain and analysis of predictors in preoperative symptoms and intraoperative events. *Surg Endosc* 1994; **8**: 90–96.

7. Joris J, Thiry E, Paris P, Weerts J, Lamy M. Pain after laparoscopic cholecystectomy: characteristics and effect of intraperitoneal bupivacaine. *Anesth Analg* 1995; **81**: 379–384.

8. Pier A, Thevissen P, Ablaßmaier B. Die Technik der laparoskopischen Cholecystektomie. Erfahrungen und Ergebnisse bei 200 Eingriffen. *Chirurg* 1991; **62**: 323–331.

9. Riedel HH, Brosche T, Fielitz J, Lehmann Willenbrock E, Semm K. Die Entwicklung der gynäkologischen Endoskopie in Deutschland – eine statistische Erhebung der Jahre 1989 bis 1993. *Zentralbl Gynakol* 1995; **117**: 402–412.

10. Smith I, Ding Y, White PF. Muscle pain after outpatient laparoscopy – influence of propofol versus thiopental and enflurane. *Anesth Analg* 1993; **76**: 1181–1184.

11. Kröhl R. Vergleichende Füllung des Pneumoperitoneums mit CO_2 und N_2O [Comparison of CO_2 and N_2O for abdominal inflation]. In: Ottenjann R (Ed.), *Fortschr Endoskop*. Stuttgart: Schattauer, 1969; pp. 247–250.

12. Lindgren L, Koivusalo A-M, Kellokumpu I. Conventional pneumoperitoneum compared with abdominal wall lift for laparoscopic cholecystectomy. *Br J Anaesth* 1995; **75**: 567–572.

13. Stanley IR, Laurence AS, Hill JC. Disappearance of intraperitoneal gas following gynaecological laparoscopy. *Anaesthesia* 2002; **57**: 57–61.

14. Fredman B, Jedeikin R, Olsfanger D, Flor P, Gruzman A. Residual pneumoperitoneum: a cause of postoperative pain after laparoscopic cholecystectomy. *Anesth Analg* 1994; **79**: 152–154.

15. Narchi P, Benhamou D, Fernandez H. Intraperitoneal local anaesthetic for shoulder pain after day-case laparoscopy. *Lancet* 1991; **338**: 1569–1570.

16. Loughney AD, Sarma V, Ryall EA. Intraperitoneal bupivacaine for the relief of pain following day case laparoscopy. *Br J Obstet Gynaecol* 1994; **101**: 449–451.

17. Helvacioglu A, Weis R. Operative laparoscopy and postoperative pain relief. *Fertil Steril* 1992; **57**: 548–552.

18. Rademaker BMP, Kalkman CJ, Odoom JA, De Wit L, Ringers J. Intraperitoneal local anaesthetics after laparoscopic cholecystectomy: effects on postoperative pain, metabolic responses and lung function. *Br J Anaesth* 1994; **72**: 263–266.

19. Scheinin B, Kellokumpu I, Lindgren L, Haglund C, Rosenburg PH. Effect of intraperitoneal bupivacaine on pain after laparoscopic cholecystectomy. *Acta Anaesthesiol Scand* 1995; **39**: 195–198.

20. Schulte-Steinberg H, Weninger E, Jokisch D *et al*. Intraperitoneal versus interpleural morphine or bupivacaine for pain after laparoscopic cholecystectomy. *Anesthesiology* 1995; **82**: 634–640.

21. Labaille T, Mazoit JX, Paqueron X, Franco D, Benhamou D. The clinical efficacy and pharmacokinetics of intraperitoneal ropivacaine for laparoscopic cholecystectomy. *Anesth Analg* 2002; **94**: 100–105.

22. Chundrigar T, Morris R, Hedges AR, Stamatakis JD. Intraperitoneal bupivacaine for effective pain relief after laparoscopic cholecystectomy. *Ann R Coll Surg Engl* 1993; **75**: 437–439.

23. Huang KC, Wolfe WM, Tsueda K, Simpson PM, Caissie KF. Effects of meclofenamate and acetaminophen on abdominal pain following tubal occlusion. *Am J Obstet Gynecol* 1986; **155**: 624–629.

24. Liu J, Ding Y, White PF, Feinstein R, Shear JM. Effects of ketorolac on postoperative analgesia and ventilatory function after laparoscopic cholecystectomy. *Anesth Analg* 1993; **76**: 1061–1066.

25. Gillberg LE, Harsten AS, Stahl LB. Preoperative diclofenac sodium reduces postlaparoscopy pain. *Can J Anaesth* 1993; **40**: 406–408.

26. Meyer R. Rofecoxib reduces perioperative morphine consumption for abdominal hysterectomy and laparoscopic gastric banding. *Anaesth Intensive Care* 2002; **30**: 389–390.

27. Shapiro MH, Duffy BL. Intramuscular ketorolac for postoperative analgesia following laparoscopic sterilisation. *Anaesth Intensive Care* 1994; **22**: 22–24.

28. Crocker S, Paech MJ. Preoperative rectal indomethacin for analgesia after laparoscopic sterilisation. *Anaesth Intensive Care* 1992; **20**: 337–340.

29. Ng A, Temple A, Smith G, Emembolu J. Early analgesic effects of parecoxib versus ketorolac following laparoscopic sterilization: a randomized controlled trial. *Br J Anaesth* 2004; **92**: 846–849.

30. Hong JY, Lee IH. Suprascapular nerve block or a piroxicam patch for shoulder tip pain after day case laparoscopic surgery. *Eur J Anaesthesiol* 2003; **20**: 234–238.

31. Koivusalo AM, Lindgren L. Effects of carbon dioxide pneumoperitoneum for laparoscopic cholecystectomy. *Acta Anaesthesiol Scand* 2000; **44**: 834–841.

32. Gillis JC, Brogden RN. Ketorolac. A reappraisal of its pharmacodynamic and pharmacokinetic properties and therapeutic use in pain management. *Drugs* 1997; **53**: 139–188.

33. Hahn TW, Mogensen T, Lund C *et al*. Analgesic effect of i.v. paracetamol: possible ceiling effect of paracetamol in postoperative pain. *Acta Anaesthesiol Scand* 2003; **47**: 138–145.

34. Van Aken H, Thys L, Veekman L, Buerkle H. Assessing analgesia in single and repeated administrations of propacetamol for postoperative pain: comparison with morphine after dental surgery. *Anesth Analg* 2004; **98**: 159–165.

35. Edwards JE, Meseguer F, Faura CC, Moore RA, McQuay HJ. Single-dose dipyrone for acute postoperative pain. *Cochrane Database Syst Rev* 2001; **3**: CD003227.

36. Chandrasekharan NV, Dai H, Roos KL *et al*. COX-3, a cyclooxygenase-1 variant inhibited by acetaminophen and other analgesic/antipyretic drugs: cloning, structure, and expression. *Proc Natl Acad Sci USA* 2002; **99**: 13926–13931.

37. Schwab JM, Schluesener HJ, Meyermann R, Serhan CN. COX-3 the enzyme and the concept: steps towards highly specialized pathways and precision therapeutics? *Prostaglandins Leukot Essent Fatty Acids* 2003; **69**: 339–343.

38. Bonnefont J, Courade JP, Alloui A, Eschalier A. Mecanisme de l'action antinociceptive du paracetamol. [Antinociceptive mechanism of action of paracetamol]. *Drugs* 2003; **63(Spec No 2)**: 1–4.

39. Courade JP, Chassaing C, Bardin L, Alloui A, Eschalier A. 5-HT receptor subtypes involved in the spinal antinociceptive effect of acetaminophen in rats. *Eur J Pharmacol* 2001; **432**: 1–7.

40. Beck DH, Schenk MR, Hagemann K, Doepfner UR, Kox WJ. The pharmacokinetics and analgesic efficacy of larger dose rectal acetaminophen (40 mg/kg) in adults: a double-blinded, randomized study. *Anesth Analg* 2000; **90**: 431–436.

41. Montgomery JE, Sutherland CJ, Kestin IG, Sneyd JR. Morphine consumption in patients receiving rectal paracetamol and diclofenac alone and in combination. *Br J Anaesth* 1996; **77**: 445–447.

42. Reuben SS, Steinberg RB, Maciolek H, Joshi W. Preoperative administration of controlled-release oxycodone for the management of pain after ambulatory laparoscopic tubal ligation surgery. *J Clin Anesth* 2002; **14**: 223–227.

43. Kong SK, Onsiong SM, Chiu WK, Li MK. Use of intrathecal morphine for postoperative pain relief after elective laparoscopic colorectal surgery. *Anaesthesia* 2002; **57**: 1168–1173.

44. Götz F, Pier A, Bacher C. Die laparoskopische Appendektomie – Alternativtherapie in allen Appendizitisstadien? [Laparoscopic appendectomy – alternative therapy in all stages of appendicitis?]. *Langenbecks Arch Chir* Supp II *Verh Dtsch Ges Chir*; 1351–1353.

45. Huskisson EC. Measurement of pain. *Lancet* 1974; **II**: 1127–1131.

46. Attwood SE, Hill AD, Mealy K, Stephens RB. A prospective comparison of laparoscopic versus open cholecystectomy. *Ann R Coll Surg Engl* 1992; **74**: 397–400.

47. Barkun JS, Barkun AN, Sampalis JS *et al.* Randomized controlled trial of laparoscopic versus mini cholecystectomy. The McGill Gallstone Treatment Group. *Lancet* 1992; **340**: 1116–1119.

48. Kunz R, Orth K, Vogel J *et al.* Laparoskopische Cholezystektomie versus Mini-Lap-Cholezystektomie. Ergebnisse einer prospektiven, randomisierten Studie. *Chirurg* 1992; **63**: 291–295.

49. Putensen-Himmer G, Putensen C, Lammer H, Lingau W, Aigner F, Benzer H. Comparison of postoperative respiratory function after laparoscopy or open laparotomy for cholecystectomy. *Anesthesiology* 1992; **77**: 675–680.

50. Rademaker BM, Ringers J, Odoom JA, de-Wit LT, Kalkman CJ, Oosting J. Pulmonary function and stress response after laparoscopic cholecystectomy: comparison with subcostal incision and influence of thoracic epidural analgesia. *Anesth Analg* 1992; **75**: 381–385.

51. Attwood SEA, Hill ADK, Murphy PG, Thornton J, Stephans RB. A prospective randomized trial of laparoscopic versus open appendectomy. *Surgery* 1992; **112**: 497–501.

52. Lejus C, Plattner V, Baron M, Guillou S, Héloury Y, Souron R. Randomized, single-blinded trial of laparoscopic versus open appendectomy in children. *Anesthesiology* 1996; **84**: 801–806.

53. McAnena OJ, Austin O, O'Connel PR, Hedermann WP, Gorey TF, Fitzpatrick J. Laparoscopic versus open appendectomy: a prospective evaluation. *Br J Surg* 1992; **79**: 818–820.

54. Ure BM, Spangenberger W, Hebebrand D, Eypasch EP, Troidl H. Laparoscopic surgery in children and adolescents with suspected appendicitis: results of medical technology assessment. *Eur J Pediat Surg* 1992; **2**: 336–340.

55. Kranke P, Eberhardt L, Roewer N, Tramer M. Single-dose parenteral pharmacological interventions for the prevention of postoperative shivering – a quantitative systematic review of randomized controlled trials. *Eur J Anaesthesiol* 2004; **21(Suppl 32)**: A37.

LAPAROSCOPIC BARIATRIC SURGERY

8

Bariatrics is the branch of medicine that deals with obese patients and their problems, but mainly with their weight itself. The term bariatics comes from the Greek βαρνσ (barys) meaning "heavy" and a derivative of the word ιατρεια (iatreia) which means "healing", as in paediatrics and geriatrics.

Morbid obesity used to be a typical relative contraindication for laparoscopic surgery. Now it is an indication of its own. The intention of bariatric surgery is to enable morbidly obese patients to lose weight that they are unable to lose by conservative means. The procedures used in bariatric surgery are not simple weight reduction methods, such as liposuction, that work by directly removing excess fatty tissue. Bariatric surgery takes a more complex approach that modifies the gastrointestinal system in such a manner as to make it almost impossible for the patient to maintain his or her weight at a high level. Weight reduction surgery has been performed since the 1960s as a measure of last resort to enable morbidly obese patients to lose weight. Conventional surgery in these patients is fraught with a wide array of potentially lethal complications ranging from pulmonary embolism and pneumonia to poor wound healing and wound infection. Laparoscopic techniques are the obvious solution to these problems and have been used in bariatric surgery since 1993.[1,2] The intraoperative course can be turbulent during laparoscopic procedures, but recovery is more rapid with fewer complications. Virtually all bariatric operations, even the technically most sophisticated, are now being performed laparoscopically.[3–6] The very indication for bariatric surgery is a prime cause of typical anaesthesiological problems and complications, which the anaesthetist has to anticipate and ultimately deal with in this type of laparoscopic surgery.

The term obesity comes from the Latin word *obesitas* that ultimately derives from the verb *obedere*, which means, "to eat away (and get fat)". It is a condition characterized by an excessive accumulation of body fat. There is no natural dividing line between obesity and normal weight and no obvious way to grade the condition, so that any classification will be arbitrary to a certain degree. An operative definition of obesity states that an individual should be considered obese when the amount of fat tissue is "increased to such an extent that physical and mental health are affected and life expectancy is reduced".[7] But, while the economic, social or psychological impact of excess adipose tissue varies widely between individuals, epidemiological studies and actuary tables of life insurance companies can give accurate estimates of its effects on morbidity and mortality, and have led to generally accepted classification systems.

There are two measures commonly used to quantify the degree of obesity. One is based on the concept of an ideal body weight (IBW), which is derived from actuary tables that give the body weight associated with the lowest overall mortality rate for a given height and gender. IBW is calculated with the following formula:

Male: IBW (kg) = height (cm) -100
Female: IBW (kg) = height (cm) -105

Long-term studies have shown that men whose weight was 100–109% of IBW had the lowest mortality rates.

The second, more widely used measure was originally described by Quetelet, a Belgian mathematician, in 1835 and is now known as the body mass index (BMI).[9] This is calculated using the following formula:

$$BMI = \frac{\text{weight (kg)}}{\text{height (m)}^2} \text{ in kg m}^{-2}$$

where normal range is 18–25 kg m^{-2}.
A person with a BMI of 25–30 kg m^{-2} is considered to be overweight, while a BMI over 30 kg m^{-2} defines obesity.[10] Above this level, the nomenclature becomes confusing, since different groups apply the same term to different cut-off points.[11] Most studies define morbid obesity as a BMI over 35 kg m^{-2}, but the limit is sometimes set at 40 kg m^{-2}. This, of course, makes it difficult to compare epidemiological surveys. A BMI over 40 kg m^{-2} is occasionally referred to as severe obesity, and one over 55 kg m^{-2} as super-morbid obesity. For comparison, the BMI of a person 170 cm tall with an ideal weight of 70 kg would be 24 kg m^{-2}.

Prevalence of obesity

Obesity has a high prevalence in most of Europe and North America, and this has been increasing steadily over the past decades.[12] The present incidence of obesity (BMI over $30 \, kg \, m^{-2}$) in the USA is between 20.9% and 30.5% depending on the survey, with the incidence of persons with a BMI over $40 \, kg \, m^{-2}$ between 2.3% and 4.7%.[13,14] This represents an increase of 74% since 1991.

The incidence of obesity in Europe exhibits marked geographical variations. In the UK in 1998, 17.3% of the men and 21.2% of the women had a BMI of more than $30 \, kg \, m^{-2}$, and 0.6% of the men and 1.9% of the women were classified as morbidly obese (BMI $> 40 \, kg \, m^{-2}$).[15] The incidence of obesity varies even within a country and between genders. In 1991, 24.5% of the female residents of former Eastern Germany were obese as opposed to 18% of Western German men.[16] The prevalence of obesity in men of both sections of the country increased during the following 10 years. During this period, the prevalence of obesity amongst West German women increased by 6.4%, while there was a 6.3% decrease in the eastern half of the country. In comparison, in 1991, only 7.0% of French women and 6.5% of French men were obese.[17] In 2000, the percentage of the adult French population with a BMI of more than $30 \, kg \, m^{-2}$ had increased to 8.2%.[18]

Obesity has an enormous impact on public health, since morbidity and mortality are greatly increased in persons with a BMI over $30 \, kg \, m^{-2}$ (Table 8.1).[10,19,20] A person with a BMI over 30 has a 50% higher risk of death than a person with normal body weight, while the risk is doubled in a person with a BMI over 35.[21] Some studies also show an increased risk of death in underweight persons.[22] In 2000, obesity accounted for nearly as many preventable deaths as tobacco smoking in the USA; 18.1% of all deaths were attributed to smoking and 16.6% to the effects of obesity.[23] In comparison,

only 3.5% of all deaths were caused by alcohol. It is likely that obesity has now passed tobacco smoking as the main ultimate cause of death in the USA.

Other terms such as severe obesity or super-morbid obesity are not unanimously defined, but generally refer to a BMI of more than $40-50 \, kg \, m^{-2}$.

Surgery is recommended in patients with a BMI over 40, or over 35 if life-threatening co-morbidity is present. To give an idea of what we are talking about: a 165-cm-tall patient with a BMI of $40 \, kg \, m^{-2}$ will weigh 108 kg (5 ft 6 in. tall and 17 stones).

Obesity predisposes to a wide variety of associated diseases and disease conditions. The most common of these are type II diabetes mellitus, ischaemic heart disease, peripheral vascular disease, heart failure, hypertension, dyslipidaemia, obstructive sleep apnoea syndrome (OSAS) and cancer (Table 8.2).[24-29] The relative risk ranges from about three for myocardial infarction and cancer of the colon up to about eight for diabetes mellitus. These risks are reversible after the patient loses weight.[30,31] Aside from these organic diseases, obesity also impinges on economic and social aspects of the individual's life.

In the UK, reports commissioned by the National Health Services (NHS) and the National Institute for Clinical Excellence (NICE) have demonstrated the cost effectiveness of bariatric surgery,[32,33] showing that it not only brings an increase in the quality-adjusted life years for the individual patient, but that it also reduces the societal costs of the co-morbidities of obesity. This insight led to the recommendation that this treatment modality be offered to persons suffering from morbid obesity as an aid to weight loss.[34,35] A similar American study also found that providing bariatric surgery to select patient populations was less costly than financing the health costs of the co-morbidities and was less expensive in the long run than medical weight reduction programmes.[36]

The generally accepted guidelines on the eligibility of patients for bariatric surgery define the weight-related indication for bariatric surgery as a BMI over $40 \, kg \, m^{-2}$

Table 8.1 Grading of obesity and its associated health risk		
Classification	**BMI** $(kg \, m^{-2})$	**Risk of early death**
Underweight	<18	Moderate
Normal weight	18–25	Lowest
Mild overweight	25–30	Moderate
Obese	>30	Significantly increased
Morbid obesity	>35 (40)	Very high

Table 8.2 Co-morbidity of obesity

- Diabetes mellitus type II
- Ischaemic heart disease
- Cancer
- Hypertension
- OSAS
- Peripheral vascular disease
- Psychosocial impairment
- Osteoarthrosis
- Heart failure

(over $35\,kg\,m^{-2}$, in patients with life-threatening co-morbidities) and failure to lose more than 5–10% of excess weight by supervised weight-loss diets, or weight gain after an initial loss. Further criteria are current intensive management in a specialized hospital obesity clinic, an age of 18 years or over, no general contraindications for anaesthesia or surgery, no specific clinical or psychological contraindications for this particular type of surgery and willingness to participate in long-term follow-up.[34,37] Patients with behavioural abnormalities, such as significant psychiatric disease (e.g. schizophrenia), mental retardation, substance abuse, self-destructive behaviour, etc., are excluded from bariatric surgery by the National Institute of Health (NIH) guidelines on the grounds that these abnormalities would probably prevent the patients from complying with the postoperative counselling necessary to obtain the greatest benefit from the operation.

The very nature of the patient selection criteria for bariatric surgical interventions defines the co-morbidity and perioperative complications with which the anaesthetist will be dealing in the management of these patients. Well-founded knowledge is required regarding the physiological changes of metabolism and drug disposition resulting from excessive body weight, the concomitant pathophysiology of the respiratory and cardiovascular systems, and their responses to increased intra-abdominal pressure (IAP) and extreme surgical positions, and the typical, but serious, postoperative complications in order to provide these patients with the best possible care.

Physiology of obesity

Respiratory system

Obesity has profound effects on the respiratory system. Functional residual capacity (FRC) decreases with increasing BMI, falling from approximately 1.5–2.5 l at a BMI of 20–25 $kg\,m^{-2}$ to 0.3–0.7 l at a BMI of 40–50 $kg\,m^{-2}$.[38] Expiratory reserve volume and total lung capacity are also decreased.[39] FRC is reduced to an extent that it falls below closing capacity (CC) leading to small airway closure, ventilation–perfusion mismatch, right-to-left shunting and arterial hypoxaemia even in the awake patient.[40–42] Intrapulmonary shunt was found to be 10–25% in the obese as compared to 2–5% in lean control persons.[43] The morphological correlate of this functional pattern is the significantly greater extent of atelectasis seen in thoracic computed tomography (CT) scans in spontaneously breathing, awake obese individuals (Figure 8.1).[44]

Obesity reduces the compliance and increases the resistance of the total respiratory system.[38] The chest

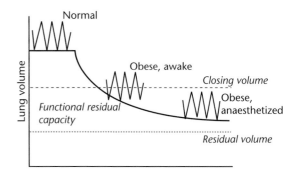

Figure 8.1 The effect of obesity on FRC. Closure of some small airways occurs at the end of expiration. This increases venous admixture and $AaDO_2$ and causes hypoxaemia. This change is aggravated by induction of general anaesthesia.

wall contributes only slightly to the changes of compliance and airway resistance caused by increasing body weight. The decrease of lung compliance is due in part to the increased pulmonary blood volume,[45,46] and partly due to the reduction of FRC with a shift of the neutral position to a flatter portion of the pressure–volume curve.[38]

The extent of the atelectatic areas seen in the CT scans increases after induction of anaesthesia in spontaneously breathing as well as mechanically ventilated patients,[47,48] but this increase is much greater in obese patients (BMI $> 35\,kg\,m^{-2}$) than in non-obese patients (BMI $< 30\,kg\,m^{-2}$). The area of roentgenologically detectable atelectasis increases from 2.1% preoperatively to 7.6% at the end of laparoscopic surgery in the obese vs. from 1.0% to 2.8%, respectively, in the non-obese patients.[44] These areas resolve completely within 24 h in lean patients, but still remain or even increase (to 9.7%) in the obese. The result of this along with the reduced FRC is that obese patients have a larger alveolar–arterial oxygen (O_2) gradient than patients with a normal BMI.[38,49] At an inspired O_2 concentration of 50%, the alveolar–arterial O_2 difference ($AaDO_2$) is 66 mmHg in non-obese patients, while it averages 160 mmHg in the morbidly obese (BMI $> 46\,kg\,m^{-2}$).

O_2 consumption and carbon dioxide (CO_2) production are increased in the obese individual due to the metabolic activity of the additional tissue and the increased workload.[45,50] However, the arterial–venous CO_2 difference is normal and the metabolic activity related to body surface area is within normal limits. Increased CO_2 production requires an increase in alveolar minute ventilation in order to maintain normocapnia. This puts an additional strain on the respiratory system and increases the O_2 cost of breathing.

OSAS occurs more frequently in obese persons.[28] A long-term consequence of OSAS is the obesity hypoventilation syndrome, an alteration in the control of breathing characterized by central apnoeic events with an increased reliance on hypoxic drive for ventilation. The end stage of this is the Pickwickian syndrome with hypersomnolence, hypoxaemia, hypercapnia, increased pulmonary artery pressure and right ventricular failure.[51] Weight reduction after bariatric surgery has been shown to improve the sleep apnoea index and arterial blood gases, and to reduce the need for supplemental O_2.[31]

Anaesthesia and pneumoperitoneum further aggravate the poor respiratory situation of the obese patient. Induction of anaesthesia reduces FRC by 50% in the obese patient as opposed to only 20% in the non-obese.[52,53] The increased IAP during pneumoperitoneum reduces FRC still further.[49] After insufflation, body position (Trendelenburg or reverse Trendelenburg) has no significant effect on respiratory mechanics or FRC (Table 8.3).[49,54] Some authors recommend ventilation with tidal volumes up to $20\,ml\,kg^{-1}$ as a method of counteracting the fall in FRC and the subsequent widening of the $AaDO_2$,[55,56] but others have shown this to be ineffective or even detrimental.[57,58] Positive end-expiratory pressure (PEEP) ventilation can increase FRC, reduce $AaDO_2$ and improve oxygenation in obese patients.[59,60] An end-expiratory pressure of $10\text{--}12\,cmH_2O$ is commonly used, but one study showed that a PEEP of $15\,cmH_2O$ increased partial pressure of O_2 in arterial blood (P_aO_2) by *ca.* 50% from 14.0 to 21.5 kPa ($F_IO_2 = 0.5$) and reduced the intrapulmonary shunt fraction from 21% to 13%.[61] At the same time, cardiac output (CO) fell by 20% from 5.5 to $4.4\,l\,min^{-1}$ so that the net effect was a reduction of O_2 delivery, since haemoglobin O_2 saturation, the primary determinant of blood O_2 content was not altered by the increase in P_aO_2. It is, therefore, important to determine the PEEP level that optimizes pulmonary mechanics without impairing CO and O_2 delivery, and to keep haemoglobin O_2 saturation at 98% or above by adjusting the inspired O_2 concentration.

Table 8.3 Respiratory effects of obesity

- Hypoxaemia
- Reduced FRC
- Ventilation–perfusion mismatch
- Reduced lung compliance
- OSAS
- Obesity hypoventilation syndrome
- Increased minute ventilation (O_2 consumption and CO_2 production increased)

Obese patients require a larger minute ventilation to maintain normocapnia[49] due to their greater CO_2 production.

Cardiovascular system

Cardiovascular disorders are common in the obese population and are a leading cause of morbidity and mortality. In one survey, 37% of the adult population with a BMI over $30\,kg\,m^{-2}$ also suffered from a cardiovascular disease, while the prevalence was only 10% in persons with a BMI under $25\,kg\,m^{-2}$.[62] Hypertension is very common in the obese. Factors contributing to this are sodium retention with expansion of extracellular and intravascular volumes, increase in CO, and the enhancement of the pressor activity of catecholamines and angiotensin II and central sympathetic nervous system stimulation by the adipocyte-derived protein leptin.[63–66] Total blood volume is increased, but the weight-adjusted volume is lower than in lean individuals ($50\,ml\,kg^{-1}$ in obese vs. $75\,ml\,kg^{-1}$ in non-obese).[67] CO increases to meet the demands of increased O_2 consumption by increasing stroke volume with a constant ejection fraction. This, combined with the increased afterload of hypertension, results in eccentric left ventricular hypertrophy: the ventricle becomes less compliant and end-diastolic pressure rises.[68]

Obesity is an independent risk factor for ischaemic heart disease and sudden death, and co-existing hypertension, diabetes mellitus and dyslipidaemia will compound this problem.[25,69,70] The concentration of high-density lipoprotein (HDL) cholesterol is decreased, while that of low- and very low-density lipoproteins (LDL and VLDL) is increased. Despite this, 40% of the patients with symptoms of angina do not have demonstrable coronary artery stenosis on catheterization.[62] Cardiac dysrhythmias are common in obese patients, and are the results of increased autonomic stimulation as well as pathological changes in the cardiac conduction system.[69,71,72] The condition can be aggravated by the hypoxaemia, hypercapnia and myocardial hypertrophy frequently present in obesity.

Obese patients frequently suffer from an impairment of cardiac function commonly referred to as "obesity-related cardiomyopathy" (Table 8.4). The earlier conception that this was a consequence of a fatty infiltration of the myocardium has been refuted. The sequence of events leading to cardiac dysfunction and, eventually, manifest heart failure are thought to begin with the increased stroke volume being pumped against an elevated afterload. End-diastolic volume increases and the ensuing increased wall tension induces eccentric left ventricular hypertrophy. The increased wall thickness of the dilated ventricle is less compliant and causes impaired diastolic function, increased left ventricular end-diastolic pressure (LVEDP), and insipient interstitial pulmonary oedema.[68,73–75] This backward failure of the left ventricle tends to chronically elevate pulmonary capillary occlusion pressure, which, together with the increased pulmonary vascular resistance resulting from hypoxic pulmonary vasoconstriction, subjects the right ventricle to an increased workload. The simple change from a sitting to a supine position increases venous return, left ventricular filling and CO, but also causes a simultaneous, significant rise in pulmonary capillary occlusion pressure and mean pulmonary artery pressure[76] which can precipitate paroxysmal dyspnoea and pulmonary oedema. These patients tolerate rapid increases of intravascular volume only very poorly. Figure 8.2 gives a summary of the events leading to "obesity-related cardiomyopathy" and cardiac failure.

Table 8.4 Cardiovascular effects of obesity

- Intravascular volume increased
- CO increased
- Systemic and pulmonary hypertension
- Left and right ventricular hypertrophy
- Obesity-related cardiomyopathy
- Reduced exercise tolerance
- Ischaemic heart disease
- Sudden death

Drug distribution and disposition in obesity

Obesity is associated with a number of changes that will have an impact on the distribution, protein binding, metabolism and renal elimination of drugs.[77] A fundamental question in anaesthesia for obese patients is therefore which drugs are least affected by these changes, and which body weight – ideal, lean or actual – should be used when calculating the required dose of intravenous drugs. It is difficult to anticipate the net effect of these changes, and monitoring clinical end points is more important than blindly following calculated doses. However, a number of approximations can be made that will help one make a rough estimate of the required dose. An overview of the factors affecting drug disposition is given in Table 8.5.

The volume of distribution is an important factor when calculating drug dosages. Factors that will affect this are the increase in adipose tissue, increased lean body mass (LBM), increased intravascular volume with a reduction of total body water, altered protein binding and increased CO. The central volume of distribution (V_{Dc}), which for practical purposes can be considered identical with intravascular volume, is a determinant of the initially required dose. The absolute value of intravascular volume increases with body weight, but to a lesser extent than weight itself.[79] Therefore, initial doses should be calculated on the basis of IBW or, more accurately, of LBM.[80,81]

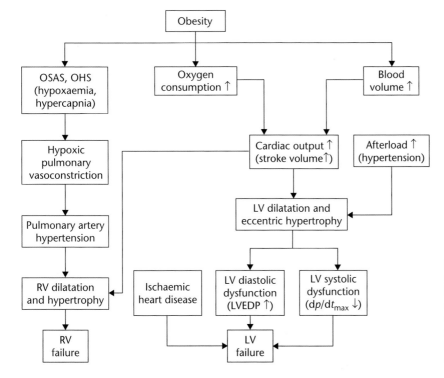

Figure 8.2 Pathogenesis of obesity-related cardiomyopathy and cardiac failure. OHS: obesity hypoventilation syndrome; LV: left ventricle; RV: right ventricle; dp/dt_{max}: measure of inotropy; ↑: increase; ↓: decrease.

Table 8.5 The effect of obesity on determinants of pharmacokinetics

Absorption	Oral drugs $\leftrightarrow$
	Unpredictable after intramuscular or subcutaneous administration
Distribution	
Body composition	Adipose and lean tissue $\uparrow$; V_D of lipophilic drugs $\uparrow$
	Blood volume $\uparrow$; V_D of hydrophilic drugs slightly $\uparrow$
Protein binding	Total protein, albumin $\leftrightarrow$; free fraction of acidic drugs $\leftrightarrow$
	Triglycerides, cholesterol, lipoproteins, free fatty acids $\uparrow$ causing displacement of acidic drugs and thus raising free fraction $\uparrow$[78]
	α1-acid glycoprotein $\uparrow$; free fraction of basic drugs $\downarrow$
Elimination	
Metabolism	Splanchnic blood flow $\uparrow$
	Phase I reactions $\leftrightarrow\uparrow$; Phase II reactions $\uparrow$ despite histological and laboratory evidence of hepatic damage
	Data on drugs with high extraction rate are conflicting, but reduction of CO and hepatic blood flow will have large impact on their elimination
Excretion	Renal blood flow, GFR, tubular secretion $\uparrow$; renal clearance $\uparrow$

$\uparrow$ increased; $\downarrow$: decreased; $\leftrightarrow$: unchanged. V_D: volume of distribution; GFR: glomerular filtration rate.

Table 8.6 How to dose intravenous anaesthetics in obese patients

Drug	Dosed on	Comments
Propofol	IBW, TBW	Calculate induction dose with IBW, but maintenance dose with TBW. Systemic clearance and V_D correlate well with TBW
Thiopental	LBM	For induction – not used for maintenance
Atracurium, Cisatracurium	TBW	Absolute V_D unchanged, but higher relative dose does not prolong effect[89,90]
Vecuronium, Rocuronium	IBW or LBM	Little distribution into adipose tissue; pharmacokinetics and pharmacodynamics unaltered in obese patients[85,86]
Fentanyl, Sufentanil	TBW	V_D correlates with TBW; clearance is unchanged, but effects can be prolonged[91,92]
Alfentanil	LBM, TBW	V_D is smaller than for sufentanil or fentanyl, but alfentanil still distributes widely into adipose tissues. Effect prolonged after continuous infusion
Remifentanil	IBW or LBM	Small V_D, similar in obese and lean patients[93]
Midazolam	TBW	Highly lipophilic; V_D increases with weight. Prolonged effect after adequate dose[84]

TBW: total body weight; V_D: volume of distribution.

LBM is higher than IBW, since approximately 20–40% of an obese individual's weight gain is due to an increase in lean tissue.

The required maintenance dose of a continuously infused drug depends on its volume of distribution at steady state (V_{Dss}), and this depends on its lipid solubility. Due to the absolute increase in adipose tissue, the volume of distribution of highly lipophilic drugs, such as barbiturates, propofol or benzodiazepines is greatly increased in obesity[82–84] and maintenance doses should be calculated on the basis of total body weight. Less lipophilic drugs, on the other hand, such as non-depolarizing neuromuscular blockers, should still be dosed on the basis of IBW or LBM.[85–87] Succinylcholine and atracurium are exceptions to this rule. Plasma cholinesterase activity increases in proportion to body weight and the dose of succinylcholine should be increased accordingly.[88] Despite the lower volume of distribution of atracurium relative to weight, its effect is not prolonged when dosed according to total body weight.[89,90] Specific data on cisatracurium is lacking, but it is virtually indistinguishable from atracurium, and its distribution and metabolism should be similar. Table 8.6

gives an overview of the weight that should be used to calculate the doses of drugs used in anaesthesia.

Fentanyl and its congeners are highly lipophilic and should thus be dosed according to total body weight, with the exception of remifentanil. The volume of distribution of fentanyl and sufentanil correlates well with total body weight, and both substances are distributed extensively in fatty as well as lean tissues.[91,92] Remifentanil, on the other hand, although also highly lipophilic, has only a small volume of distribution and its pharmacokinetics are virtually the same in obese and lean patients.[93] This is due in part to its degradation by ubiquitously present esterases. Alfentanil has a similar volume of distribution in obese and non-obese individuals, but the elimination half-life is longer in obese patients due to its reduced clearance.

The extent of protein binding will probably differ in obese patients. Total plasma protein and albumin concentrations are the same in lean and obese individuals but their binding capacity can be reduced by the higher concentrations of triglycerides, cholesterol, free fatty acids and lipoproteins in dyslipidaemia. The net effect of this would be higher free fractions of acidic drugs. The plasma concentration of $\alpha 1$-acid glycoprotein is elevated in obese patients, and this will decrease the free fraction of basic drugs.

Hepatic drug elimination is usually not affected in obese patients, despite the fact that histological abnormalities, such as fatty infiltration, parenchymal cell degeneration and periportal cellular infiltration, are nearly always present. Phase I reactions (dealkylation, oxidation, etc.) are generally normal or even slightly increased. Phase II metabolism (glucuronidation, sulfatation, alkylation, etc.) is consistently increased. The reduction of CO and hepatic perfusion as caused by the increased IAP during pneumoperitoneum can decrease the elimination of drugs with a high hepatic extraction rate (e.g. midazolam, sufentanil,[94] fentanyl,[95] methohexital[96]) and prolong their effects.

Renal elimination and clearance of drugs is increased in obese patients due to an increase in renal blood flow and glomerular filtration rate of up to 40%.[97,98] It might be necessary to increase the doses of renally excreted drugs.

Effect of obesity on drug distribution

- Volume of distribution increases with body weight for lipophilic drugs (e.g. opioids (except remifentanil), hypnotics)
- Volume of distribution does not increase with body weight for hydrophilic drugs (e.g. neuromuscular blockers)

Gastric emptying

Obese patients are thought to be at a higher risk of aspiration of gastric contents due to increased IAP, delayed gastric emptying, and an increased incidence of hiatus hernia and reflux. After an 8-h fast, 90% of obese patients had a gastric fluid volume of more than 25 ml with a pH of less than 2.5.[99] These figures are generally considered to represent a high risk of aspiration pneumonitis should the gastric fluid enter the lungs. Later studies have shown that gastric emptying is actually more rapid in obese individuals,[100] and that the lower oesophageal sphincter is as competent in obese patients without symptomatic gastro-oesophageal reflux as in non-obese individuals.[101] But since obese patients have a much greater gastric volume to begin with, the residual volume will still be larger than in non-obese individuals despite more rapid emptying. It is therefore sensible to take all precautions against aspiration of gastric contents. These include lowering gastric pH with H_2 receptor antagonists and antacids, rapid-sequence induction with cricoid pressure or even awake intubation.

Endocrine disorders

Insulin resistance and hyperinsulinaemia are consistent features of obesity and are directly related to body weight. Type 2 diabetes mellitus (non-insulin-dependent diabetes mellitus) is present despite elevated levels of insulin. This type of diabetes is virtually non-existent in individuals with a BMI of less than $22\,kg\,m^{-2}$. Long-standing diabetes leads to peripheral sensory neuropathy and autonomic dysfunction with gastroparesis, instable heart rate and silent myocardial infarctions. Autonomic dysfunction, or dysautonomia, predisposes to cardiac dysrhythmias and sudden death. Gonadal hormone levels are altered in both men and women. Testosterone levels are decreased in men, whereas androgen and/or oestrogen levels may be increased in obese females. Obesity is associated with an earlier onset of menarche, irregular and anovulatory cycles and an earlier menopause.

Laparoscopic bariatric operations

Two fundamentally different surgical approaches have been used to help patients control their caloric intake. One, referred to as restrictive, aims to restrict the absolute amount of food the individual can eat and the other, referred to as malabsorptive, aims at limiting the number of calories that can be absorbed from the ingested food. Each approach has its own devoted champions, but they are both basically the same with regard to anaesthesiological management.

In the restrictive procedures, most of the stomach is either resected or otherwise blocked off, leaving only a small pouch of about 15–35 ml. This restricts the amount of food that a patient is able to ingest per unit time. Purely restrictive procedures were formerly the most commonly performed bariatric operations, making up 95% of all cases. Weight loss after this type of operation required a high degree of patient compliance with diet guidelines. The operations were not always successful, particularly not in patients who were so addicted to food that they ingested high caloric liquid foods or sweets in order to satisfy their craving. These patients can actually gain weight after a restrictive operation.

Malabsorptive procedures are designed to overcome this shortcoming by limiting the amount of calories a patient can absorb, no matter how much he or she eats. This can be achieved by interfering with digestion or by reducing the time available for nutrient uptake, or by a combination of the two. In the latter, small intestinal flow is divided into a biliary–pancreatic conduit and a food conduit that rejoin near the ileocoecal valve. The malabsorptive procedure reduces the absorption of nutrients and calories from the ingested food by reducing the time left for complete digestion and uptake.

The current philosophy is to combine a restrictive operation with a malabsorptive modification of the small intestine to obtain the best and longest lasting results. The individual procedures are listed in Table 8.7 and shown schematically in Figure 8.3.

Table 8.7 Types of bariatric surgery

Restrictive procedures	Reduces the size of the stomach and limits the amount of food that can be ingested per unit of time
Malabsorptive procedures	Splits small intestinal flow and reduces the time available for digestion and uptake
Restrictive operations	Horizontal gastroplasty
	Vertical-banded gastroplasty (VBG)
	SBG with or without adjustable cuff
Malabsorptive operations	Jejuno-ileal bypass
Combined operations	Gastric bypass with Roux-en-Y (RNY)
	BPD with or without DS

SBG: silicone-banded gastroplasty; DS: duodenal switch. BPD: Biliopancreatic diversion.

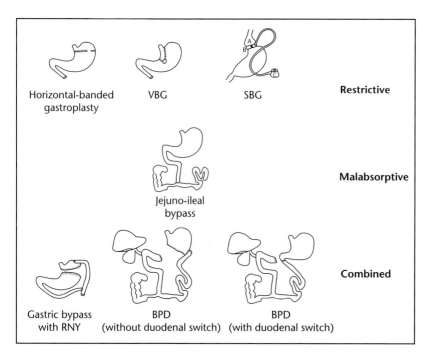

Horizontal-banded gastroplasty   VBG   SBG   **Restrictive**

Jejuno-ileal bypass   **Malabsorptive**

Gastric bypass with RNY   BPD (without duodenal switch)   BPD (with duodenal switch)   **Combined**

Figure 8.3 Schematic diagrams of various bariatric operations. (For abbreviations see Table 8.7.)

Typical long-term complications of most of these operations are protein malnutrition and vitamin, iron and calcium deficiencies. The anaesthetist dealing with patients who have undergone bariatric surgery may be confronted with the sequelae. Complications more specific for individual procedures are dumping syndrome, gastric outlet obstruction, stoma margin ulceration, slipped bands and band-related erosions.

Restrictive surgical procedures

Restrictive bariatric operations are the least invasive of the weight reducing procedures and simply reduce the holding capacity of the stomach. There are a number of methods by which this goal can be achieved, some of which are adjustable or even completely reversible.

Gastric banding

In the original silicone gastric banding (SGB) procedure, a silicone band was placed around the stomach dividing it into two portions: a small pouch adjacent to the oesophagus and the rest of the stomach.[102] The size of the resulting orifice was determined during surgery and it regulated how fast ingested food could leave the pouch. Once the band had been positioned there was no way to change the connecting passageway other than with a second operation.

In a modification of the SGB operation an adjustable portion was added to the silicone band to permit correction of the stomal diameter. This portion is connected to a subcutaneously positioned injection reservoir through which it can be inflated or deflated to narrow or widen the stoma.[2,102,103]

The main complications of gastric banding procedures are slippage or malposition of the band requiring repositioning, and gastric erosion and perforation under the band.[104]

Horizontal-banded gastroplasty

This was the original restrictive operation that became possible after the introduction of the surgical stapler. Three staples were removed from the staple cartridge that was used to partition off the stomach just distal to the oesophageal–gastric junction. This left a small opening through which food was able to pass only slowly. This operation is no longer popular.

Vertical-banded gastroplasty

The vertical-banded gastroplasty (VBG) was at one time the most popular and most commonly performed weight reducing operation, but its limitations have caused the enthusiasm for it to wane. In this operation, a circular window is made through both walls of the stomach about 10 cm below the oesophageal–gastric junction. From this hole, a vertical row of surgical staples is applied up to the His' angle to create small pouch. A polypropylene mesh band is placed through the window around the outlet of the pouch and adjusted to control the size of the outlet and to prevent it from stretching.[105]

Malabsorptive surgical procedures

Jejuno-ileal bypass

In the jejuno-ileal bypass procedure, a short length of jejunum is anastomosed to the terminal ileum a short distance from the ileocoecal valve, either as an end-to-side or end-to-end enteroenterostomy.[106] The malabsorption caused by bypassing such a long stretch of small intestine does indeed induce significant weight loss and remission of co-morbidities such as diabetes mellitus. But the procedure has a number of side effects that ranged from the subjectively unpleasant, such as abdominal bloating and arthralgia, to the life threatening. Protein malnutrition is frequent and for unknown reasons 5–10% of the patients develop liver cirrhosis.[106–108]

Combined surgical procedures

Gastric bypass with Roux-en-Y

The concept of combining a reduction of the gastric holding capacity with a diversion of the chymus past the duodenum with the purpose of inducing weight loss was introduced by Mason and Ito.[109] Various modifications of the original technique aimed at reducing the complication rate and improving the efficacy led to the bariatric procedure currently most commonly performed in the US. This is the gastric bypass with Roux-en-Y (RNY), which accounts for approximately 75% of all operations. In this operation, a small (ca. 25 ml) pouch is formed from the stomach at the entrance of the oesophagus. This blocks off the larger portion of the fundus and the antrum. The small intestine is transected and the distal end is attached to the newly formed gastric pouch with a narrow (0.7–1.2 cm) gastroenterostomy to form the food conduit. The proximal end of the transected small intestine that carries the biliary and pancreatic secretions is then reconnected to the food conduit with an enteroenterostomy.

Dumping syndrome is the typical complication of gastric bypass procedures, and occurs in two phases. Early dumping is a group of abdominal and vasomotor symptoms arising shortly after food ingestion that are triggered by osmotically induced fluid shifts into the intestinal lumen and by the release of vasoactive hormones. These symptoms include nausea, vomiting, diarrhoea, abdominal cramps, flushing and palpitations. Late dumping is caused by reactive hypoglycaemia following rapid insulin release. Anaemia is very common in patients with gastric bypass of this type, since the absorption of iron and vitamin B_{12} is poor. Poor absorption of calcium may also occur. These nutrients will have to be supplemented in the diet or given parenterally if necessary. Surgical complications include anastomotic leak, deep vein thrombosis, pulmonary embolism and respiratory failure.

Biliopancreatic diversion

The biliopancreatic diversion (BPD) resembles the jejuno-ileal bypass in that it limits the time and intestinal surface area available for the absorption of nutrients, but it avoids a number of complications, such as hepatic damage, by not defunctionalizing a section of the small intestine. BPD also resembles the RNY procedure in that food and biliopancreatic secretions are initially conducted through separate channels and then recombined through an enteroenterostomy. The biliopancreatic division procedure differs from the latter procedure in that the antrum and part of the fundus are not simply sealed off, but are actually removed. In the BPD, a limited gastrectomy is performed that removes the antrum and pylorus and closes the proximal end of the duodenum. The resulting small gastric pouch significantly limits food intake, creating the restrictive component of the procedure. The ileum is transected approximately 250 cm from the ileocoecal valve and the distal portion of the ileum is anastomosed to the gastric pouch to form the food conduit. An enteroenterostomy connects the distal end of the remaining small intestine to the distal ileum about 100 cm from the ileocoecal valve. The short remaining common alimentary channel creates the malabsorptive component of the procedure.[110] Although some complications are avoided, others such as dumping syndrome, marginal ulcers, stoma closures and blockages still occur. Removing the antrum and part of the fundus and diverting the chymus away from the duodenum and jejunum also predisposes the patient to protein malnutrition and to vitamin B_{12}, iron and calcium deficiencies.

In a modification of the BPD known as the duodenal switch,[111,112] the antrum and pylorus are not removed, but instead stomach volume is reduced by a parietal gastrectomy along the greater curvature, which maintains normal digestive function and leaves the antro-pyloroduodenal pump intact. The duodenum is stapled shut and chymus is diverted from its proximal end through an approximately 250 cm long stretch of terminal ileum. The biliopancreatic diverting limb of the small intestine is anastomosed to the ileal food conduit *ca.* 100 cm proximal to the ileocoecal valve. Proteins have already been largely digested by gastric secretions; so that the short common alimentary channel interferes primarily with the digestion and uptake of fats. This technique essentially eliminates dumping syndrome and stomal ulceration and reduces the severity of protein malnutrition and micronutrient deficiencies.

Positioning the patient for bariatric surgery

Bariatric surgery requires special operating room (OR) equipment. The gurneys and operating tables must be designed to tolerate a load of at least 400 kg and should be wider than standard OR equipment to accommodate the added width of the supine, obese patient. Electrically or hydraulically adjustable tables are preferable to manually operated ones for manoeuvring the patient into the required position. Obese patients have the tendency to slip off the operating table when it is sharply tilted, and should therefore be securely strapped on. Pressure sores and nerve injuries are common in these patients, especially in diabetics, and the danger spots should be carefully padded. Soft pads filled with tiny beads are available that mould themselves to the patient's body. Applying an external vacuum to the bag fixes it in the adapted shape. Gel pads are also available for padding critical pressure points, such as elbows, shoulder blades, heels, back of the head, sacrum, hips, buttocks, etc. Ulnar neuropathy occurs more frequently in morbidly obese patients that in the non-obese.[113] Sciatic nerve and brachial plexus palsies can also occur and are usually caused by keeping the patient in a tilted position, either sideways or Trendelenburg, for longer periods. Nerve injury may still occur in these patients despite all efforts at careful positioning and padding. This must be pointed out and discussed with the patient during the preoperative visit.

For bariatric surgery, the patient is positioned as for most other upper abdominal laparoscopic procedures. The patient lies supine, thighs fully abducted and slightly flexed in the hips. The surgeon stands between the patient's legs with one assistant on each side of the patient and the scrub nurse to the surgeon's left. The laparoscopy tower is positioned near the patient's right shoulder (for a right-handed surgeon) so that the patient's right arm lies alongside his or her body. The left arm usually remains abducted and is accessible to the anaesthetist. However, it may be adducted and covered according to the custom of the hospital or the surgeon's preference. Venous lines will then have to be extended and fitted with three-way stopcocks to allow drug administration.

During the phase in which the surgeon is manipulating the stomach, the table will be tilted into a more or less steep reversed Trendelburg position. If the procedure requires access to the small intestine, the patient will then be brought into a Trendelenburg position to give easier exposure of the operation site.

Anaesthesia

Preoperative considerations

For a comprehensive overview on obesity in anaesthesia see the excellent reviews of Adams and Murphy[55] or Ogunnaike et al.[114]

History and examination

A meticulous and exhaustive history of patients presenting for bariatric surgery is necessary in order to correctly assess the perioperative risk profile of these patients and to determine the invasiveness of monitoring required for optimal management. These patients tend to limit their own mobility and even sleep upright and will therefore not report episodes of exertional dyspnoea or angina, paroxysmal nocturnal dyspnoea or even orthopnoea. Direct questioning is required to obtain this information. The patient should be carefully evaluated for symptoms of significant involvement of the cardiorespiratory system with particular emphasis on systemic and pulmonary hypertension, signs of left and/or right ventricular strain or failure, ischaemic heart disease, gastro-oesophageal reflux, diabetic neuropathy or OSAS. The patient should be asked to walk the length of the ward and to lie supine in order to detect reduced exercise tolerance or orthopnoea.

Auscultatory signs of heart failure such as crepitant rales and additional heart sounds, jugular venous engorgement, hepatomegaly and peripheral oedema may be difficult to detect due to the large amount of subcutaneous tissue. Clinical symptoms of left or right ventricular failure such as exertional dyspnoea and fatigue indicate further evaluation by a cardiologist. Echocardiography, although frequently difficult in these patients, can yield important information such as the tricuspid regurgitation indicative of significant pulmonary hypertension, the eccentric left ventricular hypertrophy indicating incipient failure even though ventricular function might appear normal, or regional wall hypokinesia that might indicate ischaemic disease.

The mandatory preoperative electrocardiogram (ECG) can show the relatively tall R-wave in V_1 ($R \geqslant S$), right axis deviation, and the ST segment depression and T-wave inversion in the right to mid-precordial leads characteristic of right ventricular hypertension, or the tall R-waves in V_5 or V_6, the deep S-waves in V_1 together with the ST segment depression and T-wave inversion in left precordial leads that point to left ventricular strain. On the other hand, the thickness of the intervening tissue may cause low voltage in the precordial leads and thus mask the severity of existing ventricular hypertrophy.

Venous status and arterial access sites should be evaluated during the preoperative visit, and the probability of central venous and arterial cannulation discussed with the patient. Peripheral veins may be very difficult to find in obese patients and central venous catheterization, preferably the internal jugular vein, is recommended. This will allow a more efficient treatment of intraoperative complications as well as ensure better postoperative venous access and avoid repeated venipuncture. Patients with serious cardiovascular co-morbidity might profit from the placement and use of a pulmonary artery thermodilution

---

What to look for and ask about in obese patients

- *Systemic and pulmonary hypertension*: Exertional dyspnoea, additional heart sounds on auscultation, signs of strain or axis deviation in the ECG, echocardiography, have patient walk the ward or climb stairs
- *Ischaemic heart disease*: History of angina pectoris (may be negative), chronic medication, ST changes in the ECG, heart wall akinesia or hypokinesia in ultrasound
- *Congestive heart failure*: Exertional dyspnoea, paroxysmal nocturnal dyspnoea, orthopnoea, pulmonary rales on auscultation, reduced ejection fraction in echocardiography, have patient walk the ward or climb stairs, and lie flat in bed
- *Gastro-oesophageal reflux*: History of heart burn, typical self-medication, patient sleeps elevated
- *Diabetic neuropathy, including autonomic dysfunction*: History, laboratory and medication will reveal diabetes, finding neuropathy is more difficult. Valsalva manoeuvre can give evidence of dysautonomia
- *Other pre-existing sensory or motor impairment*: History, physical examination
- *Sleep apnoea*: Likely to be present, often not diagnosed, clinical suspicion warranted
- *Possible difficult intubation*: Evaluate for Mallampati score
- *Difficult venous access*: Check vascular status including neck and feet

catheter. This should be discussed with the patient during the preoperative work-up.

Classical risk predictors of difficult intubation, such as the Mallampati score[115] should be noted. One should discuss the possibility with the patient that tracheal intubation might be difficult and that alternative methods, such as fibre-optic awake intubation, although somewhat more unpleasant, might provide a greater degree of safety. These should be explained to the patient in detail.

The laboratory work-up will probably reveal signs of hepatic dysfunction, which are usually of no consequence. Cholesterol and triglyceride levels are usually elevated, and dyslipidaemia is frequently present. Blood glucose concentrations are likely to be increased in the presence of diabetes mellitus. Extremely high glucose concentrations indicating poor metabolic control could indicate postponing the operation until the diabetes is adequately treated.

One should discuss with the patient the typical risks and possible complications as well as the planned preventive or therapeutic measures on this occasion and this should be documented.

What risks and measures should be discussed with the patient

- *Difficult intubation*: Aspiration of gastric contents with all its consequences, possible dental injuries, possible necessity of awake nasal intubation
- *Respiratory problems*: Atelectasis, pneumonia, postoperative respiratory support with endotracheal tube or nasal continuous positive airway pressure (CPAP)
- *Cardiovascular problems*: Central venous catheter, pulmonary artery catheter, risk of postoperative myocardial infarction, cardiac decompensation, death
- *Deep vein thrombosis*: Risk of fatal pulmonary embolism, early mobilization mandatory
- *Pressure sores and nerve damage*: Sometimes unavoidable despite all precautions

---

Concurrent medication

There is still some controversy over whether a patient's chronic medication should be discontinued or not. In our institution, all medications with few exceptions are continued until the time of surgery. We withhold oral hypoglycaemics on the day of surgery and infuse glucose to avoid hypoglycaemia resulting from residual effects. Biguanides are discontinued 2–3 days before surgery. Patients under treatment with insulin are given one-third of their usual morning insulin dose as regular insulin together with an infusion of 5% glucose running at a rate of 125 ml h^{-1}.

Oral benzodiazepines in anxiolytic but not hypnotic doses (e.g. 7.5–10 mg midazolam or 5–10 mg diazepam) are acceptable for premedication. Absorption is unreliable after intramuscular or subcutaneous injections, and these routes of administration should be avoided. Midazolam can be titrated intravenously during the immediate preoperative period to achieve the desired level of anxiolysis. Oral H$_2$-antagonists (e.g. ranitidine or effervescent cimetidine), proton pump inhibitors (e.g. omeprazole), propulsives (e.g. metoclopramide, domperidone) and water soluble antacids (e.g. sodium citrate) can be given to reduce gastric volume and acidity, thus reducing the risk of aspiration pneumonitis and minimizing its severity should it occur (see below).

Preparing the patient for anaesthesia

Venous cannulae are best placed in the left arm or in an external jugular vein, since the right arm is positioned at the patient's side and covered by the surgical drapes. It is usually very difficult to find accessible veins in obese patients, and one should consider inserting an intravenous catheter into the brachial or internal jugular vein after induction of anaesthesia and to leave it in place for use in the postoperative period, to draw blood and administer intravenous drugs, and to avoid the need of repeated venipuncture.

The patient's arms, legs, back and head must be carefully positioned and padded to avoid pressure damage during surgery. Well-padded shoulder supports are required in procedures during which the patient will be brought into the Trendelenburg position. They must not be too near the neck in order to avoid brachial plexus damage. The shoulders and head are positioned on towels or other supports in order to bring the patient's chin anterior to the chest (see below).

Choice of anaesthetic regimen and anaesthetic drugs

General anaesthesia with endotracheal intubation is the standard anaesthetic procedure for bariatric surgery. Mechanical ventilation is absolutely indicated since the combined effects of obesity and pneumoperitoneum will otherwise lead to hypoventilation and hypoxaemia in the spontaneously breathing obese patient. This will increase pulmonary vascular resistance and put an additional load on the right ventricle and should thus be avoided. Some authors advocate the use of a thoracic epidural catheter to supplement the general anaesthetic and to provide postoperative analgesia.[116] This is definitely an option for open bariatric

Table 8.8 Standard anaesthetic for morbidly obese patients in the University Hospital, Göttingen

Preparation	Premedication with midazolam 7.5–10 mg *per os* (orally) or diazepam 10 mg *per os* Rofecoxib (50 mg) or valdecoxib (40 mg) can be given orally for pre-emptive postoperative analgesia
Induction	Induction with propofol (2 mg kg^{-1} total body weight) after a bolus dose of remifentanil (1 μg kg^{-1} LBM) (alfentanil (20 μg kg^{-1}) or sufentanil (0.3 μg kg^{-1}) are used occasionally) Diclofenac (100 mg supplement) if rofecoxib or valdecoxib has not been given
Intubation	Relaxation with rocuronium (0.6 mg kg^{-1} LBM) Orotracheal intubation with armoured endotracheal tube Endotracheal tube is fixed securely and bilateral breath sounds are rechecked after patient is in Trendelenburg position
Maintenance	Propofol infused at a rate of 5–6 mg kg^{-1} h^{-1} total body weight or target plasma concentration of 2–2.5 μg ml^{-1} if using a TCI pump *Or* Desflurane 3–4% end tidal or isoflurane 0.7–1.0% end tidal Remifentanil is infused at an initial rate of 0.2–0.5 μg kg^{-1} min^{-1}: • If alfentanil is used, the initial rate is 30–40 μg kg^{-1} h^{-1} • If sufentanil is used, the initial rate is 0.3–0.5 μg kg^{-1} h^{-1} *In all cases, the infusion rate of the opioid is increased or decreased as necessary, and as described in the chapter on anaesthesia.*
Emergence	Extubation when patient is fully awake and in semi-recumbent position O$_2$ by mask or nasal prongs until no further risk of hypoxaemia Consider nasal CPAP on third to fifth postoperative night
Pain therapy	Rofecoxib (50 mg) or valdecoxib (40 mg) given orally with the premedication, or Diclofenac suppository (100 mg) given after induction of anaesthesia Intravenous paracetamol (1000 mg) infused 15 min before the end of surgery. Repeated every 6 h Bolus injections of morphine (2 mg bolus) if requested by the patient

procedures that, likely any upper abdominal operation, have a high potential for severe postoperative pain and respiratory impairment.[117] However, an epidural catheter is probably rarely indicated in minimally invasive laparoscopic procedures, since there is much less interference with postoperative pulmonary function, atelectasis is less extensive, arterial oxygenation is better, and there is less pain compared to the same operation, gastric bypass with RNY, performed in the conventional, open fashion.[118]

A balanced anaesthetic is the method of choice for general anaesthesia in the morbidly obese. The hypnotics, analgesics and muscle relaxants used for the anaesthetic should be chosen on the basis of their pharmacokinetics, particularly the context-sensitive half-time (see Chapter 5), as well as metabolism and elimination.

Remifentanil is the obvious choice for the analgesic component, due to its unique pharmacokinetics and lack of cumulation. Remifentanil in a dose of 1 μg kg^{-1} is as effective as 1 μg kg^{-1} fentanyl or 10 μg kg^{-1} alfentanil in suppressing cardiovascular responses to intubation in morbidly obese patients.[119] It is dosed according to lean body weight.

The hypnotic component of the balanced anaesthetic can be either propofol or a volatile anaesthetic with low lipid solubility, such as desflurane, isoflurane or sevoflurane (Table 8.8). Propofol is distributed extensively in the body, and the pharmacokinetics of propofol used as a component of total intravenous anaesthesia in the morbidly obese do not differ from those in lean patients.[83] However, there was no sign of cumulation, even when the drug was dosed according to total body weight. This makes propofol a suitable choice for the hypnotic component of a balanced anaesthetic. A direct comparison of a total intravenous technique using propofol with inhalational anaesthesia with sevoflurane (end-tidal concentration 1–2%) showed both methods to be similar with regard to haemodynamic stability and recovery characteristics.[120] One can avoid overdosing propofol by using a target-controlled infusion (TCI) pump, ideally with neuromonitoring of the depth of anaesthesia. There are no studies that show that obese patients differ from the non-obese with regard to the plasma concentration of propofol required to produce loss of consciousness and intraoperative awareness, and a targeted concentration of 2.0–2.5 μg ml^{-1} will be adequate for the vast majority of the patients.

Of the volatile anaesthetics, desflurane is probably the agent of choice for use in laparoscopic bariatric surgery due to its physicochemical properties and its consistently rapid recovery profile.[121] Recovery is slightly more rapid after 2 h of anaesthesia with remifentanil–desflurane than after remifentanil–sevoflurane for laparoscopic gastroplasty. The times to extubation and orientation were 5.9 and 6.6 min, respectively, in the desflurane group, and 7.9 and 9.0 min, respectively, in the sevoflurane group.[122]

Emergence and recovery times were slightly shorter after a monoanaesthetic with sevoflurane than after isoflurane in morbidly obese patients.[123,124] The time to extubation was 6 min in morbidly obese patients undergoing gastric banding with sevoflurane anaesthesia as compared to 10 min in patients given isoflurane.[123] Wash-in times are somewhat faster for sevoflurane than for isoflurane, and the F_A/F_I ratio was higher in the patients given sevoflurane during the first 30 min.[125] This is of no great import, since the required alveolar concentration can be achieved just as rapidly with isoflurane by simply increasing the inspiratory concentration. Wash-out of sevoflurane was significantly faster than that of isoflurane during the first 60 s after discontinuation of the inhalational agent. On the other hand, isoflurane maintains splanchnic blood flow better than does sevoflurane, and this might be a more important aspect in laparoscopic surgery than a gain of a few minutes after several hours of surgery. Halothane should probably be avoided altogether because of its high lipid solubility with slow recovery, and also because obesity is possibly a risk factor for halothane-induced hepatic injury.[126,127]

The choice of the muscle relaxant is not critical, and nearly all currently available drugs with a short to medium duration of action can be used to advantage. We prefer rocuronium for its very rapid onset of action that allows rapid intubation, but atracurium, cisatracurium, vecuronium or even mivacurium are suitable. Pancuronium, pipecuronium or even tubocurarine would not be optimal choices, but if nothing else is available they can be used. Residual effects of the muscle relaxant should be reversed at the end of surgery. Succinylcholine should be given to facilitate intubation if a muscle relaxant with a slower onset is used.

Induction of anaesthesia

Anaesthesia should be induced with an intravenous hypnotic and not by inhalation, since there is a higher incidence of gastro-oesophageal reflux in obese patients, and this is a risk factor for regurgitation and aspiration of gastric contents. In fact, one should consider using a rapid-sequence induction regimen in obese patients. Some authors, reluctant to abandon their tried ways, recommend inhalational induction with sevoflurane with the patient in a lateral decubitus position in order to avoid aspiration of gastric content should he or she regurgitate or vomit.[128] While this method is obviously possible, mechanics argues against it: positioning awake, obese patients on their sides on a narrow operating table is no mean feat, while repositioning them on their back again once anaesthesia has been induced is positively daunting.

Intubation

There is still controversy over the question of whether the incidence of difficult tracheal intubation is higher in obese patients,[129–131] but although there does not seem to be a direct correlation between body weight or BMI and grade of difficulty, it does appear that difficult intubation is more common in patients with moderate to morbid obesity.[129,131] In studies correlating classical risk predictors for difficult intubation, such as the Mallampati score,[115] thryomental distance, mobility of head and neck, interincisor gap and mandibular recession with difficult visualization of the larynx[132] and difficult intubation, the single independent risk factor that could be found was a Mallampati score of 3 or higher.[129–131] The positive predictive value of 66.7% with a sensitivity of 88.9–100% was higher in obese patients than in the general population.[131] In one study, neck circumference was also found to be an independent risk factor for difficult laryngoscopy; a Cormack–Lehane class III or higher was found in 5% of patients with a neck circumference of 40 cm while the incidence increased to 35% in patients with a

---

Anaesthesia for bariatric surgery: basic considerations

- *General anaesthesia with endotracheal intubation and mechanical ventilation*
  - Calculate minute ventilation on basis of lean body weight
  - Avoid extreme tidal volumes
  - Add slight PEEP to improve oxygenation
- *Balanced anaesthetic with propofol or desflurane and remifentanil*
  - Propofol dosed according to total body weight
  - Isoflurane or sevoflurane acceptable alternatives
  - Remifentanil dosed according to IBW or LBM
  - Alfentanil or sufentanil possible alternatives to remifentanil
- *Choice of muscle relaxant not critical (except for long-acting agents)*
  - Relaxants cumulate in same manner in obese and lean patients
  - Effects can be reversed

neck circumference of 60 cm.[130] A barrel-chest or voluminous breasts are occasional extrathoracic impediments to intubation that can be circumvented by proper positioning of the patient or by the use of a short-handled laryngoscope.

A number of authors have advocated awake intubation in all morbidly obese patients. This is an unpleasant procedure for the patient, and as studies have shown, only truly indicated in a minority of all cases. A pragmatic approach is to apply topical anaesthesia to pharynx, supralaryngeal area and tongue and to take an "awake look". If the epiglottis and dorsal larynx cannot be visualized using gentle pressure of the laryngoscope, one should resort to awake, fibre-optic nasotracheal intubation. This is performed in the usual manner using only the barest minimum of sedative and analgesic drugs; preferably propofol and remifentanil or alfentanil.

In order to facilitate intubation, the obese patient should be positioned with pads or towels under the shoulders with the head elevated and the neck extended in order to bring the chin anterior to the chest (Figure 8.4). The patient should breathe 100% O_2 through a tight-fitting face mask for a minimum of 3 min or until the end-expiratory O_2 concentration is 85% or above. Obese patients tolerate hypoventilation and apnoea much worse and O_2 saturation tends to fall more rapidly after cessation of respiration than in the non-obese. This is likely to be a consequence of their reduced FRC.[55] During apnoea after a period of pre-oxygenation that brought the end-tidal O_2 concentration to 95% or higher, arterial O_2 saturation dropped below 90% more than twice as fast in morbidly obese patients than in lean individuals (163 vs. 364 s).[133]

A rapid-sequence induction using succinylcholine for muscle relaxation is recommended to minimize the risk of aspiration pneumonitis. This will also permit one to await the return of spontaneous respiration should all attempts at intubation fail. Some authors recommend inserting a laryngeal mask airway as a temporary ventilatory device when initial attempts at intubation have failed.[134] In the reported series, placement of the airway was successful in all cases, but tracheal intubation ultimately failed in 3% of the patients. In these patients, surgery was carried out uneventfully using the laryngeal mask airway. A second option is to use an intubating laryngeal mask airway as a ventilatory device through which the endotracheal tube can be inserted with less risk of hypoxemic episodes.[135] In any case, care must be taken to position the tip of the endotracheal tube correctly in relation to the carina, and to detect and, if

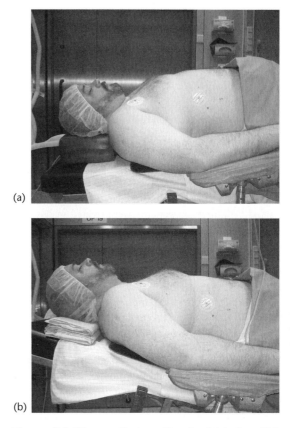

(a)

(b)

Figure 8.4 Obese patient position for intubation. This patient is 175 cm tall with a BMI of 51. With the patient in the normal supine Jackson position (a) the chin is lower than the chest, and one will probably encounter difficulties in inserting the laryngoscope. Slightly elevating the upper body and reclining the head (b) brings the chin higher than the chest and facilitates mouth opening and insertion of the laryngoscope.

Intubation of obese patients

- Intubation frequently more difficult than in lean patients
  - None of the commonly used indicators of difficult intubation are very specific or selective
  - Mallampati score most closely associated with difficult intubation
- Neck should be extended and chin anterior to chest:
  - Voluminous breasts or barrel-chest can interfere with the introduction of the laryngoscope
- Effective pre-oxygenation, rapid intubation:
  - O_2 saturation falls rapidly in obese patients
- Laryngeal mask airway as temporary device if intubation fails

necessary, to amend any changes. The tip of the endo-tracheal tube was found to descend in 50% of morbidly obese patients undergoing laparoscopic gastric banding and to enter the right bronchus in one-third of these patients.[136]

Intraoperative considerations

Faced with a patient presenting with such current and potential problems, one would intuitively tend to opt for maximum monitoring and postoperative care. This may not always be necessary as a study comparing the outcome after gastric reduction surgery demonstrated.[137] Thirty-six patients were treated in hospital A with high intensity intraoperative monitoring and routine postoperative ventilation on an intensive care unit. The patients were equipped with an arterial line, two intravenous lines and a urinary catheter. The anaesthetic was with 0.7 MAC isoflurane, 53% nitrous oxide, pancuronium (13.2 mg, reversed in only five patients) and sometimes fentanyl (only 26 of the patients, and only a moderate dose of 0.7 mg). On average, the patients had a 46.5-h stay in the intensive care unit and a 9.7-day postoperative stay in the hospital. The 50 patients in hospital B, on the other hand, were equipped only with one intravenous line, no arterial line, no urinary catheter, and postoperative ventilation was not planned. The anaesthetic was with nitrous oxide (64%), fentanyl (1.3 mg) and pancuronium (9.7 mg). Isoflurane was only given to 14 patients, and then in a low dose of 0.3 MAC. Respiratory depression and muscle relaxation were routinely reversed with naloxone and pyridostigmine allowing extubation in the operating theatre. The patients spent 1.7 h in the recovery room and 9.6 postoperative days in the hospital. The outcome was the same in both hospitals, but the costs differed significantly.

The data are interesting and thought provoking, but we believe, nonetheless, that state-of-the-art anaesthetic management of morbidly obese patients frequently requires invasive intraoperative monitoring and intensive postoperative respiratory care. Cardiovascular and respiratory co-morbidity is so frequent, and the functional reserves of these patients so slim that lack of attention to perioperative care can have catastrophic consequences.

Maintenance of anaesthesia

Anaesthesia is maintained as a balanced technique with remifentanil infused at a rate adequate to suppress autonomic responses to noxious stimuli. This is usually between 0.2 and 0.5 $\mu g\,kg^{-1}min^{-1}$ based on LBM.

Unconsciousness is maintained with propofol, desflurane or isoflurane. Propofol is infused at a rate of 5–6 $mg\,kg^{-1}h^{-1}$ based on total body weight. Alternatively, a TCI system can be used with the propofol plasma concentration set at 2.0–2.5 $\mu g\,ml^{-1}$. The volatile anaesthetic is given at an end-tidal concentration of 0.5 MAC. Complete muscle relaxation is crucial during all laparoscopic surgery, but this is particularly the case for bariatric procedures in order to maintain an adequate intra-abdominal working space with the preset inflation pressure. Relaxometry is desirable, but not always possible in the obese patient. A reduction of the space in the pneumoperitoneum should be taken as a clinical sign that the effects of the muscle relaxant are waning. For further details refer to the chapter on anaesthesia.

Monitoring

Intraoperative monitoring for bariatric surgery should include continuous ECG, preferably with continuous ST evaluation, continuous or intermittent blood pressure measurement, pulse oximetry, capnometry and relaxometry. Patients with severe cardiopulmonary disease might benefit from CO and pulmonary artery pressure monitoring.

Except for all but minor procedures and in otherwise healthy obese patients, blood pressure should be monitored invasively through an intra-arterial catheter. Most of these patients have one or several cardiovascular risk factors. Laparoscopic procedures compromise CO and blood pressure should be closely monitored. Non-invasive pressure measurements are difficult to obtain due to the poor fit of blood pressure cuffs on the conical shape of the upper arms. If one decides to use non-invasive blood pressure measurements, one must be certain that the bladder in the cuff is long enough to encircle at least 75% of the circumference of the arm. Blood pressure measurements with a constant, predictable bias can be obtained from the wrist, and this method could be an acceptable alternative.[138]

Technical assistance

The anaesthetist is frequently requested to place a bougie, nasogastric tube or intragastric balloon during surgery that the surgeon will use to size the gastric pouch or to calibrate the diameter of the stoma. The anaesthetist might also be asked to help perform the leak test by injecting air, methylene blue, etc. into the gastric tube to assess anastomotic integrity. This must be done carefully in order not to disrupt the staple line. Care must be taken to prevent introduction of methylene blue into the patient's lungs. All endo-gastric tubes must be removed completely before gastroplasty or gastric diversion is performed to avoid stapling or transecting these objects. Once the pouch has been formed, great care must be exercised when reintroducing the nasogastric tube.

Postoperative considerations

Extubation

The trachea should be extubated postoperatively only when the patient is fully awake and in a semi-recumbent position. Supplemental O_2 should be administered and pulse oximetric monitoring continued until it is certain that there is no longer a risk of alveolar hypoxia and hypoxaemia that would increase pulmonary vascular resistance. A course of nasal CPAP might be beneficial, particularly during the third to fifth night when rapid eye movement (REM) sleep rebound and sleep apnoea phases reach a maximum even when opioids are avoided.[139]

Postoperative analgesia

It is important to provide not only adequate pain relief at rest, but also to allow deep breathing and coughing. This is of particular importance in the obese patient due to the higher likelihood of alveolar collapse and atelectasis. The pain potential of laparoscopic operations is much lower than that of their conventional open counterparts. Regimens for postoperative pain therapy will have to take this into account and rely more on minor analgesics than on opiates.

We take a multimodal approach to postoperative pain therapy. Our first line analgesic is a more or less specific cyclo-oxygenase (Cox) 2 inhibitor. This can be diclofenac, naproxen, rofecoxib, valdecoxib or something similar. Ibuprofen is more specific for Cox-1, as is acetylsalicylic acid, and will inhibit thrombocyte function to a greater degree and cause more bleeding. Our initial analgesic is diclofenac 100 mg given as a suppository after induction of anaesthesia, or rofecoxib 50 mg or valdecoxib 40 mg given orally together with the premedication. The latter alternative is easier to comply with, less likely to be forgotten and thus preferable. The effect of the first agent is augmented postoperatively with intravenous paracetamol (acetaminophen). This combination is frequently sufficient to reduce the postoperative pain to a tolerable level and to make the patient comfortable. If not, the residual pain is treated by intravenous bolus injections of morphine (2 mg) as requested by the patient. Subcutaneous injections should be avoided, since absorption is extremely unreliable.

Continuous epidural analgesia is sometimes considered to be better than conventional pain therapy with intravenous opioids, involving less impairment of gastrointestinal function or sensorial obtundation. However, a study comparing epidural analgesia with bupivacaine and fentanyl to patient-controlled analgesia (PCA) with intravenous morphine after gastric bypass surgery was unable to confirm this.[140] There was no difference between the groups with regard to pain control, time to ambulation, time to first flatus, occurrence of nausea or pruritus, and length of hospital stay. Wound infection was 85% in the epidural group, but only 38% in the PCA group ($P < 0.01$). Epidural analgesia is not warranted in laparoscopic bariatric surgery, since there is only little pain and the procedures are designed to be minimally invasive and permit earliest possible ambulation.

Thromboprophylaxis

Morbid obesity is a major independent risk factor for death from postoperative pulmonary embolism on the basis of deep vein thrombosis.[141] Subcutaneously administered heparin (5000 IU every 12 h) reduces the incidence of thrombosis. Low molecular weight heparins are as effective as non-fractionated heparin in reducing postoperative deep vein thrombosis but more cost effective and with fewer side effects.[142] Both enoxaparin and nadroparin were effective in randomized studies.[143,144] A recent survey of the preferred method used to prevent thromboembolism in a large association for bariatric surgery showed that 50% used subcutaneous unfractionated heparin, 5000 IU every 8–12 h, 33% used pneumatic compression stockings and 13% used low molecular weight heparin.[145] Although the main responsibility of thromboprophylaxis rests with the surgeon, the anaesthetist can contribute to the efforts by giving an anaesthetic that allows earliest possible mobilization of the patient.

References

1. Wittgrove AC, Clark GW, Schubert KR. Laparoscopic gastric bypass, Roux-en-Y: technique and results in 75 patients with 3–30 months follow-up. *Obes Surg* 1996; **6**: 500–504.

2. Belachew M, Jacqet P, Lardinois F, Karler C. Vertical banded gastroplasty vs adjustable silicone gastric banding in the treatment of morbid obesity: a preliminary report. *Obes Surg* 1993; **3**: 275–278.

3. Chua TY, Mendiola RM. Laparoscopic vertical banded gastroplasty: the Milwaukee experience. *Obes Surg* 1995; **5**: 77–80.

4. Lonroth H, Dalenback J, Haglind E, Lundell L. Laparoscopic gastric bypass. Another option in bariatric surgery. *Surg Endosc* 1996; **10**: 636–638.

5. Wittgrove AC, Clark GW. Laparoscopic gastric bypass, Roux-en-Y- 500 patients: technique and results, with 3–60 month follow-up. *Obes Surg* 2000; **10**: 233–239.

6. Schauer PR, Ikramuddin S, Gourash W, Ramanathan R, Luketich J. Outcomes after laparoscopic Roux-en-Y gastric bypass for morbid obesity. *Ann Surg* 2000; **232**: 515–529.

7. National Institutes of Health Consensus Development Conference Statement. Health implications of obesity. *Ann Intern Med* 1985; **1013**: 147–151.

8. Pai MP, Paloucek FP. The origin of the "ideal" body weight equations. *Ann Pharmacother* 2000; **34**: 1066–1069.

9. Quetelet LAJ. Sur l'homme et le développement de ses facultés, essai d'une physique sociale. Paris; 1835.

10. Bray GA. Pathophysiology of obesity. *Am J Clin Nutr* 1992; **55**: 488S–494S.

11. International Obesity Task Force. About obesity: classification. 18 March 2004 18 www.iotf.org.

12. Mokdad AH, Serdula M, Dietz W. The spread of the obesity epidemic in the United States. *J Am Med Assoc* 1999; **282**: 1519–1522.

13. Mokdad AH, Ford ES, Bowman BA *et al*. Prevalence of obesity, diabetes, and obesity-related health risk factors, 2001. *J Am Med Assoc* 2003; **289**: 76–79.

14. Flegal KM, Carroll MD, Ogden CL, Johnson CL. Prevalence and trends in obesity among US adults, 1999–2000. *J Am Med Assoc* 2002; **288**: 1723–1727.

15. Erens B, Primatesta P (Eds), *Health Survey for England: Cardiovascular disease '98. Vol. 1. Findings.* London: Stationery Office, 1999.

16. Bergmann KE, Mensink GB. Anthropometrische Daten und Adipositas [Anthropometric data and obesity]. *Gesundheitswesen* 1999; **61**: S115–S120.

17. Maillard G, Charles MA, Thibult N *et al*. Trends in the prevalence of obesity in the French adult population between 1980 and 1991. *Int J Obes Relat Metab Disord* 1999; **23**: 389–394.

18. Charles MA, Basdevant A, Eschwege E. Prévalence de l'obésité de l'adulte en France. La situation en 2000. *Ann Endocrinol (Paris)* 2002; **63**: 154–158.

19. Garrison RJ, Castelli WP. Weight and thirty-year mortality of men in the Framingham study. *Ann Intern Med* 1985; **103**: 1006–1009.

20. Jonsson S, Hedblad B, Engstrom G, Nilsson P, Berglund G, Janzon L. Influence of obesity on cardiovascular risk. Twenty-three-year follow-up of 22,025 men from an urban Swedish population. *Int J Obes Relat Metab Disord* 2002; **26**: 1046–1053.

21. Manson JE, Willett WC, Stampfer MJ *et al*. Body weight and mortality among women. *New Engl J Med* 1995; **333**: 677–685.

22. Calle EE, Thun MJ, Petrelli JM, Rodriguez C, Heath Jr CW. Body-mass index and mortality in a prospective cohort of U.S. adults. *New Engl J Med* 1999; **341**: 1097–1105.

23. Mokdad AH, Marks JS, Stroup DF, Gerberding JL. Actual causes of death in the United States, 2000. *J Am Med Assoc* 2004; **291**: 1238–1245.

24. Chan JM, Rimm EB, Colditz GA, Stampfer MJ, Willett WC. Obesity, fat distribution, and weight gain as risk factors for clinical diabetes in men. *Diabet Care* 1994; **17**: 961–969.

25. Manson JE, Colditz GA, Stampfer MJ *et al*. A prospective study of obesity and risk of coronary heart disease in women. *New Engl J Med* 1990; **322**: 882–889.

26. Rimm EB, Stampfer MJ, Giovannucci E *et al*. Body size and fat distribution as predictors of coronary heart disease among middle-aged and older US men. *Am J Epidemiol* 1995; **141**: 1117–1127.

27. Brown CD, Higgins M, Donato KA *et al*. Body mass index and the prevalence of hypertension and dyslipidemia. *Obes Res* 2000; **8**: 605–619.

28. Young T, Palta M, Dempsey J, Skatrud J, Weber S, Badr S. The occurrence of sleep-disordered breathing among middle-aged adults. *New Engl J Med* 1993; **328**: 1230–1235.

29. Bergström A, Pisani P, Tenet V, Wolk A, Adami HO. Overweight as an avoidable cause of cancer in Europe. *Int J Cancer* 2001; **91**: 421–430.

30. Bacci V, Basso MS, Greco F *et al*. Modifications of metabolic and cardiovascular risk factors after weight loss induced by laparoscopic gastric banding. *Obes Surg* 2002; **12**: 77–82.

31. Boone KA, Cullen JJ, Mason EE, Scott DH, Doherty C, Maher JW. Impact of vertical banded gastroplasty on respiratory insufficiency of severe obesity. *Obes Surg* 1996; **6**: 454–458.

32. National Institute for Clinical Excellence. Final Appraisal Determination: Surgery to aid weight reduction for people with morbid obesity. 15 March 2004 http://www.nice.org.uk/article.asp?a = 32081.

33. Clegg A, Sidhu MK, Colquitt J, Royle P, Loveman E, Walker AM. Clinical and cost effectiveness of surgery for people with morbid obesity. 14 March 2004 http://www.nice.org.uk/pdf/surgicalobesityassessmentreport.pdf.

34. National Institute for Clinical Excellence. Guidance on the use of surgery to aid weight reduction for people with morbid obesity. London: NICE, 19 July 2002.

35. National Institutes of Health. NIH conference: gastrointestinal surgery for severe obesity. Consensus development conference panel. *Ann Intern Med* 1991; **115**: 956–961.

36. Martin LF, Tan TL, Horn JR *et al*. Comparison of the costs associated with medical and surgical treatment of obesity. *Surgery* 1995; **118**: 599–606.

37. National Institutes of Health. *Clincal Guidelines on the Identification, Evaluation, and Treatment of Overweight and Obesity in Adults. The Evidence Report.* Bethesda: National Heart, Lung, and Blood Institute, September 1998.

38. Pelosi P, Croci M, Ravagnan I *et al*. The effects of body mass on lung volumes, respiratory mechanics, and gas exchange during general anesthesia. *Anesth Analg* 1998; **87**: 654–660.

39. Biring MS, Lewis MI, Liu JT, Mohsenifar Z. Pulmonary physiologic changes of morbid obesity. *Am J Med Sci* 1999; **318**: 293–297.

40. Hakala K, Mustajoki P, Aittomaki J, Sovijarvi AR. Effect of weight loss and body position on pulmonary function

and gas exchange abnormalities in morbid obesity. *Int J Obes Relat Metab Disord* 1995; **19**: 343–346.

41. Santesson J, Nordenstrom J. Pulmonary function in extreme obesity. Influence of weight loss following intestinal shunt operation. *Acta Chir Scand Suppl* 1978; **482**: 36–40.

42. Hedenstierna G, Santesson J, Norlander O. Airway closure and distribution of inspired gas in the extremely obese, breathing spontaneously and during anaesthesia with intermittent positive pressure ventilation. *Acta Anaesthesiol Scand* 1976; **20**: 334–342.

43. Söderberg M, Thomson D, White T. Respiration, circulation and anaesthetic management in obesity. Investigation before and after jejunoileal bypass. *Acta Anaesthesiol Scand* 1977; **21**: 55–61.

44. Eichenberger A, Proietti S, Wicky S *et al.* Morbid obesity and postoperative pulmonary atelectasis: an underestimated problem. *Anesth Analg* 2002; **95**: 1788–1792.

45. Luce JM. Respiratory complications of obesity. *Chest* 1980; **78**: 626–631.

46. Pelosi P, Croci M, Ravagnan I, Vicardi P, Gattinoni L. Total respiratory system, lung, and chest wall mechanics in sedated-paralyzed postoperative morbidly obese patients. *Chest* 1996; **109**: 144–151.

47. Strandberg A, Tokics L, Brismar B, Lundquist H, Hedenstierna G. Atelectasis during anaesthesia and in the postoperative period. *Acta Anaesthesiol Scand* 1986; **30**: 154–158.

48. Hedenstierna G, Strandberg Å, Tokics L, Lundqvist H, Brismar B. Correlation of gas exchange impairment to development of atelectasis during anesthesia and muscle paralysis. *Acta Anaesthesiol Scand* 1986; **30**: 183–191.

49. Sprung J, Whalley DG, Falcone T, Warner DO, Hubmayr RD, Hammel J. The impact of morbid obesity, pneumoperitoneum, and posture on respiratory system mechanics and oxygenation during laparoscopy. *Anesth Analg* 2002; **94**: 1345–1350.

50. de Divitiis O, Fazio S, Petitto M, Maddalena G, Contaldo F, Mancini M. Obesity and cardiac function. *Circulation* 1981; **64**: 477–482.

51. Burwell CS, Robin Ed, Whaley RD, Bickelman AG. External obesity associated with alveolar hypoventilation – a Pickwickian syndrome. *Am J Med* 1956; **25**: 815–820.

52. Damia G, Mascheroni D, Croci M, Tarenzi L. Perioperative changes in functional residual capacity in morbidly obese patients. *Br J Anaesth* 1988; **60**: 574–578.

53. Wahba RW. Perioperative functional residual capacity. *Can J Anaesth* 1991; **38**: 384–400.

54. Casati A, Comotti L, Tommasino C *et al.* Effects of pneumoperitoneum and reverse Trendelenburg position on cardiopulmonary function in morbidly obese patients receiving laparoscopic gastric banding. *Eur J Anaesthesiol* 2000; **17**: 300–305.

55. Adams JP, Murphy PG, Carroll MD. Obesity in anaesthesia and intensive care. *Br J Anaesth* 2000; **85**: 91–108.

56. Shenkman Z, Shir Y, Brodsky JB. Perioperative management of the obese patient. *Br J Anaesth* 1993; **70**: 349–359.

57. Bardoczky GI, Yernault JC, Houben JJ, d'Hollander AA. Large tidal volume ventilation does not improve oxygenation in morbidly obese patients during anesthesia. *Anesth Analg* 1995; **81**: 385–388.

58. Sprung J, Whalley DG, Falcone T, Wilks W, Navratil JE, Bourke DL. The effects of tidal volume and respiratory rate on oxygenation and respiratory mechanics during laparoscopy in morbidly obese patients. *Anesth Analg* 2003; **97**: 268–274.

59. Salem MR, Dalal FY, Zygmunt MP, Mathrubhutham M, Jacobs HK. Does PEEP improve intraoperative arterial oxygenation in grossly obese patients? *Anesthesiology* 1978; **48**: 280–281.

60. Pelosi P, Ravagnan I, Giurati G *et al.* Positive end-expiratory pressure improves respiratory function in obese but not in normal subjects during anesthesia and paralysis. *Anesthesiology* 1999; **91**: 1221–1231.

61. Santesson J. Oxygen transport and venous admixture in the extremely obese. Influence of anaesthesia and artificial ventilation with and without positive endexpiratory pressure. *Acta Anaesthesiol Scand* 1976; **20**: 387–392.

62. Lean MEJ. Obesity and cardiovascular disease: the waisted years. *Br J Cardiol* 1999; **6**: 269–273.

63. Suter PM, Locher R, Hasler E, Vetter W. Is there a role for the ob gene product leptin in essential hypertension? *Am J Hypertens* 1998; **11**: 1305–1311.

64. Uckaya G, Ozata M, Sonmez A *et al.* Plasma leptin levels strongly correlate with plasma renin activity in patients with essential hypertension. *Horm Metab Res* 1999; **31**: 435–438.

65. Hall JE, Hildebrandt DA, Kuo J. Obesity hypertension: role of leptin and sympathetic nervous system. *Am J Hypertens* 2001; **14**: 103S–115S.

66. Mikhail N, Golub MS, Tuck ML. Obesity and hypertension. *Prog Cardiovasc Dis* 1999; **42**: 39–58.

67. Backman L, Freyschuss U, Hallberg D, Melcher A. Cardiovascular function in extreme obesity. *Acta Med Scand* 1973; **193**: 437–446.

68. Alpert MA, Lambert CR, Terry BE *et al.* Interrelationship of left ventricular mass, systolic function and diastolic filling in normotensive morbidly obese patients. *Int J Obes Relat Metab Disord* 1995; **19**: 550–557.

69. Hubert HB, Feinleib M, McNamara PM, Castelli WP. Obesity as an independent risk factor for cardiovascular disease: a 26-year follow-up of participants in the Framingham heart study. *Circulation* 1983; **67**: 968–977.

70. Duflou J, Virmani R, Rabin I, Burke A, Farb A, Smialek J. Sudden death as a result of heart disease in morbid obesity. *Am Heart J* 1995; **130**: 306–313.

71. Bharati S, Lev M. Cardiac conduction system involvement in sudden death of obese young people. *Am Heart J* 1995; **129**: 273–281.

72. Valensi P, Thi BN, Lormeau B, Paries J, Attali JR. Cardiac autonomic function in obese patients. *Int J Obes Relat Metab Disord* 1995; **19**: 113–118.

73. Alpert MA, Lambert CR, Terry BE *et al.* Influence of left ventricular mass on left ventricular diastolic filling

in normotensive morbid obesity. *Am Heart J* 1995; **130**: 1068–1073.

74. Berkalp B, Cesur V, Corapcioglu D, Erol C, Baskal N. Obesity and left ventricular diastolic dysfunction. *Int J Cardiol* 1995; **52**: 23–26.

75. de Simone G, Devereux RB, Mureddu GF *et al.* Influence of obesity on left ventricular midwall mechanics in arterial hypertension. *Hypertension* 1996; **28**: 276–283.

76. Paul DR, Hoyt JL, Boutros AR. Cardiovascular and respiratory changes in response to change of posture in the very obese. *Anesthesiology* 1976; **45**: 73–78.

77. Blouin RA, Kolpek JH, Mann HJ. Influence of obesity on drug disposition. *Clin Pharm* 1987; **6**: 706–714.

78. Noctor TA, Wainer IW, Hage DS. Allosteric and competitive displacement of drugs from human serum albumin by octanoic acid, as revealed by high-performance liquid affinity chromatography, on a human serum albumin-based stationary phase. *J Chromatogr* 1992; **577**: 305–315.

79. Messerli FH, Christie B, DeCarvalho JG *et al.* Obesity and essential hypertension. Hemodynamics, intravascular volume, sodium excretion, and plasma renin activity. *Arch Intern Med* 1981; **141**: 81–85.

80. Leslie K, Crankshaw DP. Lean tissue mass is a useful predictor of induction dose requirements for propofol. *Anaesth Intens Care* 1991; **19**: 57–60.

81. Bouillon T, Shafer SL. Does size matter? *Anesthesiology* 1998; **89**: 557–560.

82. Jung D, Mayersohn M, Perrier D, Calkins J, Saunders R. Thiopental disposition in lean and obese patients undergoing surgery. *Anesthesiology* 1982; **56**: 269–274.

83. Servin F, Farinotti R, Haberer JP, Desmonts JM. Propofol infusion for maintenance of anesthesia in morbidly obese patients receiving nitrous oxide. A clinical and pharmacokinetic study. *Anesthesiology* 1993; **78**: 657–665.

84. Greenblatt DJ, Abernethy DR, Locniskar A, Harmatz JS, Limjuco RA, Shader RI. Effect of age, gender, and obesity on midazolam kinetics. *Anesthesiology* 1984; **61**: 27–35.

85. Schwartz AE, Matteo RS, Ornstein E, Halevy JD, Diaz J. Pharmacokinetics and pharmacodynamics of vecuronium in the obese surgical patient. *Anesth Analg* 1992; **74**: 515–518.

86. Pühringer FK, Keller C, Kleinsasser A, Giesinger S, Benzer A. Pharmacokinetics of rocuronium bromide in obese female patients. *Eur J Anaesthesiol* 1999; **16**: 507–510.

87. Beemer GH, Bjorksten AR, Crankshaw DP. Pharmacokinetics of atracurium during continuous infusion. *Br J Anaesth* 1990; **65**: 668–674.

88. Rose JB, Theroux MC, Katz MS. The potency of succinylcholine in obese adolescents. *Anesth Analg* 2000; **90**: 576–578.

89. Varin F, Ducharme J, Theoret Y, Besner JG, Bevan DR, Donati F. Influence of extreme obesity on the body disposition and neuromuscular blocking effect of atracurium. *Clin Pharmacol Ther* 1990; **48**: 18–25.

90. Weinstein JA, Matteo RS, Ornstein E, Schwartz AE, Goldstoff M, Thal G. Pharmacodynamics of vecuronium and atracurium in the obese surgical patient. *Anesth Analg* 1988; **67**: 1149–1153.

91. Schwartz AE, Matteo RS, Ornstein E, Young WL, Myers KJ. Pharmacokinetics of sufentanil in obese patients. *Anesth Analg* 1991; **73**: 790–793.

92. Slepchenko G, Simon N, Goubaux B, Levron JC, Le Moing JP, Raucoules Aime M. Performance of target-controlled sufentanil infusion in obese patients. *Anesthesiology* 2003; **98**: 65–73.

93. Egan TD, Huizinga B, Gupta SK *et al.* Remifentanil pharmacokinetics in obese versus lean patients. *Anesthesiology* 1998; **89**: 562–573.

94. Lange H, Stephan H, Zielmann S, Sonntag H. Hepatic disposition of sufentanil in patients undergoing coronary bypass surgery. *Acta Anaesthesiol Scand* 1993; **37**: 154–158.

95. Koren G, Barker C, Goresky G *et al.* The influence of hypothermia on the disposition of fentanyl – human and animal studies. *Eur J Clin Pharmacol* 1987; **32**: 373–376.

96. Lange H, Stephan H, Brand C, Zielmann S, Sonntag H. Hepatic disposition of methohexitone in patients undergoing coronary bypass surgery. *Br J Anaesth* 1992; **69**: 478–481.

97. Ribstein J, du Cailar G, Mimran A. Combined renal effects of overweight and hypertension. *Hypertension* 1995; **26**: 610–615.

98. Brochner-Mortensen J, Rickers H, Balslev I. Renal function and body composition before and after intestinal bypass operation in obese patients. *Scand J Clin Lab Invest* 1980; **40**: 695–702.

99. Vaughan RW, Bauer S, Wise L. Volume and pH of gastric juice in obese patients. *Anesthesiology* 1975; **43**: 686–689.

100. Gryback P, Naslund E, Hellstrom PM, Jacobsson H, Backman L. Gastric emptying of solids in humans: improved evaluation by Kaplan–Meier plots, with special reference to obesity and gender. *Eur J Nucl Med* 1996; **23**: 1562–1567.

101. Zacchi P, Mearin F, Humbert P, Formiguera X, Malagelada JR. Effect of obesity on gastroesophageal resistance to flow in man. *Dig Dis Sci* 1991; **36**: 1473–1480.

102. Kuzmak LI. A review of seven years' experience with silicone gastric banding. *Obes Surg* 1991; **1**: 403–408.

103. Belachew M, Zimmermann JM. Evolution of a paradigm for laparoscopic adjustable gastric banding. *Am J Surg* 2002; **184**: 21s–25s.

104. Favretti F, Cadiere GB, Segato G *et al.* Laparoscopic banding: selection and technique in 830 patients. *Obes Surg* 2002; **12**: 385–390.

105. Mason EE. Vertical banded gastroplasty for obesity. *Arch Surg* 1982; **117**: 701–706.

106. Baddeley RM. The management of gross refractory obesity by jejuno-ileal bypass. *Br J Surg* 1979; **66**: 525–532.

107. Schmeisser W, Schrader CP, Greim H, von Oldershausen HF. Leberschaden nach intestinaler

Kurzschlussoperation zur Gewichtsreduktion [Liver damage following intestinal by-pass surgery for weight reduction]. *Z Gastroenterol* 1975; **13**: 619–628.

108. Solhaug JH, Grundt I. Metabolic changes after jejuno-ileal bypass for obesity. *Scand J Gastroenterol* 1978; **13**: 169–175.

109. Mason EE, Ito C. Gastric bypass in obesity. *Surg Clin North Am* 1967; **47**: 1345–1351.

110. Scopinaro N, Gianetta E, Adami GF *et al.* Biliopancreatic diversion for obesity at eighteen years. *Surgery* 1996; **119**: 261–268.

111. Marceau P, Biron S, Bourque RA, Potvin M, Hould FS, Simard S. Biliopancreatic diversion with a new type of gastrectomy. *Obes Surg* 1993; **3**: 29–35.

112. Hess DS, Hess DW. Biliopancreatic diversion with a duodenal switch. *Obes Surg* 1998; **8**: 267–282.

113. Warner MA, Warner ME, Martin JT. Ulnar neuropathy. Incidence, outcome, and risk factors in sedated or anesthetized patients. *Anesthesiology* 1994; **81**: 1332–1340.

114. Ogunnaike BO, Jones SB, Jones DB, Provost D, Whitten CW. Anesthetic considerations for bariatric surgery. *Anesth Analg* 2002; **95**: 1793–1805.

115. Mallampati SR, Gatt SP, Gugino LD *et al.* A clinical sign to predict difficult tracheal intubation: a prospective study. *Can Anaesth Soc J* 1985; **32**: 429–434.

116. Buckley FP, Robinson NB, Simonowitz DA, Dellinger EP. Anaesthesia in the morbidly obese. A comparison of anaesthetic and analgesic regimens for upper abdominal surgery. *Anaesthesia* 1983; **38**: 840–851.

117. Michaloudis D, Fraidakis O, Petrou A *et al.* Continuous spinal anesthesia/analgesia for perioperative management of morbidly obese patients undergoing laparotomy for gastroplastic surgery. *Obes Surg* 2000; **10**: 220–229.

118. Nguyen NT, Lee SL, Goldman C *et al.* Comparison of pulmonary function and postoperative pain after laparoscopic versus open gastric bypass: a randomized trial. *J Am Coll Surg* 2001; **192**: 469–476.

119. Salihoglu Z, Demiroluk S, Demirkiran, Kose Y. Comparison of effects of remifentanil, alfentanil and fentanyl on cardiovascular responses to tracheal intubation in morbidly obese patients. *Eur J Anaesthesiol* 2002; **19**: 125–128.

120. Salihoglu Z, Karaca S, Kose Y, Zengin K, Taskin M. Total intravenous anesthesia versus single breath technique and anesthesia maintenance with sevoflurane for bariatric operations. *Obes Surg* 2001; **11**: 496–501.

121. Juvin P, Vadam C, Malek L, Dupont H, Marmuse JP, Desmonts JM. Postoperative recovery after desflurane, propofol, or isoflurane anesthesia among morbidly obese patients: a prospective, randomized study. *Anesth Analg* 2000; **91**: 714–719.

122. De Baerdemaeker LE, Struys MM, Jacobs S *et al.* Optimization of desflurane administration in morbidly obese patients: a comparison with sevoflurane using an 'inhalation bolus' technique. *Br J Anaesth* 2003; **91**: 638–650.

123. Torri G, Casati A, Albertin A *et al.* Randomized comparison of isoflurane and sevoflurane for laparoscopic gastric banding in morbidly obese patients. *J Clin Anesth* 2001; **13**: 565–570.

124. Sollazzi L, Perilli V, Modesti C *et al.* Volatile anesthesia in bariatric surgery. *Obes Surg* 2001; **11**: 623–626.

125. Torri G, Casati A, Comotti L, Bignami E, Santorsola R, Scarioni M. Wash-in and wash-out curves of sevoflurane and isoflurane in morbidly obese patients. *Minerva Anestesiol* 2002; **68**: 523–527.

126. Fee JP, Black GW, Dundee JW *et al.* A prospective study of liver enzyme and other changes following repeat administration of halothane and enflurane. *Br J Anaesth* 1979; **51**: 1133–1141.

127. Bentley JB, Vaughan RW, Gandolfi AJ, Cork RC. Halothane biotransformation in obese and nonobese patients. *Anesthesiology* 1982; **57**: 94–97.

128. Aono J, Ueda K, Ueda W, Manabe M. Induction of anaesthesia in the lateral decubitus position in morbidly obese patients. *Br J Anaesth* 1999; **83**: 356.

129. Juvin P, Lavaut E, Dupont H *et al.* Difficult tracheal intubation is more common in obese than in lean patients. *Anesth Analg* 2003; **97**: 595–600.

130. Brodsky JB, Lemmens HJ, Brock Utne JG, Vierra M, Saidman LJ. Morbid obesity and tracheal intubation. *Anesth Analg* 2002; **94**: 732–736.

131. Voyagis GS, Kyriakis KP, Dimitriou V, Vrettou I. Value of oropharyngeal Mallampati classification in predicting difficult laryngoscopy among obese patients. *Eur J Anaesthesiol* 1998; **15**: 330–334.

132. Cormack RS, Lehane J. Difficult tracheal intubation in obstetrics. *Anaesthesia* 1984; **39**: 1105–1111.

133. Jense HG, Dubin SA, Silverstein PI, O'Leary-Escolas U. Effect of obesity on safe duration of apnea in anesthetized humans. *Anesth Analg* 1991; **72**: 89–93.

134. Keller C, Brimacombe J, Kleinsasser A, Brimacombe L. The laryngeal mask airway ProSeal(TM) as a temporary ventilatory device in grossly and morbidly obese patients before laryngoscope-guided tracheal intubation. *Anesth Analg* 2002; **94**: 737–740.

135. Frappier J, Guenoun T, Journois D *et al.* Airway management using the intubating laryngeal mask airway for the morbidly obese patient. *Anesth Analg* 2003; **96**: 1510–1515.

136. Ezri T, Hazin V, Warters D, Szmuk P, Weinbroum AA. The endotracheal tube moves more often in obese patients undergoing laparoscopy compared with open abdominal surgery. *Anesth Analg* 2003; **96**: 278–282.

137. Ledgerwood AM, Harrigan C, Saxe JM, Lucas CE. The influence of an anesthetic regimen on patient care, outcome, and hospital charges. *Am Surg* 1992; **58**: 527–533.

138. Emerick DR. An evaluation of non-invasive blood pressure (NIBP) monitoring on the wrist: comparison with upper arm NIBP measurement. *Anaesth Intens Care* 2002; **30**: 43–47.

139. Cronin AJ, Keifer JC, Davies MF, King TS, Bixler EO. Postoperative sleep disturbance: influences of opioids and pain in humans. *Sleep* 2001; **24**: 39–44.

140. Charghi R, Backman S, Christou N, Rouah F, Schricker T. Patient controlled i.v. analgesia is an acceptable pain management strategy in morbidly

obese patients undergoing gastric bypass surgery. A retrospective comparison with epidural analgesia. *Can J Anaesth* 2003; **50**: 672–678.

141. Blaszyk H, Wollan PC, Witkiewicz AK, Bjornsson J. Death from pulmonary thromboembolism in severe obesity: lack of association with established genetic and clinical risk factors. *Virchows Arch* 1999; **434**: 529–532.

142. Hull RD, Pineo GF, Raskob GE. The economic impact of treating deep vein thrombosis with low-molecular-weight heparin: outcome of therapy and health economy aspects. low-molecular-weight heparin versus unfractionated heparin. *Haemostasis* 1998; **28(Suppl S3)**: 8–16.

143. Kalfarentzos F, Stavropoulou F, Yarmenitis S *et al.* Prophylaxis of venous thromboembolism using two different doses of low-molecular-weight heparin (nadroparin) in bariatric surgery: a prospective randomized trial. *Obes Surg* 2001; **11**: 670–676.

144. Scholten DJ, Hoedema RM, Scholten SE. A comparison of two different prophylactic dose regimens of low molecular weight heparin in bariatric surgery. *Obes Surg* 2002; **12**: 19–24.

145. Wu EC, Barba CA. Current practices in the prophylaxis of venous thromboembolism in bariatric surgery. *Obes Surg* 2000; **10**: 7–13.

Minimally invasive endoscopic surgery of thoracic organs can be performed by bronchoscopy, mediastinoscopy or thoracoscopy and usually involves the lungs, the pericardium, the oesophagus, the thymus, the thoracic part of the sympathetic nervous system and occasionally the thoracic spine. The following, noninclusive list gives an idea of the scope of present indications for endoscopic thoracic surgery (Table 9.1).

Bronchoscopy

Bronchoscopy is possibly the oldest endoscopic procedure used in the diagnosis and treatment of intrathoracic disease processes. In 1897, Gustav Killian used a Mikulicz-Rosenheim oesophagoscope to extract a bone lodged in the right main bronchus of a 63-year-old man.[1] Chevalier Jackson and Victor Negus were instrumental in the introduction of the technique in the US and the UK. Innovations in fibre-optics led to the development of a flexible bronchoscope and its introduction into clinical practice by Shijeto Ikeda in 1968. The rise of the field of interventional pneumonology is directly related to improvements of bronchoscopic instruments. There is considerable overlap of the departments of otorhinolaryngology and interventional pneumonology in the treatment of airway tumours (see Chapter 10).

The modern rigid bronchoscope is a metal tube, available in various sizes, with a bevelled, slightly flared distal end, and a proximal end with a side-arm for attaching the anaesthetic breathing system (Figure 9.1). The open proximal end can be occluded with an eyepiece or a port, which allows the introduction of the rod telescope and permits simultaneous bronchoscopy and ventilation. Since the bronchoscope does not have a snug fit in the trachea there is always a gas leak of variable magnitude. Some bronchoscopes incorporate a channel to allow Venturi jet ventilation. Rigid bronchoscopy causes significant surgical stimulation and requires hyperextension of the neck, and is therefore routinely performed in general anaesthesia. The rigid bronchoscope in combination with a rod telescope gives a very detailed view and permits extensive endobronchial instrumentation, such as removal of foreign bodies, placement of stents and resection of airway tumours. Lasers are frequently used

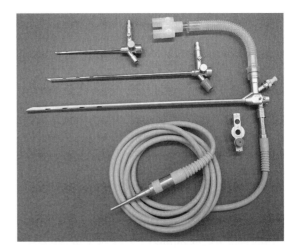

Figure 9.1 Rigid bronchoscopes in various sizes for patients ranging from the neonate to the adult. The instrument for the adult patient is equipped with a fibre-optic cable to the light source and has an attachment for connecting it to the anaesthesia machine. The end piece with a slider containing a closed glass observation port, an open aperture for inserting instruments and a self-sealing port for inserting the rod telescope is seen below the adult instrument.

Table 9.1 Techniques and indications in endoscopic thoracic surgery

Bronchoscopy

Rigid
- Removal of foreign bodies, stent placement, resection of airway tumours, diagnosis and treatment of haemoptysis, removal of granulations

Flexible
- Diagnostic, bronchial alveolar lavage, removal of secretions in intensive care patients

Mediastinoscopy
- Diagnostic biopsies (e.g. lung malignancies, lymphomas), treatment of retrosternal masses (e.g. thymus, thyroid gland)

Thoracoscopy
- Diagnostic, lung resection, (segment, lobe), pericardectomy, thoracic sympathectomy, oesophagus resection, resection of masses in lower mediastinum, spinal surgery

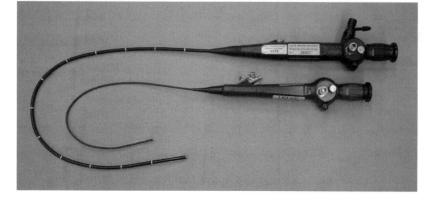

Figure 9.2 Flexible broncho-scopes for adult and paediatric patients. The thumb lever for manipulating the bronchoscope tip is seen at the lower edge of the headpiece adjacent to the eyepiece. The port for the instrument channel is visible on the upper distal edge of the headpiece. The larger instrument has a separate side-port for attaching and activating suction.

for the latter indication (see Chapter 10). The rigid bronchoscope is the instrument of choice in small children and in patients with massive endobronchial bleeding. Rigid bronchoscopy was displaced by flexible bronchoscopy in the 1970s and early 1980s, but the work of Jean-François Dumon in France brought about a renaissance of the technique in Europe.

The flexible bronchoscope consists of a long, tubular structure, available in various diameters, with a tip that can be moved up and down in one plane. Bundles of glass fibres are incorporated into this structure which conduct light from a cold-light source for illuminating the field under observation, and transmit the picture to the eyepiece. Larger instruments have a suction channel, which can also be used to introduce instruments, apply drugs or remove secretions. The view obtained with the flexible bronchoscope is not as defined as that of the telescopes used in rigid bronchoscopy, and the thinner the bronchoscope the poorer the view. One is also limited in the manipulations that are possible through the instrument channel. On the other hand, flexible bronchoscopy can be performed on the awake patient under topical anaesthesia. Flexible bronchoscopy is typically performed as an initial measure to inspect the airways and to obtain specimens for further assessment when airway pathology is suspected. It has a number of indications in the intensive care unit, such as removal of retained secretions from the bronchi of intubated and ventilated patients, confirmation of correct endotracheal tube position, and protected collection of specimens for the diagnosis of ventilator-associated infections.[2–6]

Preparing the patient for bronchoscopy

Children are commonly referred for bronchoscopy for removal of foreign bodies from the airway, diagnosis of airway stenosis (e.g. tracheomalacia) or for surgical treatment of tracheal papillomatosis. These patients are usually otherwise healthy. Adult patients presenting

for bronchoscopy other than for removal of a foreign body frequently have a long history of cigarette smoking, and consequently a hyper-reactive bronchial system, impaired pulmonary function and probably concomitant cardiovascular disease.

The preoperative assessment of these patients should be aimed at determining the severity of their cardiopulmonary impairment, and whether it can be improved. The routine preoperative investigation includes a standard laboratory work-up, 12-lead electrocardiogram (ECG) and chest radiograph. The latter may reveal atelectatic or consolidated areas, pneumothorax, pleural effusions, or a localized hyperinflated area indicative of a foreign body obstructing a bronchus in a ball-valve fashion (Figure 9.5(b)). Pulmonary function testing and a preoperative blood gas analysis are frequently indicated.

Rigid bronchoscopy requires hyperextension of the neck and the preoperative examination should include an assessment of the mobility of the cervical spine. Patients with cervical ankylosis, or micro- or retrognathism may not be suited for rigid bronchoscopy. Cervical involvement of chronic polyarthritis predisposes to luxation of the first and second cervical vertebrae with the risk of damage to the cervical spinal cord.

Premedication for bronchoscopy might include a short-acting benzodiazepine such as midazolam to relieve anxiety, but heavy sedation should be avoided in patients

---

Characteristics of patients presenting for bronchoscopy

- Foreign body removal
  - Usually children, usually healthy, atelectasis possible

- Pulmonary or bronchial pathology
  - Chronic obstructive lung disease (COLD), ischaemic heart disease, arterial hypertension, atelectasis, pleural effusions, pneumothorax, bronchus occlusion, hyper-reactive airways

with suspected airway obstruction. An anticholinergic drug, such as glycopyrrolate or atropine, is frequently given in the endeavour to reduce bronchial secretions and aid visualization.[7] But studies have shown that they are possibly ineffective in this respect,[8] and might increase the incidence of hypertension and cardiac dysrhythmias.[9] Patients should be given their regular antihypertensive, antidysrhythmic and bronchodilatory medication.

Cardiopulmonary complications are common during both flexible and rigid bronchoscopy[10–13] and monitoring should take this into account. Monitoring should include continuous ECG and pulse oximetry, non-invasive blood pressure measurement and capnometry during general anaesthesia. Measuring end-tidal carbon dioxide (CO_2) concentrations is difficult during rigid bronchoscopy due to the air leak around the instrument. Transcutaneous measurement of arterial carbon dioxide tension, as mentioned in Chapter 4, would be a suitable alternative during lengthy procedures. Airway pressure (P_{AW}) and expiratory gas flow should be monitored closely, since the bronchial irritation associated with the procedure can provoke bronchospasm.

Anaesthesia for bronchoscopy

Flexible bronchoscopy

Flexible bronchoscopy is commonly performed as an outpatient procedure on the awake, spontaneously breathing patient. General anaesthesia is reserved for patients unable to co-operate or otherwise unable to tolerate the procedure. The bronchoscope can be introduced through the mouth or the nose. If the latter is chosen, the nasal mucosa is anaesthetized with a topically applied local anaesthetic combined with a vasoconstrictor as a decongestant. The pharynx and hypopharynx can be anaesthetized by direct application of a local anaesthetic spray. The local anaesthetic can be applied to the larynx and lower airways by transcricothyroid injection, nebulization or application under direct vision through the instrument channel of the bronchoscope.[14] Considerable amounts of local anaesthetic are required for adequate anaesthesia, and plasma concentrations can reach toxic, and occasionally lethal levels.[15,16] One must be aware of this and observe the patient for signs of local anaesthetic toxicity.

If required, sedation can be provided by the intravenous application of midazolam or propofol. Propofol is more

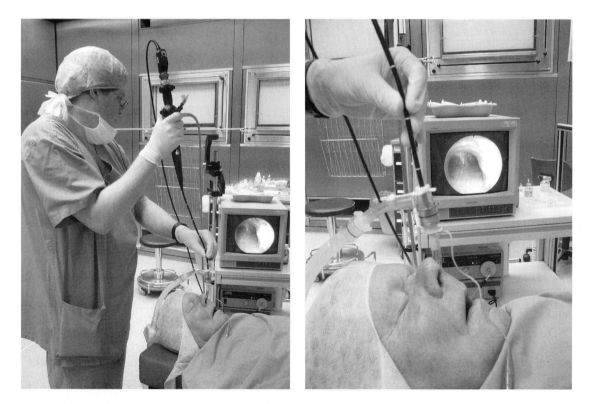

Figure 9.3 Flexible bronchoscopy through the endotracheal tube. The right picture shows the bronchoscope in the self-sealing adapter that allows simultaneous bronchoscopy and ventilation. The carina is visible on the video screen in the background.

expensive than midazolam but allows better control over the depth of sedation.[17,18] An opioid may be added to provide better analgesia and suppress the cough reflex to a certain degree, but one must keep the synergistic depressive effects on respiration in mind.

During general anaesthesia, the bronchoscope can be inserted through a self-sealing port in the angle piece connected to the endotracheal tube allowing ventilation to continue (Figure 9.3). The largest possible endotracheal tube must be used, since the bronchoscope significantly reduces the open cross section. Resistance to gas flow is increased in the endotracheal tube and the ventilatory pattern must be adapted accordingly with prolongation of the expiratory phase. Neuromuscular relaxation is not mandatory, but if desired, a short-acting agent should be used. Flexible bronchoscopy can also be performed through a laryngeal mask airway. The stem of the mask airway normally has a larger diameter than the endotracheal tube, and the increase in gas flow resistance caused by the bronchoscope will be less. Spontaneous respiration might be a feasible alternative in this case. Another alternative is to insert the bronchoscope through the aperture of a suitably modified face mask, such as the Patil mask (Figure 9.4).[19] There is no obstruction of airway tubing and little impairment of spontaneous respiration.

Rigid bronchoscopy

Rigid bronchoscopy is performed under general anaesthesia, usually with controlled ventilation. The patient is positioned with the upper body slightly elevated and the neck strongly retroflexed to give straight access to the larynx (Figure 9.5). Any general anaesthetic regimen is possible, but intravenous techniques are preferred, since the gas leak around the bronchoscope leads to a high level of workspace air pollution when volatile anaesthetics are used. A total intravenous technique with propofol and an opioid, such as remifentanil or alfentanil as described in Chapter 5, gives optimal control of the depth of anaesthesia. The plane of anaesthesia must be sufficiently deep to prevent airway responses such as bronchospasm, laryngospasm, or bucking and coughing. Neuromuscular relaxation is not mandatory, but with its judicious use the amount of anaesthetic can be reduced considerably. For short procedures lasting not longer than 10–15 min, intermittent bolus doses of propofol, methohexital or etomidate can be given. There is a certain risk of intraoperative awareness with this method when signs of awakening are used to guide the administration of the anaesthetic. Propofol administered by continuous infusion prevents awareness more

reliably, and should be used for all longer procedures. Muscle relaxation can be provided during very short procedures with the repetitive administration of succinylcholine, but a longer acting agent, such as mivacurium, atracurium, vecuronium or rocuronium, should be used if a duration of more than 10–15 min is anticipated in order to avoid prolonged competitive block from succinylcholine metabolites.[20]

Anaesthesia for rigid bronchoscopy of short duration

- Oral (or intravenous) premedication with short-acting benzodiazepine
- Alfentanil (20 μg kg^{-1}) or other suitable opioid. Wait for effect to set in (90 s)
- Induction with propofol, methohexital or etomidate (thiopental gives slower recovery)
- Relaxation with succinylcholine (1.5 mg kg^{-1}) after low-dose precurarization, if desired
- Maintenance with repeated doses of hypnotic and succinylcholine as required

---

Rigid bronchoscopy can be performed under inhalational anaesthesia on the spontaneously breathing patient, and this is still the method of choice in some centres. A deep plane of anaesthesia is required to abolish airway reflexes, and the line between excessive depth with hypoventilation on the one hand, and bronchospasm or laryngospasm due to inadequate anaesthesia, on the other, is narrow. Sevoflurane is superior to halothane with regard to incidence of complications and to recovery time.[21]

There are number of ways to manage ventilation during rigid bronchoscopy, among which are apnoeic oxygenation, use of the ventilating bronchoscope, and various methods of jet ventilation. The apnoeic technique and jet ventilation are described in detail in Chapter 10. The ventilating bronchoscope can be compared to an unblocked endotracheal tube with an undefined and changing volume of gas leakage around the distal end. Large leaks can be reduced by packing the posterior pharynx, mouth and nose with gauze. The proximal end of the bronchoscope has a cap with a slide that can occlude the opening with an eyepiece or allow introduction of the telescope through a self-sealing port (see Figure 9.1). The slide also has an opening through which instruments can be introduced for suctioning or removing material. The efficacy of ventilation with the ventilating bronchoscope is difficult to assess, since end-tidal gas contains an unknown amount of dead-space air and capnometry consistently yields values that are too low. There is thus a high risk of hypoventilation and hypercapnia, which is

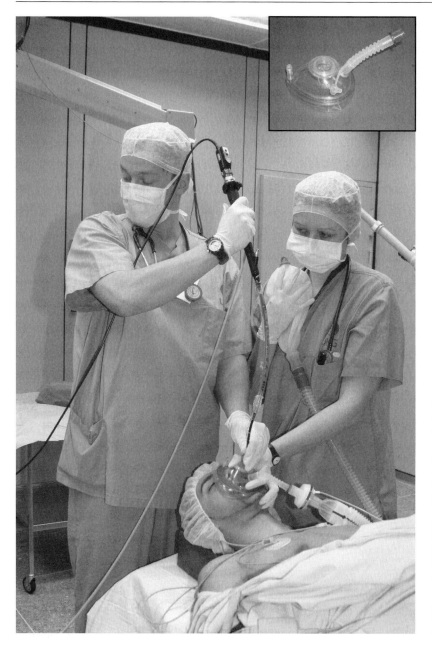

Figure 9.4 Flexible bronchoscopy through the self-sealing membrane in a face mask. The anaesthetist controls the airway and ventilation while the endoscopist performs the bronchoscopy. Both can follow the procedure on the video screen. The bronchoscope can be inserted either orally or through the nasal passage. A bite guard is used if the instrument is inserted through the mouth. (Photograph courtesy of Dr Arnd Timmermann, Department of Anaesthesiology, Emergency and Intensive Care Medicine, University of Göttingen.)

compounded by the interruption of ventilation that occurs whenever the slide is opened.

The pharynx should be inspected at the end of the procedures performed under general anaesthesia to remove secretions and blood. Neuromuscular block is reversed if necessary, the bronchoscope is removed and the airway is managed with a face mask and oropharyngeal tube. A laryngeal mask airway or endo–tracheal tube may also be inserted to maintain airway

patency. Patients with persisting haemorrhage or purulent infection in one lung should be positioned on their sides with the affected lung down in order to prevent contamination of the healthy lung.

Complications of bronchoscopy

The rigid bronchoscope can cause structural damage to the tracheobronchial system resulting in haemorrhage, oedema or mucosal perforation with subsequent

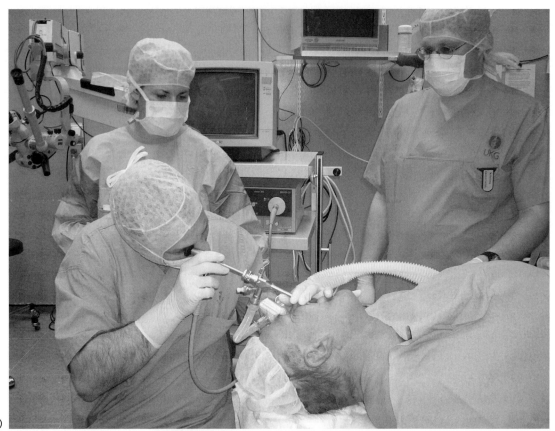

(a)

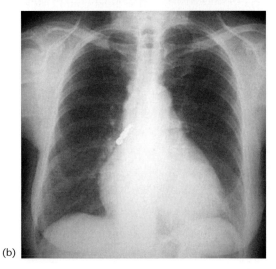

(b)

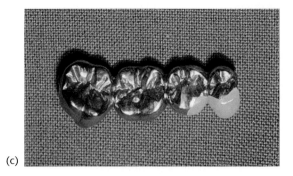

(c)

Figure 9.5 Rigid bronchoscopy. (a) Patient undergoing rigid bronchoscopy to remove foreign object. The bronchoscope is in place and the surgeon is inspecting the right bronchus with a rod telescope inserted through the bronchoscope. The flexible connection of the anaesthesia machine with the rigid bronchoscope is readily visible. (b) Foreign object visible in projection on the right main bronchus. The right upper lobe appears hyperinflated, which would be the case if the foreign object obstructed the right upper lobe bronchus. (c) Dental bridge removed from the right main bronchus of the patient. (Chest X-ray and photograph of bridge courtesy of Dr Ralph Rödel, Department of Otorhinolaryngology, University of Göttingen.)

Table 9.2 Complications of bronchoscopy

Mechanical effects
- Damage to teeth, larynx or vocal cords on insertion, bronchial or tracheal perforation, pneumothorax, subcutaneous emphysema, barotrauma, haemorrhage, airway obstruction

Physiological reactions
- Subglottic oedema, bronchospasm, laryngospasm, hypoxaemia, arterial hypertension, cardiac dysrhythmias, tachycardia

Foreign substances
- Local anaesthetic toxicity, loss of swabs or other material

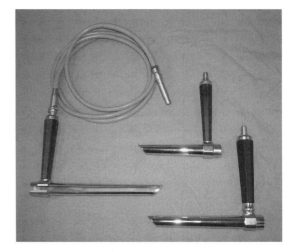

Figure 9.6 Mediastinoscopes of different sizes. The coiled flexible lightguide is connected to the fibre-optic light conductor integrated into the inner wall of the instrument.

subcutaneous emphysema or pneumothorax. Incorrectly applied jet ventilation can cause pulmonary barotrauma and pneumothorax (see Chapter 10).

Significant cardiovascular reactions with considerable increases of heart rate and arterial pressure and signs of myocardial ischaemia can occur during rigid bronchoscopy.[22,23] The magnitude and severity of the response is reduced when propofol is employed instead of thiopental. One might consider the intravenous administration of a beta-adrenergic antagonist, such as esmolol, atenolol or metoprolol, to improve cardiovascular stability. Cardiac dysrhythmias are common during rigid and flexible bronchoscopy. The intense vagal stimulation can induce bradycardia which occasionally requires treatment with atropine or glycopyrrolate. Other dysrhythmias are caused by sympathetic stimulation, and can be aggravated by hypoventilation with hypoxia and hypercapnia.[24,25] This should be corrected before pharmacological therapy is instituted.

Airway obstruction due to laryngeal oedema or laryngospasm can occur after completion of rigid bronchoscopy. Relaxation and reintubation of the trachea may be required in severe cases.

Mediastinoscopy

Carlens introduced cervical mediastinoscopy in 1959 as a method to obtain biopsy material from the superior mediastinum posterior to the great vessels without having to perform a thoracotomy.[26] In this procedure, a small transverse incision is made cephalad to the jugulum through which the mediastinoscope (Figure 9.6) is inserted behind the manubrium into the mediastinum. In the less common approach known as the Chamberlain procedure, or anterior mediastinoscopy, the instrument is inserted through a transverse

parasternal incision in the second intercostal interspace, usually on the left side. This approach gives access to the lower mediastinum on the side of the incision. During cervical mediastinoscopy the instrument is in direct contact with the great vessels of the upper thorax, with the oesophagus, the trachea and the recurrent laryngeal nerve (Figure 9.7).

Mediastinoscopy is primarily a procedure used to obtain tissue for the histological diagnosis of a mediastinal mass. This is crucial for planning therapy, since lymphomas, metastatic lung malignancies, sarcoidosis, thymomas or tuberculosis – to list the most commonly detected diseases – will each require a different therapeutic management. Improved resolution of magnetic resonance imaging and computed tomography has reduced the need for mediastinoscopy in many cases.

Mediastinoscopy is a relatively safe procedure with an incidence of major complications of approximately 0.5%[27] and an operative mortality of 0.1% in a series of more than 6000 patients.[28] There is little postoperative discomfort,[29] and the procedure is commonly performed on an outpatient basis. The unscheduled postoperative hospital admission rate is between 1% and 4%.[30–32] Mediastinoscopy is contraindicated as a repeat procedure since the plane of dissection is obliterated by scarring. Superior vena cava syndrome, severe tracheal deviation and thoracic aortic aneurysm are relative contraindications to the procedure.

Preparing the patient for mediastinoscopy

Patients scheduled for mediastinoscopy can present with a wide variety of clinical symptoms. They can

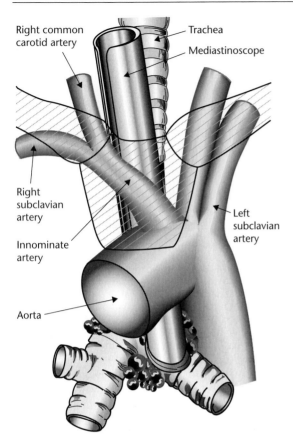

Figure 9.7 Topographical anatomy of upper mediastinum during mediastinoscopy. The mediastinoscope is in direct contact with the innominate artery, aorta and trachea. The innominate artery can be completely occluded by pressure with the instrument, which will cause loss of radial artery pulse in the right arm and right-sided cerebral ischaemia. (Adapted from Ref [26].)

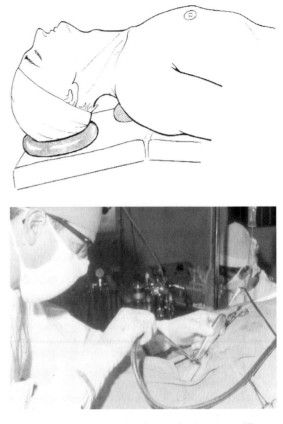

Figure 9.8 Patient position for mediastinoscopy. (Illustrations by courtesy of Dr Hilmar Dörge, Department of Cardiothoracic Surgery, University of Göttingen.) (a) The upper body is elevated and the neck is extended to give direct access to the manubrium and jugulum. (b) The surgeon makes a small transverse incision and inserts the mediastinoscope after blunt digital dissection of the correct plane.

range from the totally asymptomatic patient with a mediastinal mass discovered on a routine chest X-ray, to the dyspoeic, cyanotic patient with superior vena cava obstruction. Numerous diseases requiring a mediastinoscopy for ultimate diagnostic clarification are associated with clinically relevant, and typical, co-morbidities. Patients with small-cell lung cancer can suffer from a paraneoplastic syndrome with symptoms including hypercalcaemia, hyponatraemia, hypercortisolaemia, acromegaly, encephalitis, para- or quadriplegia secondary to necrotizing myelitis and Lambert–Eaton myasthenic syndrome. Thymoma is a common cause of an anterior mediastinal mass, and is frequently associated with myasthenia gravis. Approximately 5% of patients with sarcoidosis have significant cardiac dysfunction, with dysrhythmias, conduction disturbances, pericarditis, and congestive heart failure. The anaesthetist must be aware of the possibility of these co-existing diseases and actively search for signs or symptoms. Figure 9.8a illustrates the positioning of patient for mediastinoscopy.

> **Co-existing diseases in patients presenting for mediastinoscopy**
>
> - *Lung cancer*: paraneoplastic syndromes, dyspnoea, atelectasis, tracheal infiltration
> - *Thymoma*: myasthenia gravis
> - *Sarcoidosis*: myocardial dysfunction, cardiac dysrhythmias, congestive heart failure, pulmonary fibrosis

Mediastinoscopy carries a definite risk of haemorrhage, and at least two units of blood should be typed and cross-matched before the operation.

Anaesthetic management

An oral benzodiazepine can be given as premedication, but caution is advised in the patient with respiratory impairment or with myasthenia gravis. Two large-bore venous cannulae are inserted, one in the upper and one in the lower extremity. Blood pressure monitoring should be on the right arm, in order to detect compression of the innominate artery (see below). Some authors recommend measuring blood pressure on the left arm and monitoring blood flow in the right arm by radial artery cannulation, continuous palpation of the radial pulse, or pulse oximetry on a finger of the right hand. This will make it easier to differentiate between a spurious decrease in blood pressure due to vascular compression and hypotension resulting from blood loss, while still allowing early detection of innominate artery compression.

Mediastinoscopy has been performed under local anaesthesia[33] (not recommended) but general anaesthesia with endotracheal intubation and controlled ventilation is preferable; surgery can proceed with fewer interruptions, and the risk of pulmonary air embolism is reduced. In patients without respiratory obstruction, anaesthesia is induced with propofol, etomidate or a short-acting barbiturate after adequate pre-oxygenation and administration of an opioid. Tracheal intubation is facilitated by the administration of a neuromuscular blocking agent. The effect and duration of action of these agents is enhanced in patients with myasthenia. The dose must be reduced in these patients and neuromuscular transmission must be monitored. Fibre-optic awake intubation or inhalation induction and tracheal intubation in deep anaesthesia should be considered in patients with significant airway obstruction.

A balanced anaesthetic technique with a combination of an opioid and propofol or a volatile anaesthetic, such as isoflurane, desflurane or sevoflurane, is used for maintenance. Nitrous oxide should be avoided due to the potential risk of pulmonary air embolism (see Chapter 6).

Complications

Although the incidence of complications of mediastinoscopy is fairly low, those that do occur can be sudden, severe and life threatening.[28,34] Massive haemorrhage from an injured or transected large, intrathoracic vessel is the most serious acute complication. Access to the vessels through the mediastinoscope is difficult at best, and transected ends tend to retract out of reach. The initial treatment is therefore to pack the mediastinum with a gauze tamponade, which can

be left in place at least overnight. If this does not stop the bleeding and vital signs begin to deteriorate, a thoracotomy is necessary. The posterolateral approach is most commonly used, but a median sternotomy is sometimes required.[35] The role of the anaesthetist is to replace blood losses, preferably with blood, ensure adequate perfusion pressure pharmacologically, treat cardiac dysrhythmias, and, if required, induce deliberate hypotension to reduce blood loss. It is not advisable to lose precious time in replacing the initially inserted endotracheal tube with a double-lumen tube. Transpleural surgical access can be facilitated by temporarily disconnecting the anaesthesia machine, and compressing and retracting the lung before resuming ventilation. Fluids and blood should be infused through the venous cannula in the lower extremity, since it might simply drain from the injured vessel into the mediastinum before reaching the right atrium if infused into an arm vein.

Pneumothorax is the second most common major complication of mediastinoscopy. It is usually not detected until the postoperative period, and rarely requires decompression,[28] but all patients should have a postoperative chest X-ray. Tension pneumothorax, occasionally even bilateral, can occur intraoperatively, causing an increase in P_{AW}, hypotension, arterial desaturation and reduced breath sounds on the affected side. This complication requires immediate treatment with a chest tube.[36]

Compression of the innominate artery can critically reduce blood flow in the right carotid artery leading to cerebral ischaemia with cerebral oedema and transient or even permanent hemiparesis. Since compression of the innominate artery also causes loss of the right radial pulse, this complication can be detected by continuous blood pressure measurement in the right arm.[37]

In a series of over 2000 patients undergoing mediastinoscopy, Puhakka found three cases of tracheal rupture and two cases of pericardial damage.[27] P_{AW} must be monitored closely, since compression of the trachea can impair ventilation. Pressure on the aorta can induce reflex bradycardia. Recurrent laryngeal nerve paralysis, if it occurs, is permanent in about 50% of the cases.[28] Pulmonary air embolism can occur if intrathoracic veins are opened, and the incidence of this complication is likely to be higher in the spontaneously breathing patient.

Thoracoscopy

As at the inception of laparoscopy, a cystoscope was used to perform the first recorded thoracoscopy. In 1910, Hans Christian Jacobeus, a Swedish internist

Table 9.3 Complications of mediastinoscopy[28,34]

- Haemorrhage, occasionally exsanguinating
- Pneumothorax
- Recurrent laryngeal nerve paralysis
- Infection
- Phrenic nerve injury
- Left hemiparesis following compression of the innominate artery
- Reflex bradycardia due to pressure on aorta
- Oesophageal injury
- Chylothorax
- Pulmonary air embolism
- Tracheal rupture, tracheal compression
- Pericardial injuries

Table 9.4 Selected operations in thoracoscopic surgery

Lungs and pleura
- Wedge resection, segmental resection, atypical resections
- Excision of bullae
- Lobectomy
- Pneumonectomy
- Removal of pulmonary metastases
- Diagnosis and treatment of pleural diseases

Heart
- Pericardectomy, pericardiocentesis
- Coronary artery surgery
- Implantation of AICD devices

Oesophagus
- Oesophagectomy
- Suture of oesophageal perforations

Mediastinum
- Removal of mediastinal masses

Thoracic spine
- Disc herniation
- Instrumentation and correction of spinal deformities

Miscellaneous
- Thoracic sympathectomy for hyperhidrosis
- Vagotomy

AICD: automatic implantable cardioverter defibrillator.

working in a tuberculosis sanatorium, performed a thoracoscopic lysis of pleural adhesions as preparation for lung collapse therapy.[38] In the following years, he gathered considerable experience in the use of thoracoscopy in the diagnosis of intrathoracic tumours.[39] Thoracoscopy was commonly used early on to avoid the risks of general anaesthesia and thoracotomy in patients with severe co-morbidity. The procedures were very short and were performed on the spontaneously breathing patient under local anaesthesia, perhaps with the instillation of local anaesthetic into the pleural cavity. The reader is referred to Braimbridge[40] for an intimate account of the early history of the technique.

Although not the sole indication, treatment of pulmonary tuberculosis was the primary indication for thoracoscopy, and the technique was largely abandoned following the advent of tuberculostatic drugs. It was resurrected in Europe in the following decades as an elegant, minimally invasive procedure for the diagnosis of pleural tumours and treatment of pleural effusions and later adopted in the US.[41–43]

The development of video-assisted thoracoscopic surgery (VATS) and the introduction of laser surgery led to an explosive diversification of the indications for thoracoscopic surgery in the past 10–15 years, which now include procedures lasting several hours and making great demands on the physiological reserves of the patient and the skill of the anaesthetist. The first reports of a video-assisted thoracoscopic lobectomy by Kirby in 1993[44] were followed shortly after by the report of a thoracoscopic pneumonectomy by Walker.[45] VATS has been used for operations ranging from the treatment of recurrent pneumothorax and bullous lung disease, to oesophageal resection and aortocoronary bypass surgery, thoracic sympathectomy, invasive assessment and therapy of thoracic injuries in trauma patients to operations on the thoracic spine[46–51] (Table 9.4).

Physiology of the lateral decubitus position and open chest

Thoracoscopic operations are performed with the patient in the lateral decubitus position, and the lung on the affected side is allowed to collapse to optimize surgical access. This combination has considerable adverse effects on respiratory physiology, and dealing with it in a competent manner is one of the primary anaesthesiological concerns during thoracoscopic surgery.

The lateral decubitus position itself has little effect on the ventilation–perfusion ratio or on oxygenation in the spontaneously breathing patient with a closed chest. The effects of gravity dictate that blood flow is greater in the dependent lung, while ventilation of the dependent lung is also greater as a result of the cephalad shift of the dependent hemidiaphragm, which shifts the respiratory mechanics of the dependent hemithorax onto the steep slope of the pulmonary pressure–volume curve (Figure 9.9(a)). Both blood flow and perfusion are reduced in the non-dependent lung, and the ventilation–perfusion ratio is approximately unity in both lungs. Negative pressure in the

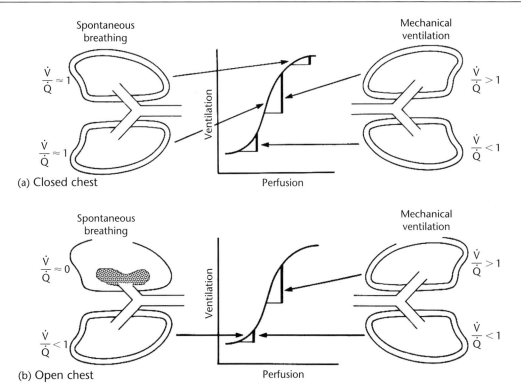

Figure 9.9 Schematic illustration of the changes in the ventilation–perfusion and pressure–volume relationships in a patient with closed or open thorax and spontaneous breathing or mechanical ventilation in the lateral decubitus position. (Modified from Ref [52].)

non-dependent pleura prevents a downward shift of the mediastinum.

Induction of anaesthesia and institution of mechanical ventilation in the patient in the lateral decubitus position does not alter the distribution of the pulmonary blood flow in the dependent and non-dependent lungs. The distribution of ventilation, on the other hand, changes radically. The reduction in functional residual capacity (FRC) that occurs after induction of anaesthesia causes each lung to move to a different position on the pressure–volume curve. The dependent lung moves down from the efficient, steep part of the curve onto the flat, non-compliant part, while the non-dependent lung shifts to a more compliant volume (Figure 9.9(a)). This increases the venous admixture in the dependent lung and the dead-space ventilation (V_D/V_T) in the non-dependent lung.

Opening the non-dependent hemithorax removes the negative intrathoracic pressure and causes the mediastinum to shift downward in the spontaneously breathing patient under the influence of gravity and the negative intrapleural pressure in the dependent hemithorax. Descent of the hemidiaphragm during active inspiration increases the negative pressure in the dependent hemithorax causing a further downward shift of the mediastinum. Tidal volume is reduced by the amount of the mediastinal shift. This can not only impair ventilation, but also venous return to the right heart. Loss of negative intrathoracic pressure allows the non-dependent lung to collapse under the influence of its unopposed elastic recoil. During spontaneous breathing with an open chest, gas is essentially sucked from the non-dependent lung during inspiration causing it to collapse still further. During expiration, air exiting the dependent lung enters the non-dependent lung inducing a slight re-inflation of the latter. This reversal of normal lung movement is referred to as "paradoxical respiration" (Figure 9.10). The ventilation–perfusion ratio falls below unity in both lungs with a subsequent increase in shunt perfusion and venous admixture (Figure 9.9(b)).

Positive pressure ventilation of the patient with an open chest in the lateral decubitus position can alleviate some of the problems arising in the spontaneously breathing patient. Mediastinal shift and paradoxical respiration are reduced, but the patient may still have a considerable ventilation–perfusion mismatch with

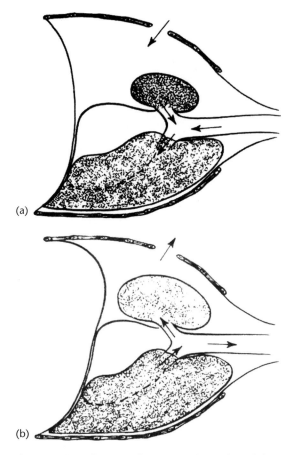

(a)

(b)

Figure 9.10 Schematic illustration of paradoxical lung movement in a patient with an open chest breathing spontaneously in the lateral decubitus position. (Adapted from Ref [53].) (a) During inspiration, the non-dependent, collapsed lung in the open hemithorax collapses further as air moves from it into the dependent lung. (b) During expiration, the collapsed lung expands as exhaled air enters it from the dependent lung.

Table 9.5 Cardiovascular effects of artificial pneumothorax with CO_2[55]	
Inflation pressure	**Effects (%)**
5 mmHg	
CI	−36
SV	−34
LVSWI	−49
15 mmHg	
MAP	−64
CI	−81
LVSWI	−95

CI: cardiac index; SV: stoke volume; MAP: mean arterial pressure; LVSWI: left ventricular stroke work index.

clinically relevant venous admixture and hypoxia. Perfusion remains higher in the dependent lung, but ventilation is now greater in the non-dependent lung. The ventilation–perfusion ratio changes to shunt perfusion in the dependent and V_D/V_T in the non-dependent lung (Figure 9.9(b)). The impairment of surgical access and progress of the operation caused by the inflated non-dependent lung can be avoided by allowing this lung to collapse and ventilating only the dependent lung, a technique known as one-lung ventilation (OLV). Attempts have occasionally been made to improve visibility even more by insufflating the pleural cavity with CO_2, but this has been shown to cause significant haemodynamic compromise in animal studies[54] as well as in patients[55] (Table 9.5).

One-lung ventilation

Although thoracoscopy was originally only considered a relative indication for OLV, the ventilatory technique has now become a virtual standard for all intrathoracic procedures, including thoracoscopic surgery. It is not absolutely indicated – thoracoscopy can be performed with two-lung ventilation in a pinch – but it has a very high priority.

Lung separation

OLV requires separation of the right and left lungs, and the standard method for achieving this is the double-lumen endotracheal tube. Bronchial blockers can be used in certain situations, and endobronchial intubation with a suitably long, single-lumen tube can be used to selectively ventilate one lung if other methods are not available.

A double-lumen endotracheal tube is essentially two tubes connected side by side, each with its own inflatable cuff and its own connector for the anaesthesia machine (Figure 9.11). One tube is intended to enter a bronchus, while the other is considerably shorter and ends in the trachea. Double-lumen endotracheal tubes are available as right- or left-sided models, depending on which main bronchus the tip is intended to enter. Both models permit separate inflation of each lung, but the left-sided tube is usually preferred. The peculiar anatomy of the bronchial tree makes it difficult to avoid occluding the right upper lobe bronchus when a right-sided tube is used. The right-sided tube has a separate opening at the tip ("Murphy eye") and a modification of the cuff designed to prevent obstruction of the right upper lobe bronchus.

The correct position is initially determined by auscultation of the chest while selectively ventilating each lung. This alone is not sufficient, and the proper position

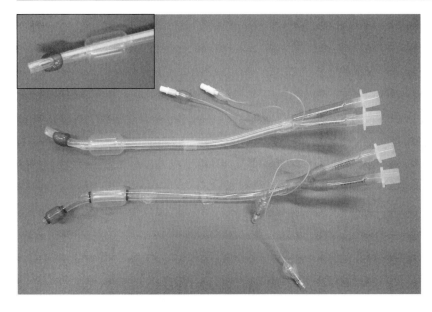

Figure 9.11 Double-lumen endotracheal tubes. The deviation of the tips of the endobronchial portion is readily visible. The right-sided tube is at the top and the left-sided tube below. The inset shows the "Murphy eye", an opening at the tip of the endobronchial catheter with a modification of the cuff of the right-sided double-lumen endotracheal tube. This is to prevent occlusion of the right upper lobe bronchus when the tip is in position.

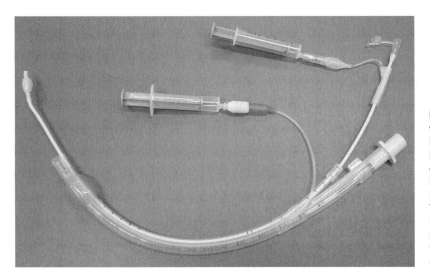

Figure 9.12 Endotracheal tube with integrated endobronchial blocker. This is positioned in the bronchus to be blocked under direct vision through a flexible bronchoscope and the cuff inflated to occlude the bronchus. The blocking catheter has an internal lumen through which the lung can be deflated, secretions can be removed and CPAP applied.

must be confirmed by fibre-optic bronchoscopy, since studies have shown the tube to be malpositioned in up to almost half of the cases even though clinical signs had been positive.[56] If not confirmed by bronchoscopy and corrected if necessary, troubles with intraoperative separation of the lungs and selective ventilation can arise in up to 25% of the patients.[57] The correct position is verified after intubation in the supine patient and then reaffirmed after the patient has been brought into the lateral decubitus position. The bronchoscope must remain available during surgery, since dislocation of the endobronchial tip is not infrequent, particularly during surgical manipulation of intrathoracic organs.

Lung separation can be achieved in small patients, for whom the smallest double-lumen tube is too large, with a bronchial blocker, an implement that is not essentially different from a Fogarty catheter. In fact, Fogarty catheters are still frequently used for this purpose. The bronchial blocker is introduced into the trachea alongside the endotracheal tube and is advanced into the desired position under direct vision through a fibre-optic bronchoscope. Endotracheal tubes have been developed with a separate channel in their wall through which the bronchial blocker can be passed[58] (Figure 9.12). Bronchial blockade with a simple catheter has a number of disadvantages compared with the double-lumen endotracheal tube for lung separation, among which are incomplete collapse of the non-dependent lung, and no way to effectively suction or independently ventilate the non-dependent lung. Modern blocking catheters have an internal lumen that allows suctioning and application of continuous positive airway pressure (CPAP) to the non-ventilated lung. In a recent study no difference was seen in effectiveness of lung collapse, or oxygen (O_2) saturation and fraction of inspired O_2 between a double-lumen endotracheal tube and a bronchial blocker for minimally invasive coronary artery surgery.[59]

Physiology of OLV

After collapse of the non-dependent lung, there is an obligatory transpulmonary right-to-left shunt of blood past non-ventilated alveoli that increases venous admixture and lowers arterial O_2 tension. The alveolar–arterial O_2 tension difference ($P_AO_2 - P_aO_2$) is larger during OLV than when both lungs are ventilated. But there are a number of factors that prevent arterial oxygen tension from decreasing to dangerous levels as precipitously as one would expect based on calculations of blood flow and ventilation.[60] The most important of these is the increase in vascular resistance in the non-ventilated lung known as hypoxic pulmonary vasoconstriction (HPV), which was first described by von Euler and Liljestrand.[61] This autoregulatory mechanism acts to divert blood flow away from non-ventilated areas to the ventilated lung, thereby preserving adequate arterial oxygen tension despite pulmonary atelectasis. The effects of HPV are enhanced by the influence of gravity in the lateral decubitus position. Cross-clamping the vessels of the non-ventilated lung will completely abolish shunt perfusion and increase arterial oxygen tension.

Most volatile anaesthetics have been shown to impair HPV and to cause arterial desaturation in an experimental setting.[62–65] In an elegant study using perfusion scans and separate lung ventilation with a double-lumen endotracheal tube, Bjertnæs showed that halothane inhibited HPV in humans in clinically relevant concentrations.[66] This effect is difficult to demonstrate in patients undergoing thoracic surgery due to the confounding effects of the anaesthetic on the circulation, but studies seem to indicate that isoflurane has less effect on arterial oxygenation and HPV than other volatiles.[67,68] Propofol and opioids have no effect on HPV or oxygenation,[69–72] in fact, propofol might even enhance HPV.[73] Yet, strangely enough, many authors still recommend inhalational anaesthesia as the anaesthetic of choice for thoracoscopic surgery,

even though all volatile anaesthetics have a detrimental effects on arterial oxygenation during one-lung anaesthesia. Volatile anaesthetics do have the theoretical advantage over intravenous agents of inducing bronchodilatation, a desired effect in patients with COLD. However, airway narrowing and closure in the typical COLD patient presenting for thoracoscopic surgery is more likely to be due to inflammation and loss of elasticity than to increased bronchomotor tone, and the theoretical benefit of the volatiles would be unlikely to outweigh the impaired oxygenation.

Practical management of OLV

OLV induces an obligatory right-to-left shunt of varying magnitude through the non-ventilated lung with a consequent fall in arterial O_2 saturation (S_aO_2). The primary goal of optimal management of OLV is to maintain S_aO_2 at a safe level above 90%. Further, secondary, goals are to ensure adequate elimination of CO_2 and, finally, to provide good operating conditions for the surgeon, in that order. If S_aO_2 is too low, the first measure is to confirm the correct position of the endobronchial tip, and to increase the inspiratory O_2 fraction, even to 1.0, if necessary. Faced with significant shunt perfusion, the latter measure will often not be sufficient to solve the problem, since blood flowing through the ventilated lung will not be able to take up enough O_2 to compensate for the venous admixture in the non-ventilated lung. However, the benefits of even a slight increase in P_aO_2 will outweigh the theoretical adverse effects of inspiring 100% O_2, such as O_2 toxicity. The dependent lung is ventilated with a tidal volume of about $10\,ml\,kg^{-1}$ body weight and with a respiratory rate sufficient to maintain partial pressure of arterial CO_2 (P_aCO_2) near $40\,mmHg$.

If hypoxia persists, the next step is to apply $5–10\,cmH_2O$ of CPAP to the non-ventilated lung. This is the single, most effective measure to improve arterial oxygenation and can substantially increase arterial oxygen tension.[74] Continuous pressure maintains airway patency in the non-ventilated lung, counteracts the development of atelectasis to a certain extent, and allows a degree of apnoeic oxygenation of the blood still perfusing this lung. Clinical studies have shown that this does not interfere with the progress of surgery.

The FRC is also decreased in the dependent lung during OLV in the lateral decubitus position, and a certain amount of venous blood will flow around non-ventilated alveoli and add to the total amount of venous admixture in the pulmonary veins. One can attempt to increase FRC over closing capacity by applying positive end-expiratory pressure (PEEP) to the ventilated lung. When doing this, however, one must remember that PEEP can compress peri-alveolar vessels, increasing pulmonary vascular resistance and thus diverting blood flow from the ventilated to the non-ventilated lung. The positive effects of PEEP ventilation of the dependent lung in increasing FRC might thus be offset by the diversion of blood flow to the non-ventilated lung with a net increase in total shunt perfusion. If fact, this can be observed clinically: adding PEEP to the dependent lung can increase or decrease arterial oxygen tension, or have absolutely no effect at all.

The pragmatic way to proceed is to apply a CPAP of $5-10\,cmH_2O$ with 100% O_2 to the non-ventilated lung. If that is not effective in bringing S_aO_2 over 90%, a PEEP of $5-10\,cmH_2O$ is added to the ventilated lung. If S_aO_2 is still below 90%, then CPAP is increased in the non-ventilated lung to $10-15\,cmH_2O$. A further increase in PEEP to between 10 and $15\,cmH_2O$ is the final step in the endeavour to raise S_aO_2 from potentially hazardous low levels.

If none of these measures succeed in bringing the S_aO_2 to around 90%, one must remember that the fastest and most successful way to improve oxygenation is to resume two-lung ventilation. One should not hesitate to remove the cross-clamp and ventilate the non-dependent lung if the patient is threatened by severe hypoxaemia.

Practical management of OLV

- Insert double-lumen endotracheal tube and verify correct position by auscultation and flexible bronchoscopy
- Cross-clamp correct connector and disconnect from endotracheal tube to allow the lung to collapse. Arterial saturation will fall
- If arterial saturation falls below 90%, increase inspiratory O_2 fraction to 1.0
- If saturation remains under 90%, add static positive pressure of $5-10\,cmH_2O$ to non-ventilated lung (CPAP)
- If saturation is still lower than 90%, add PEEP of $5-10\,cmH_2O$ to ventilated lung. Saturation may fall after PEEP ventilation is started
- If saturation remains under 90%, sequentially increase CPAP and PEEP by $5-10\,cmH_2O$
- If none of these measures are successful in raising arterial saturation to at least 85–90%, reinstate two-lung ventilation

---

Preparing the patient for thoracoscopy

The approach to the patient presenting for thoracoscopic surgery depends on the nature of the underlying disease, the planned intervention and the patient's general clinical condition. Determining the status of the cardiovascular and respiratory systems is the anaesthetists' primary concern, since many thoracoscopic procedures are performed with the aim of evaluating and treating diseases of the lungs. The wide variety of thoracoscopic procedures means that there will not be a "typical" patient profile. A young adult scheduled for treatment of recurrent pneumothorax or a patient with hyperhidrosis scheduled for thoracoscopic sympathectomy will probably be otherwise healthy and require a different preoperative work-up than an older patient with a long history of smoking scheduled for thoracoscopic lobectomy. The young patient presenting for thoracoscopic correction of kyphoscoliosis, on the other hand, might have chronic cor pulmonale with severe pulmonary hypertension and a right ventricle on the verge of decompensation.

Preoperative evaluation includes a meticulous history, physical examination, 12-lead ECG, chest X-ray, standard laboratory tests and pulmonary function testing. The latter might include peak flow measurements before and after administering a bronchodilator. The medical history focuses on smoking, occupational exposure to pulmonary irritants, exercise tolerance, episodes of angina pectoris, paroxysmal episodes of dyspnoea, muscular weakness, and current and previous medication. The physical examination might reveal rhonchi and wheezing, prolonged expiration, engorged jugular veins, cutaneous signs of emphysema or cyanosis. The ECG is useful to detect signs of ischaemic or hypertensive heart disease, pre-existing dysrhythmias or intracardial conduction defects, while the chest radiogram could reveal pulmonary infiltrates, pleural effusions, atelectatic areas, pneumothorax, radiolucent areas indicating hyperinflation or signs of congestive heart disease.

Conditions to look for in patients presenting for thoracoscopy

- *Coronary artery disease*: history, ECG, echocardiography
- *Obstructive lung disease*: history, examination, pulmonary function, X-ray
- *Restrictive lung disease*: history, examination, pulmonary function, X-ray
- *Pulmonary hypertension*: auscultation, ECG, echocardiography
- *Paraneoplastic syndrome*: history, physical examination

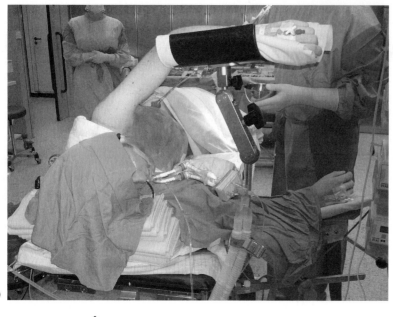

(a)

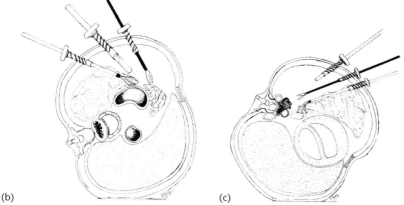

(b)   (c)

Figure 9.13 Positioning the patient for thoracoscopy. The amount of tilt of the upper body depends on the intrathoracic location of the surgical site. (a) Patient being prepared for thoracoscopic treatment of recurrent pneumothorax. Note the double-lumen endotracheal tube, the position of the arms and the venous cannulae. (b) Surgery in the anterior mediastinum. (c) Surgery of the thoracic spine, oesophagus, posterior mediastinum, hilus, etc. (Schematic illustrations by courtesy of Dr Hilmar Dörge, Department of Cardiothoracic Surgery, University of Göttingen.)

Anaesthesia

Positioning the patient

For thoracoscopy, the patient is in the lateral decubitus position with the affected side uppermost. The arm on the affected side is flexed at the elbow and abducted to about the level of the ear. The arm of the dependent side is either fixed alongside the patient's body or brought forward in the sagittal plane until it points directly away from the body (see Chapter 3). The patient is often not positioned in the classic lateral decubitus position, but only tilted about 45°, depending on the location of the surgical site – anterior or posterior thorax (Figure 9.13).

Monitoring

S_aO_2 is the single most important parameter during OLV, and pulse oximetry is therefore mandatory. Five-lead ECG, preferably with automated ST segment analysis, capnometry and arterial cannulation for invasive blood pressure monitoring and serial blood gas sampling are standard. Depth of relaxation monitoring is useful if continuous neuromuscular block is required. Transoesophageal echocardiography (TEE) might be useful to monitor cardiac function and surgical progress involving the pericardium. If the radial artery is to be cannulated, this should be done in the elevated arm, since it is usually more easily accessible, and there is less risk of arterial compression. A large-bore venous cannula is inserted into a vein of the elevated arm. A central venous catheter can be introduced through the brachiocephalic vein of either arm or the jugular vein on the non-dependent side.

Essential monitoring for thoracoscopic surgery

- Pulse oximetry, perhaps with additional serial blood gas analyses
- Five-lead ECG, preferably with automated ST segment analysis
- Continuous blood pressure measurement (non-invasive or radial artery cannulation)
- Capnometry

Useful additional monitoring

- Relaxometry
- Temperature
- TEE

Induction and maintenance of anaesthesia

Brief diagnostic thoracoscopic procedures can be performed safely under local anaesthesia in the awake, spontaneously breathing patient.[75] The port insertion sites in the chest wall and the parietal pleura can be simply infiltrated with local anaesthetic, but intercostal nerve blocks or thoracic epidural anaesthesia provide more complete analgesia. The cough reflex, which is triggered by manipulations of the hilum, can be suppressed by an ipsilateral stellate ganglion block. Supplementary O_2 should be administered via face mask or nasal prongs to prevent hypoxia consequent to collapse of the non-dependent lung and paradoxial respiration in the spontaneously breathing patient.

However, general anaesthesia (preferably a total intravenous technique) and mechanical ventilation is the method of choice for all more complicated or lengthier procedures, since the positive intrapulmonary pressure counteracts the changes associated with lung collapse and mediastinal shift, and helps minimize pulmonary shunt perfusion. One study has shown that the combination of thoracic epidural analgesia with general anaesthesia reduces pulmonary shunt perfusion and yields better arterial oxygenation.[76] Lung separation with a double-lumen endotracheal tube and OLV is required, since it is not possible to retract the lung as during thoracotomy. Except for certain exceptions a left-sided double-lumen tube is used. The tip is placed in the left main bronchus and the correct position is verified by flexible bronchoscopy (see above). The position is confirmed again after the patient has been brought into the lateral decubitus position.

Anaesthesia is induced with a short-acting barbiturate, propofol or etomidate after an initial injection of an opioid (for details see Chapter 5). Neuromuscular relaxation is achieved with a non-depolarizing agent of suitable duration. Anaesthesia is maintained with an infusion of propofol, since this does not interfere with HPV (see above), and continuing administration of the opioid. The non-dependent lung is allowed to collapse after introduction of the trocars and instruments into the pleural cavity. This is done by cross-clamping the tube the connecting the ventilator to the lumen of the double-lumen endotracheal tube supplying the non-dependent lung and disconnecting it altogether (Figure 9.14).

Excellent postoperative pain relief can be achieved with intercostal blocks in addition to intravenous opioids. If a thoracic epidural catheter was inserted for anaesthesia, it can be used to great advantage in the postoperative period to reduce intraoperative opioid requirements and provide postoperative analgesia.

Anaesthetic management of thoracoscopic surgery

- Anxiolytic premedication with short-acting benzodiazepine
- Large-bore venous cannula in arm of affected side (this arm remains accessible). Occasionally advisable: radial artery cannulation, central venous catheter (jugular vein)
- Induction with intravenous hypnotic agent
- Intubate with double-lumen endotracheal tube (confirm position with flexible bronchoscope, check again when patient in lateral decubitus position)
- Total intravenous anaesthesia with propofol and suitable opioid (see Chapter 5 for details)
- OLV. $F_IO_2 = 1.0$. Add CPAP to collapsed lung and PEEP to ventilated lung if P_aO_2 is too low

---

Complications of thoracoscopic surgery

Hypoxia is a common occurrence during thoracoscopic surgery as described above. Treatment consists in minimizing intrapulmonary shunt perfusion, optimizing ventilation–perfusion ratios by differential lung ventilation (see above), increasing inspiratory O_2 concentration, or, ultimately, resuming two-lung ventilation.

Haemorrhage is not common during thoracoscopy, but can be profuse and severely impair visualization of the surgical site, as well as lead to circulatory collapse. Large-bore venous cannulae should be inserted as part of patient preparation, and blood should be typed and cross-matched.

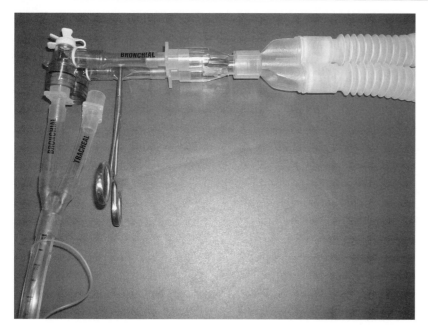

Figure 9.14 Disconnecting the lung from the ventilator to provide one-lung anaesthesia. This illustration shows a left-sided double-lumen endotracheal tube cross-clamped and disconnected to ventilate the left lung (lumen marked "bronchial") and allow the right lung (lumen marked "tracheal") to collapse.

Intraoperative hypotension during thoracoscopy not secondary to exsanguinating haemorrhage is usually due to cardiac manipulations impairing atrial filling, or cardiac dysrhythmias. The incidence and severity of the latter can be increased by hypoxia. Blood pressure improves rapidly when the surgeon eases compression on the heart. Positive intrathoracic pressure can also severely compromise cardiovascular function[55] and should be relieved immediately, if present.

In a humorous, but nonetheless deadly serious tone, Braimbridge lists kebab lung syndrome, clotted haemothorax, artificial lunchothorax and aorto-pleuro-cutaneous fistula as major surgical complications of thoracoscopy.[40] All of these involve damage to internal organs – lung, liver, stomach, and heart or aorta, respectively – with the trocar, the thoracoscope or the surgical instruments.

Minimally invasive cardiac surgery

Conventional cardiac surgery involves a median sternotomy to access an ischaemic heart in cardioplegic stillstand on cardiopulmonary bypass (CPB), all of which are principal determinants of perioperative morbidity and mortality that contribute directly to the enormous costs of cardiac surgery. Sternotomy is associated with rib fractures, sternal dehiscence, chest wall instability, wound infections and brachial plexus injuries, and a prolonged rehabilitation period to

Table 9.6 Advantages of various methods of minimally invasive coronary artery bypass surgery

OPCAB	No CPB, median sternotomy, complete coronary re-vascularization possible
PACAP	CPB via femoral artery and vein, no sternotomy, coronary artery and valve procedures possible
MIDCAB	No CPB, no sternotomy, reserved for single-vessel disease (left anterior descending artery, right coronary artery)

regain use of the arms. CPB induces a large-scale systemic inflammatory response syndrome (SIRS) with its associated complications and is a primary factor in the occurrence of perioperative stroke, myocardial infarction and mental dysfunction. Avoiding these factors amounts to a major reduction in the invasiveness of cardiac surgery.

For once, economic pressure to reduce the cost of treatment and medical efforts to improve patient outcome worked in the same direction, and a number of minimally invasive procedures have been developed that avoid median sternotomy, CPB or both. The best established methods are off-pump coronary artery bypass (OPCAB), port-access coronary artery bypass (PACAB or PortCAB) and minimally invasive direct coronary artery bypass (MIDCAB). Each of these methods has its advantages and limitations (see Table 9.6). A 1999 study in the US found that OPCAB and MIDCAB were both less expensive than conventional coronary bypass surgery: the total costs of OPCAP and MIDCAB were lower by 21% and 11%, respectively.[77] Although studies have documented the advantages of minimally invasive cardiac surgery, these procedures are not standard, at present, and are only performed in specialized centres. Of the 70,000 coronary bypass operations performed annually in Germany, only 4–5% were done with minimally invasive methods in 2001.[78] The statistics in other countries will be similar.

As Cooley points out in his contribution to the discussion of the pros and cons of minimally invasive surgery, coronary artery bypass grafting without CPB is not a new technique, but one that was used before the general acceptance of cardioplegic stillstand.[79] The technique was essentially re-introduced as OPCAB surgery in the 1970s. With this method, the heart and the coronary arteries are approached through a median sternotomy, and the target artery is occluded and stabilized mechanically to facilitate suturing the anastomosis. The first report of larger series of treated patients was published in 1975.[80] A later report gives a mortality rate of 2.5% in a series of nearly 1300 patients with an incidence of neurological complications and cardiac dysrhythmias lower than for the conventional procedure.[81] This was also the case for patients at high risk of adverse outcome due to advanced age or impaired left ventricular function.[82] OPCAB has been shown to be superior to conventional coronary artery surgery with regard to duration of ventilation (6 vs. 10 h), length of hospital stay (6 vs. 9 days) and incidence of postoperative neurological deficits (0% vs. 7.5%).[83]

MIDCAB, first described in 1994,[84] is performed through a small incision directly over the target artery. This technique met with initial enthusiasm, but as with all new techniques that have been employed beyond the range of their usefulness, there has been a certain rollback and a wave of scepticism. Access to the heart is limited, and the technique is now accepted as a standard for one-vessel bypass, occasionally in combination with interventional cardiology for angioplasty and stenting of other coronaries. The left anterior descending artery is approached through a left parasternal minithoracotomy for re-vascularization with the left internal mammary artery, and the right coronary artery is accessed through a xiphoidal incision and grafted to the gastroepiploic artery.

PACAB is performed with full CPB, but without median sternotomy. The femoral vein and femoral artery are cannulated for CPB and a ballon-tipped catheter is placed in the aorta for aortic occlusion and delivery of cardioplegia solution.

Monitoring

Standard monitoring during minimally invasive cardiac surgery should include direct arterial and central venous pressure recordings, ECG with ST segment analysis, pulse oximetry, body temperature and relaxometry. TEE is desirable to detect regional wall motion abnormalities during coronary occlusion in procedures without CPB. Some method for determining cardiac output (CO) is useful in patients with borderline myocardial function. Monitoring myocardial function can be difficult during OPCAB procedures when the heart is rotated to access the circumflex artery.

Anaesthesia for minimally invasive cardiac surgery

Anaesthesia for minimally invasive cardiac surgery requires a radical departure from the standard management of conventional cardiosurgery. The demands on intraoperative haemodynamic stability remain unaltered, but postoperative management focuses on early extubation (fast-track anaesthesia). General anaesthesia is preferred, but off-pump cardiac surgery has been successfully performed on the spontaneously breathing patient with high thoracic epidural anaesthesia.[85,86] A combination of general anaesthesia with thoracic epidural anaesthesia can provide intraoperative haemodynamic stability and facilitate effective postoperative analgesia.[76]

Patients are premedicated with an oral benzodiazepine. Anaesthesia is induced in the usual manner with an opioid and propofol, a short-acting barbiturate or etomidate. We prefer etomidate, or propofol administered with a target-controlled infusion pump to avoid high peak plasma concentrations with peripheral vasodilatation and a phase of profound hypotension. Remifentanil is given as a slow bolus injection for induction ($2\,\mu g\,kg^{-1}$) and a continuous infusion ($0.5\,\mu g\,kg^{-1}\,min^{-1}$) for maintenance as the opioid component of a totally intravenous technique combined with a propofol infusion. It reduces myocardial O_2 uptake by 42%, which should provide a degree of ischaemia protection during coronary occlusion.[87] Recovery after this regimen is shorter and more predictable than when alfentanil is used.[88]

Tracheal intubation is facilitated with a nondepolarizing muscle relaxant. A double-lumen endotracheal tube is required if the procedure is to assisted by thoracoscopy. Off-pump coronary surgery, as well as MIDCAB and PACAB procedures that do not intentionally breach the pleura only require a single-lumen endotracheal tube.

Coronary artery bypass grafting without CPB requires an alternative method to stabilize the target artery and minimize movement during the anastomosis. Surgical retractor systems have been developed for this purpose, which render the formerly used pharmacological induction of bradycardia with beta-adrenergic or calcium channel blockers, adenosine or cholinesterase inhibitors less of a concern. Anastomosis also requires occlusion of the target artery to prevent anterograde and retrograde flow. The regional ischaemia that occurs during the occlusion period can have severe effects on myocardial function, such as hypotension, reduced CO, pulmonary congestion with elevated pulmonary capillary wedge pressure, or ECG signs of ischaemia. Occlusion of the right coronary artery can induce atrial dysrhythmias or bradycardia, while occlusion of the left anterior descending artery can precipitate acute left ventricular failure requiring resuscitation and an intra-aortic balloon pump. A trial occlusion phase is frequently performed prior to grafting to detect and deal with any adverse effects. Some regard this period itself as therapeutic in the sense that it might contribute to ischaemic preconditioning.[89] Other authors have not been able to demonstrate a beneficial effect of a 5-min preconditioning period on the occurrence of segmental wall motion abnormalities.[90] Institution of CPB or conversion to the conventional procedure may be necessary if the haemodynamic derangements are severe and prolonged.

PACAB surgery requires a pulmonary artery catheter to vent the left ventricle and a coronary sinus catheter for retrograde cardioplegia if the aortic occlusion catheter does not have a lumen for anterograde cardioplegia. The aortic occlusion balloon can migrate into the aortic arch during surgery and block the innominate artery and stop blood flow in the right carotid artery. Continuous pressure recordings in the right radial artery will help detect this complication.

Pain therapy

The severity of pain following minimally invasive cardiac surgery have not been quantified in a systematic manner. One study suggests that the standard MIDCAB is not less painful than conventional coronary artery bypass surgery. There is no median sternotomy, but trauma to the costal cartilage and the rib segment resection are probably potent stimuli, since MIDCAB with endoscopic artery dissection is less painful.[91] Thoracic epidural anaesthesia is effective for analgesia, but other methods, such as continuous paravertebral block, continuous intrapleural local anaesthetic infusion or intercostal blocks are as effective, and have fewer complications.[92–94] An effective postoperative pain control regimen will incorporate local anaesthetic techniques, intravenous opioids and non-opiate analgesics in a rational combination.

References

1. Killian G. Über die direkte Bronchoskopie. *Munch Med Wochenschr* 1898; **27**: 845–847.
2. Bonten MJ, Bergmans DC, Stobberingh EE *et al.* Implementation of bronchoscopic techniques in the diagnosis of ventilator-associated pneumonia to reduce antibiotic use. *Am J Respir Crit Care Med* 1997; **156**: 1820–1824.
3. Bellomo R, Tai E, Parkin G. Fibreoptic bronchoscopy in the critically ill: a prospective study of its diagnostic and therapeutic value. *Anaesth Intens Care* 1992; **20**: 464–469.
4. Shoemaker WC, Velmahos GC, Demetriades D. *Procedures and Monitoring for the Critically Ill*. Philadelphia: W.B. Saunders, 2001.
5. Raoof S, Mehrishi S, Prakash UB. Role of bronchoscopy in modern medical intensive care unit. *Clin Chest Med* 2001; **22**: 241–261, vii.
6. Liebler JM, Markin CJ. Fiberoptic bronchoscopy for diagnosis and treatment. *Crit Care Clin* 2000; **16**: 83–100.
7. Gronnebech H, Johannson G, Smedebol M, Valentin N. Glycopyrrolate vs atropine during anaesthesia for laryngoscopy and bronchoscopy. *Acta Anaesthesiol Scand* 1993; **37**: 454–457.
8. Cowl CT, Prakash UB, Kruger BR. The role of anticholinergics in bronchoscopy. A randomized clinical trial. *Chest* 2000; **118**: 188–192.
9. Lyew MA, Behl SP. Aticholinergic pre-treatment in rigid bronchoscopy. Effect on heart rate, arterial blood pressure and cardiac arrhythmias. *Acta Anaesthesiol Belg* 1990; **41**: 25–31.
10. Lukomsky GI, Ovchinnikov AA, Bilal A. Complications of bronchoscopy. Comparison of rigid bronchoscopy under general anesthesia and flexible fiberoptic bronchoscopy under topical anesthesia. *Chest* 1981; **79**: 316–321.
11. Pereira WJ, Kovnat DM, Snider GL. A prospective cooperative study of complications following flexible fibreoptic bronchoscopy. *Chest* 1978; **73**: 813–816.
12. Lindholm CE, Ollman B, Snyder JV, Millen EG, Grenvik A. Cardiorespiratory effects of flexible fiberoptic bronchoscopy in critically ill patients. *Chest* 1978; **74**: 362–368.
13. Matot I, Kramer MR, Glantz L, Drenger B, Cotev S. Myocardial ischemia in sedated patients undergoing fiberoptic bronchoscopy. *Chest* 1997; **112**: 1454–1458.
14. Isaac PA, Barry JE, Vaughan RS, Rosen M, Newcombe RG. A jet nebuliser for delivery of topical anaesthesia to the respiratory tract. A comparison with cricothyroid puncture and direct spraying for fibreoptic bronchoscopy. *Anaesthesia* 1990; **45**: 46–48.
15. Jones DA, McBurney A, Stanley PJ, Tovey C, Ward JW. Plasma concentrations of lignocaine and its metabolites during fibreoptic bronchoscopy. *Br J Anaesth* 1982; **54**: 853–857.

16. Suratt PM, Smiddy JF, Gruber B. Deaths and complications associated with fiberoptic bronchoscopy. *Chest* 1976; **69**: 747–751.

17. Crawford M, Pollock J, Anderson K, Glavin RJ, MacIntyre D, Vernon D. Comparison of midazolam with propofol for sedation in outpatient bronchoscopy. *Br J Anaesth* 1993; **70**: 418–422.

18. Gonzalez R, De La Rosa Ramirez I, Maldonado Hernandez A, Dominguez Cherit G. Should patients undergoing a bronchoscopy be sedated? *Acta Anaesthesiol Scand* 2003; **47**: 411–415.

19. Patil V, Stehling LC, Zander HL, Koch JP. Mechanical aids for fiberoptic endoscopy. *Anesthesiology* 1982; **57**: 69–70.

20. Whittaker R. On the neuromuscular blocking action of succinylmonocholine in the rat. *J Pharm Pharmacol* 1972; **24**: 340–341.

21. Meretoja OA, Taivainen T, Raiha L, Korpela R, Wirtavuori K. Sevoflurane–nitrous oxide or halothane–nitrous oxide for paediatric bronchoscopy and gastroscopy. *Br J Anaesth* 1996; **76**: 767–771.

22. Wark KJ, Lyons J, Feneck RO. The haemodynamic effects of bronchoscopy. Effect of pretreatment with fentanyl and alfentanil. *Anaesthesia* 1986; **41**: 162–167.

23. Hill AJ, Feneck RO, Underwood SM, Davis ME, Marsh A, Bromley L. The haemodynamic effects of bronchoscopy. Comparison of propofol and thiopentone with and without alfentanil pretreatment. *Anaesthesia* 1991; **46**: 266–270.

24. Katz AS, Michelson EL, Stawicki J, Holford FD. Cardiac arrhythmias. Frequency during fiberoptic bronchoscopy and correlation with hypoxaemia. *Arch Intern Med* 1981; **141**: 603–606.

25. Schrader DL, Lakshminarayan S. The effect of fiberoptic bronchoscopy on cardiac rhythm. *Chest* 1978; **73**: 821–824.

26. Carlens E. Mediastinoscopy: a method for inspection and tissue biopsy in the superior mediastinum. *Chest* 1959; **36**: 343–352.

27. Puhakka HJ. Complications of mediastinoscopy. *J Laryngol Otol* 1989; **103**: 312–315.

28. Ashbaugh DG. Mediastinoscopy. *Arch Surg* 1970; **100**: 569–573.

29. Goldstraw P. Mediastinal exploration by mediastinoscopy and mediastinotomy. *Br J Dis Chest* 1988; **82**: 111–120.

30. Bonadies J, D'Agostino RS, Ruskis AF, Ponn RB. Outpatient mediastinoscopy. *J Thorac Cardiovasc Surg* 1993; **106**: 686–688.

31. Cybulsky IJ, Bennett WF. Mediastinoscopy as a routine outpatient procedure. *Ann Thorac Surg* 1994; **58**: 176–178.

32. Venuta F, Rendina EA, Pescarmona EO *et al.* Ambulatory mediastinal biopsy for hematologic malignancies. *Eur J Cardiothorac Surg* 1997; **11**: 218–221.

33. Morton JR, Guinn GA. Mediastinoscopy using local anesthesia. *Am J Surg* 1971; **122**: 696–698.

34. Benumof JL. Anesthesia for special elective diagnostic procedures. In: *Anesthesia for Thoracic Surgery.* Philadelphia: W.B. Saunders, 1995; pp. 491–512.

35. Albage A, Henriksson G, Lindblom D. Repair of acute mediastinoscopic injury to the pulmonary artery using an intravascular approach and deep hypothermic circulatory arrest. *Interact Cardiovasc Thorac Surg* 2004; **3**: 368–369.

36. Furgang RA, Saidman LJ. Bilateral tension pneumothorax associated with mediastinoscopy: a case report. *J Thorac Cardiovasc Surg* 1972; **63**: 329–331.

37. Petty C. Right radical pressure during mediastinoscopy. *Anesth Analg* 1979; **58**: 428–430.

38. Jacobeus HC. Ueber die Möglichkeit die Zystoskopie bei Untersuchung seröser Höhlungen anzuwenden [On the possibility of using cystoscopy for the investigation of serous cavities]. *Münch Med Wochenschr* 1910; **57**: 2090–2098.

39. Jacobeus HC. The practical importance of thoracoscopy in surgery of the chest. *Surg Gynec Obstet* 1922; **34**: 289–296.

40. Braimbridge MV. The history of thoracoscopic surgery. *Ann Thorac Surg* 1993; **56**: 610–614.

41. Swierenga J, Wagenaar JP, Bergstein PG. The value of thoracoscopy in the diagnosis and treatment of diseases affecting the pleura and the lung. *Pneumologie* 1974; **151**: 11–18.

42. Miller JL, Hatcher CRJ. Thoracoscopy: a useful tool in the diagnosis of thoracic disease. *Ann Thorac Surg* 1978; **26**: 68–72.

43. Newhouse MT. Thoracoscopy: diagnostic and therapeutic indications. *Pneumologie* 1989; **43**: 48–52.

44. Kirby TJ, Rice TW. Thoracoscopic lobectomy. *Ann Thorac Surg* 1993; **56**: 784–786.

45. Walker WS, Carnochan FM, Mattar S. Video-assisted thoracoscopic pneumonectomy. *Br J Surg* 1994; **81**: 81–82.

46. Hazelrigg SR, Landreneau RJ, Mack M *et al.* Thoracoscopic stapled resection for spontaneous pneumothorax. *J Thorac Cardiovasc Surg* 1993; **105**: 389–392.

47. Graeber GM, Jones DR. The role of thoracoscopy in thoracic trauma. *Ann Thorac Surg* 1993; **56**: 646–648.

48. Gossot D, Fourquier P, Celerier M. Thoracoscopic esophagectomy: technique and initial results. *Ann Thorac Surg* 1993; **56**: 667–670.

49. Sato M, Kosaka S. Minimally invasive diagnosis and treatment of traumatic rupture of the right hemidiaphragm with liver herniation. *Jpn J Thorac Cardiovasc Surg* 2002; **50**: 515–517.

50. Khoo LT, Beisse R, Potulski M. Thoracoscopic-assisted treatment of thoracic and lumbar fractures: a series of 371 consecutive cases. *Neurosurgery* 2002; **51(Suppl 5)**: 104–117.

51. Regan JJ, Mack MJ, Picetti GDI. A technical report of video-assisted thoracoscopy in thoracic spinal surgery. *Spine* 1995; **20**: 831–837.

52. Benumof JL, Alfery DD. Anesthesia for thoracic surgery. In: Miller RD (Ed.), *Anesthesia.* New York: Churchill Livingstone, 1986; pp. 1371–1462.

53. Tarhan S, Moffitt EA. Principles of thoracic anesthesia. *Surg Clin North Am* 1973; **53**: 813–826.

54. Hill RC, Jones DR, Vance RA, Kalantarian B. Selective lung ventilation during thoracoscopy: effects of

insufflation on hemodynamics. *Ann Thorac Surg* 1996; **61**: 945–948.

55. Jones DR, Graeber GM, Tanguilig GG, Hobbs G, Murray GF. Effects of insufflation on hemodynamics during thoracoscopy. *Ann Thorac Surg* 1993; **55**: 1379–1382.

56. Smith G, Hirsch N, Ehrenwerth J. Placement of double-lumen endobronchial tubes. Correlation between clinical impressions and bronchoscopic findings. *Br J Anaesth* 1986; **58**: 1317–1320.

57. Read R, Friday C, Eason C. Prospective study of the Robertshaw endobronchial catheter in thoracic surgery. *Ann Thorac Surg* 1977; **24**: 156–161.

58. Inoue H, Shohtsu A, Ogawa J, Kawada S, Koide S. New device for one lung anesthesia: endotracheal tube with moveable blocker. *J Thorac Cardiovasc Surg* 1982; **83**: 940–941.

59. Ender J, Bury AM, Raumanns J *et al.* The use of a bronchial blocker compared with a double-lumen tube for single-lung ventilation during minimally invasive direct coronary artery bypass surgery. *J Cardiothorac Vasc Anesth* 2002; **16**: 452–455.

60. Marshall BE, Marshall C, Benumof JL, Saidman LJ. Hypoxic pulmonary vasoconstriction in dogs: effects of lung segment size and alveolar oxygen tension. *J Appl Physiol* 1981; **51**: 1543–1551.

61. von Euler US, Liljestrand G. Observations on the pulmonary arterial blood pressure in the cat. *Acta Physiol Scand* 1946; **12**: 301–312.

62. Marshall C, Lindgren L, Marshall BE. Effects of halothane, enflurane, and isoflurane on hypoxic pulmonary vasoconstriction in rat lungs in vitro. *Anesthesiology* 1984; **60**: 304–308.

63. Ishibe Y, Gui X, Uno H, Shiokawa Y, Umeda T, Suekane K. Effect of sevoflurane on hypoxic pulmonary vasoconstriction in the perfused rabbit lung. *Anesthesiology* 1993; **79**: 1348–1353.

64. Loer SA, Scheeren TW, Tarnow J. Desflurane inhibits hypoxic pulmonary vasoconstriction in isolated rabbit lungs. *Anesthesiology* 1995; **83**: 552–556.

65. Karzai W, Haberstroh J, Priebe HJ. Effects of desflurane and propofol on arterial oxygenation during one-lung ventilation in the pig. *Acta Anaesthesiol Scand* 1998; **42**: 648–652.

66. Bjertnæs LJ. Hypoxia-induced pulmonary vasoconstriction in man: inhibition due to diethyl ether and halothane anaesthesia. *Acta Anaesthesiol Scand* 1978; **22**: 570–578.

67. Benumof JL, Augustine SD, Gibbons JA. Halothane and isoflurane only slightly impair arterial oxygenation during one-lung ventilation in patients undergoing thoracotomy. *Anesthesiology* 1987; **67**: 910–915.

68. Carlsson AJ, Bindslev L, Hedenstierna G. Hypoxia-induced pulmonary vasoconstriction in the human lung: the effect of isoflurane anesthesia. *Anesthesiology* 1987; **66**: 312–316.

69. Van Keer L, Van Aken H, Vendermeersch E, Vermaut G. Propofol does not inhibit HPV in humans. *J Clin Anaesth* 1989; **1**: 284–288.

70. Kellow NH, Scott AD, White SA, Feneck RO. Comparison of the effects of propofol and isoflurane anaesthesia on right ventricular function and shunt fraction during thoracic surgery. *Br J Anaesth* 1995; **75**: 578–582.

71. Abe K, Shimizu T, Takashina M, Shiozaki H, Yoshiya I. The effects of propofol, isoflurane, and sevoflurane on oxygenation and shunt fraction during one-lung ventilation. *Anesth Analg* 1998; **87**: 1164–1169.

72. Spies C, Zaune U, Pauli MH, Boeden G, Martin E. Vergleich von Enfluran und Propofol bei thoraxchirurgischen Eingriffen [A comparison of enflurane and propofol in thoracic surgery]. *Anaesthesist* 1991; **40**: 14–18.

73. Nakayama M, Murray PA. Ketamine preserves and propofol potentiates hypoxic pulmonary vasoconstriction compared with the conscious state in chronically instrumented dogs. *Anesthesiology* 1999; **91**: 760–771.

74. Capan LM, Turndorf H, Patel C, Ramanathan S, Acinapura A, Chalon J. Optimization of arterial oxygenation during one-lung anesthesia. *Anesth Analg* 1980; **59**: 847–851.

75. Menzies R, Charbonneau M. Thoracoscopy for the diagnosis of pleural disease. *Ann Intern Med* 1991; **14**: 271–276.

76. Von Dossow V, Welte M, Zaune U *et al.* Thoracic epidural anesthesia combined with general anesthesia: the preferred anesthetic technique for thoracic surgery. *Anesth Analg* 2001; **92**: 848–854.

77. Arom KV, Emery RW, Flavin TF, Petersen RJ. Cost-effectiveness of minimally invasive coronary artery bypass surgery. *Ann Thorac Surg* 1999; **68**: 1562–1566.

78. Cremer J, Boning A, Fraund S. Minimalinvasive Koronarchirurgie [Minimally invasive coronary artery surgery]. *Herz* 2002; **27**: 402–406.

79. Cooley DA. Con: beating-heart surgery for coronary revascularization: is it the most important development since the introduction of the heart–lung machine? *Ann Thorac Surg* 2000; **70**: 1779–1781.

80. Trapp WS, Bisarya R. Placement of coronary artery bypass graft without pump oxygenator. *Ann Thorac Surg* 1975; **19**: 1–9.

81. Buffolo E, de Andrade CS, Branco JN, Teles CA, Aguiar LF, Gomes WJ. Coronary artery bypass grafting without cardiopulmonary bypass. *Ann Thorac Surg* 1996; **61**: 63–66.

82. Del Rizzo DF, Boyd WD, Novek RJ. Safety and cost effectiveness of MIDCAB in high risk CABG patients. *Ann Thorac Surg* 1998; **66**: 1002–1007.

83. Kilger E, Weis FC, Goetz AE *et al.* Intensive care after minimally invasive and conventional coronary surgery: a prospective comparison. *Intens Care Med* 2001; **27**: 534–539.

84. Benetti FJ, Ballester C, Sani G, Boonstra PW, Grandjean JG. Video assisted coronary artery bypass surgery. *J Card Surg* 1995; **10**: 620–625.

85. Kessler P, Neidhart G, Bremerich DH *et al.* High thoracic epidural anesthesia for coronary artery bypass grafting using two different surgical approaches in conscious patients. *Anesth Analg* 2002; **95**: 791–797.

86. Charkravarthy M, Jawali V, Patil TA, Jayaprakash K, Shivananda NV. High thoracic epidural anesthesia as

the sole anesthetic for performing multiple grafts in off-pump coronary artery surgery. *J Cardiothorac Vasc Anesth* 2003; **17**: 160–164.

87. Kazmaier S, Hanekop GG, Buhre W *et al.* Myocardial consequences of remifentanil in patients with coronary artery disease. *Br J Anaesth* 2000; **84**: 578–583.

88. Ahonen J, Olkkola KT, Verkkala K, Heikkinen L, Jarvinen A, Salmenpera M. A comparison of remifentanil and alfentanil for use with propofol in patients undergoing minimally invasive coronary artery bypass surgery. *Anesth Analg* 2000; **90**: 1269–1274.

89. Pavie A, Lima L, Bonnet N, Regan M, Aktar R, Gandjbakhch I. Perioperative management in minimally invasive coronary surgery. *Eur J Cardiothorac Surg* 1999; **16(Suppl 2)**: S53–S57.

90. Heres EK, Marquez J, Malkowski MJ, Magovern JA, Gravlee GP. Minimally invasive direct coronary artery bypass: anesthetic, monitoring, and pain control considerations. *J Cardiothorac Vasc Anesth* 1998; **12**: 385–389.

91. Bucerius J, Metz S, Walther T *et al.* Endoscopic internal thoracic artery dissection leads to significant reduction of pain after minimally invasive direct coronary artery bypass graft surgery. *Ann Thorac Surg* 2002; **73**: 1180–1184.

92. Dhole S, Mehta Y, Saxena H, Juneja R, Trehan N. Comparison of continuous thoracic epidural and paravertebral blocks for postoperative analgesia after minimally invasive direct coronary artery bypass surgery. *J Cardiothorac Vasc Anesth* 2001; **15**: 288–292.

93. Mehta Y, Swaminathan M, Mishra Y, Trehan N. A comparative evaluation of intrapleural and thoracic epidural analgesia for postoperative pain relief after minimally invasive direct coronary artery bypass surgery. *J Cardiothorac Vasc Anesth* 1998; **12**: 162–165.

94. Behnke H, Geldner G, Cornelissen J *et al.* Postoperative Schmerztherapie bei minimal-invasiver direkter koronararterieller Bypass-Chirurgie (MID-CAB). I.v.-Opioid-PCA versus Interkostalblockaden. *Anaesthesist* 2002; **51**: 175–179.

The upper aerodigestive tract is a collective term designating the region from the nasal passages to the level of the bronchi. It encompasses the oropharynx and hypopharynx, the tongue, epiglottis and glottis, the larynx and trachea, the oral cavity and the nasal passages. Any and all of these structures can be approached by laser surgery, but the most common localization of pathological processes is the larynx.

Lasers were introduced into the treatment of laryngeal lesions in the early 1970s by Jako and Strong.[1] Surgeons such as Burian in Austria, Frèche in France, and Oswal and Howard in the UK helped to establish the technique in Europe. Pioneers such as Wolfgang Steiner in Germany were instrumental in taking the technique to new frontiers so that nowadays nearly every pharyngolaryngological operation, including curative and palliative resection of bulky tumours, can be performed transorally with the laser. Management of anaesthesia for these procedures has been a challenge since their very introduction. The interdependence between anaesthesia and surgery for the development of the field is illustrated by the fact that studies on the best methods of anaesthesia coincided with the surgical reports and were even co-authored by surgeons.[2–4] Further research helped to optimize working conditions for the surgeon while providing the patient with a greater degree of perioperative safety and comfort.

The use of lasers as a surgical cutting instrument provides an elegant and minimally invasive approach to surgery. With the laser beam one can operate in nearly inaccessible areas with a precision not possible with other surgical instruments. From major resections of gross tumourous growths to pinpoint removal of vocal cord papillomas, the entire palette of upper and lower airway procedures is possible with this technique. The indications for laryngeal and tracheal laser surgery are usually neoplasms – malignant or benign – such as carcinomas, papillomas, nodules or cysts. Laryngeal webs, tracheal stenosis or even a Zenker's diverticulum are fair game for the laser. Laser surgery of laryngeal cancer avoids or at least postpones the otherwise unavoidable tracheotomy with its social stigmatization – an enormous improvement of the quality of life for the patients. Surgical procedures above the level of the larynx include tonsillectomy, removal of epiglottal, glossal, buccal or retropharyngeal tumours, opening of choanal atresia, surgery of hyperplastic nasal turbinates, etc. For an excellent survey of the field, see the textbooks by Steiner and Ambrosch[5] or Davis.[6]

Laser surgery causes minimal bleeding and oedema, and little collateral tissue destruction thus preserving surrounding anatomical structures. This leads to reduced pain and more rapid healing. But this technique also confronts the anaesthetist with a number of unexpected problems that arise from the competition with the surgeon for control of the airway and also from the properties of the laser beam itself.

Laser physics

The word "laser" is an acronym that stands for *l*ight *a*mplification by *s*timulated *e*mission of *r*adiation. The light from a laser behaves the same as light from a normal light bulb, and can be reflected by mirrors, focussed with lenses or be diffracted. But in certain crucial characteristics it is completely different. A beam of laser light is highly monochromatic and contains a very narrow band of wavelengths. The light waves are coherent, or in identical phase, and show little dispersion since they are narrowly collimated.

A laser device consists of an energy source used to excite (or pump) atoms in a so-called lasing medium. The applied energy raises electrons in the atoms of the medium from a low-energy orbital to a higher-energy orbital by a process called *stimulated absorption* (Figure 10.1(a)). An electron can spontaneously drop from the higher- to the lower-energy level emitting a photon with an energy exactly equal to the difference in the energy between the two orbitals. This is called *spontaneous emission* (Figure 10.1(b)).

The frequency of the emitted light is directly proportional to the energy of the emitted photon:

$$f = \frac{E}{h}$$

where f is the frequency in hertz, E is the energy difference between the two orbitals in joules and h is the

Planck's constant, 6.626×10^{-34} J s. The wavelength λ of the emitted light:

$$\lambda = \frac{c}{f}$$

can be calculated from the frequency (f) and the speed of light (c).

Light with a wavelength between 400 and 800 nm is visible to humans (1 nm = 10^{-9} m). Ultraviolet light has a shorter wavelength, while infrared light has a longer wavelength.

If a photon with a particular energy (wavelength) collides with an atom containing an electron in a higher-energy orbital that is posed to emit a photon with the same energy by spontaneous emission, the collision will stimulate immediate emission. The colliding photon and the emitted photon leave the atom together with identical wavelength, phase and direction. The external energy source ensures that many electrons will be in a "pumped up" state, waiting for an emitted photon to trigger a chain reaction of *stimulated emission* (Figure 10.1(c)). Parallel mirrors at each end of

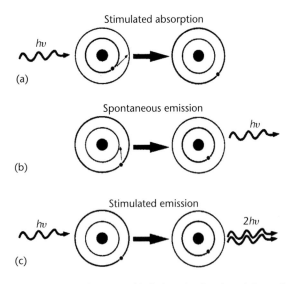

Stimulated absorption

Spontaneous emission

Stimulated emission

Figure 10.1 Electron orbitals in stimulated emission of light. (a) A photon with sufficient energy can raise an electron from a low-energy orbital to a higher-energy orbital (pumping). (b) The excited electron can spontaneously drop from the higher-energy level, emitting a photon with an energy exactly equal to the energy difference between the two orbitals. (c) If a photon with exactly this energy (wavelength) collides with an excited atom, it will stimulate the emission of a photon. The colliding photon and the emitted photon leave the atom together with identical wavelength, phase and direction.

the medium, one of which is semi-transparent, reflect the emitted light back and forth through the medium, stimulating more atoms to emit photons with every passage, thereby amplifying the original stimulus. One of the mirrors is semi-transparent and the light beam, whose light waves are now in phase, will eventually exit the medium through this mirror. It follows from the equation for the energy of a photon, that although a laser beam can be extremely powerful, the laser does not increase the energy of the individual photon but only increases the number of photons per unit of area and time.

The lasers used in surgery employ a variety of laser media and energy sources. The laser most commonly used for surgery of the upper aerodigestive tract is the carbon dioxide (CO_2) laser, while an argon laser is frequently employed in ophthalmologic surgery. Both of these use a gaseous medium that is "pumped" by an electric discharge through the gas-filled tube. Their beams can be either continuous or pulsed. The lasing medium can also be a rod of laser-passive material doped with ionic impurities. A monocrystal of the synthetic gem yttrium–aluminium–garnet (YAG) is commonly used as the laser-passive host matrix and is doped with neodymium (Nd) or holmium. The Nd–YAG laser is "pumped" with high-energy light from xenon flash lamps and only emits a pulsed laser beam. The conversion of electrical energy into light is very inefficient: a laser with an energy output of 10 W requires more than 1 kW input.

The CO_2 laser emits light in the far infrared with a wavelength of 10,600 nm, whereas the Nd–YAG laser emits light in the near-infrared spectrum with a wavelength of 1060 nm and the argon laser emits visible blue–green light with a wavelength of approximately 500 nm. The emitted laser beam can be passed through a frequency doubler that converts its light to a different wavelength. A beam of laser light passed through a crystal of potassium–titanium–phosphate (KTP) will emerge as a mixture of light with the original wavelength and light with half the wavelength (equivalent to double the original frequency). This is referred to as the KTP laser and is most commonly used in a medical setting with the Nd–YAG laser. Excimer (excited dimer) lasers use a noble gas halide such as argon fluoride (ArF) or xenon chloride (XeCl) as lasing medium and emit high-energy photons in the ultraviolet spectrum. The wavelength of the ArF laser is 193 nm. The common laser pointer uses a laser diode that emits a beam with a wavelength of 650 nm. For normal surgery of the upper aerodigestive tract the power of the CO_2 laser beam is set between 5 and 25 W. For comparison, the beam of a laser pointer has a maximum power of 5 mW.

The wavelength of the emitted light determines both how the beam can be conducted from the source to the surgical field and also what effects it has on the target tissue. Visible and near-infrared light can be sent from the source to the tissue through flexible plastic or glass fibre conduits. The long-wave infrared light from the CO_2 laser cannot be guided in this manner but must be reflected with front-surface mirrors along articulated tubes (Figure 10.2). Once the beam is near the surgical field the light can either be sharply focussed in an operating microscope, applied directly to the surgical site with the waveguide bundle or diffused through a contact probe onto the tissue to be destroyed.

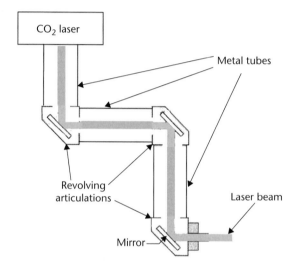

Figure 10.2 Waveguide used for the beam from CO_2 lasers.

Laser surgery of the upper aerodigestive tract is usually performed with the beam of a CO_2 laser applied through an operating microscope. A confocal, low-power, visible laser beam from a helium–neon laser that is sent through the waveguide and the microscope together with the CO_2 laser is used to aim the invisible surgical beam. The beam can be sharply focussed to a spot of only 0.03 cm in diameter corresponding to an area of about 0.001 cm². A 10 W laser beam with an original cross section of 1 cm² would have a power density of approximately 10,000 W cm⁻² when focussed on such a tiny spot. This power density would deliver 2500 cal s⁻¹ to the target, causing it to heat up at a rate of up to several thousand degrees per second depending on the degree of light absorption.

The wavelength of the CO_2 laser is readily absorbed by water (Figure 10.3), of which human tissue is largely made up. The beam penetrates only to a depth of about 0.01 mm, but since its energy is almost entirely absorbed in this short distance, the beam heats the water almost instantaneously, denaturing the proteins and causing almost explosive vaporization of the tissue. The heat transmitted to the immediately surrounding tissue cauterizes the capillaries and prevents bleeding. For example, this property along with the ability to focus the beam to a precisely defined point allows minute papillomas to be removed from the delicate vocal cords while causing nearly no damage to the surrounding tissue.

The shorter wavelength light from the Nd–YAG laser is less strongly absorbed by water and penetrates deeper into the tissue (Figure 10.4). Its energy is distributed to a volume of tissue which is at least two

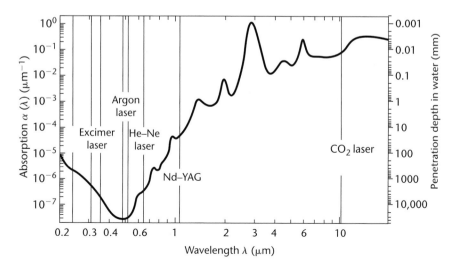

Figure 10.3 Absorption spectrum of water. Light of longer wavelength is more readily absorbed than visible light.

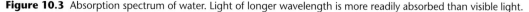

orders of magnitude larger than that affected by the CO_2 laser and causes much less vaporization and more thermal coagulation. This effect is sometimes not apparent until much later with shrinking and scarring of the treated tissue. For example, the Nd–YAG laser is used for reduction of hypertrophied nasal turbinates. These are irradiated under topical anaesthesia and shrink due to subsequent scarring and sloughing. The coagulating properties of the Nd–YAG laser can be used to treat bleeding vascular malformations such as in Morbus Osler.

The argon laser with its light in the blue–green visible spectrum is not commonly used in otorhinological surgery. The light is absorbed poorly by water and can therefore penetrate tissue to a greater depth than the beams from CO_2 or Nd–YAG lasers. However, it is strongly absorbed by haemoglobin and melanin and can thus be used to coagulate or obliterate blood vessels without destroying the overlying tissue (Figure 10.4). For an overview of the surgical use of lasers the reader is referred to monographs on the subject.[6,7]

Diode or semiconductor lasers have been recently introduced into routine clinical use. They are no longer restricted to low-power applications but can deliver up to 50 W of continuous power. Diode lasers have the advantage of being smaller and less expensive than the Nd–YAG or argon lasers, which they are slowly replacing. Most diode lasers are based on gallium–arsenide, and the wavelength of the light emitted by the diode depends on its exact composition and construction. The most commonly used wavelengths are 810, 940 and 980 nm. The shorter wavelength is absorbed by water to an extent between that of the Nd–YAG and the argon laser and has a wide variety of uses from ophthalmology to dermatology. The 810 nm wavelength light is optimal for pumping an Nd–YAG laser instead of xenon lamps. After passing the beam through a KTP frequency doubler, the resulting light with a wavelength of 534 nm can replace the argon laser in ophthalmological surgery. The light from the longer wavelength lasers more closely resembles that of the Nd–YAG laser, which they are now replacing. Table 10.1 gives a summary of commonly used lasers and their characteristics.

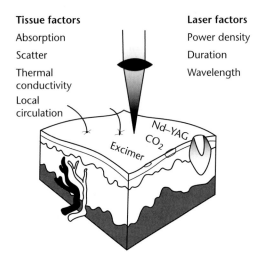

Tissue factors

Absorption

Scatter

Thermal conductivity

Local circulation

Laser factors

Power density

Duration

Wavelength

Figure 10.4   The effects of different types of laser beams on tissue.

Table 10.1 Characteristics of laser beams used in surgery

Laser type	Wavelength (nm)	Comments
CO_2	10,600	Far infrared; beam invisible; strongly absorbed by water and PVC; superficial tissue penetration (10 μm); carbonizes and vaporizes tissue, cutting laser
Nd–YAG	1060	Near infrared; beam invisible; absorbed less well by water; absorbed by haemoglobin (penetration 200 μm); tissue penetration depends on blood flow; PVC is transparent at this wavelength; beam can be applied through flexible waveguide
Argon	488/515	Visible light; poorly absorbed by water (penetrates 12 m!); strongly absorbed by haemoglobin (penetrates 30 μm); tissue penetration depends on blood flow; passes through cornea and vitreous humour but coagulates retina
Gallium–arsenide diodes	810, 940, 980	Red to infrared light; poorly absorbed by water; absorbed by haemoglobin
KTP frequency doubler		Effects depend on the resulting wavelengths

Technical aspects of the procedures

The large majority of these laser operations are performed by microlaryngoscopy with the surgeon viewing the operating site through a binocular microscope, guiding the laser beam with a micromanipulator, which is basically a joystick, with his right hand and grasping the tissue with long forceps held in the left hand (Figure 10.5). During laser surgery of the upper aerodigestive tract, the patient's head is maximally reflected and the operation site is visualized using either a closed laryngoscope (Kleinsasser laryngoscope) or a distending laryngopharyngoscope (Figure 10.6). After the instrument has been introduced it is attached to a chest support and fixed in the

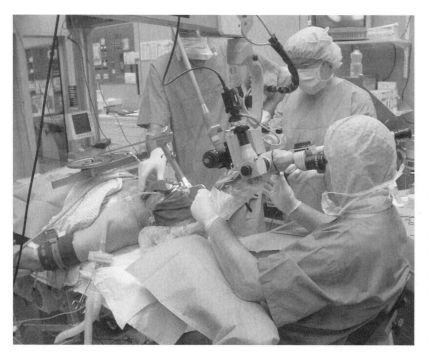

Figure 10.5 Picture of surgeon performing laser surgery of the pharynx. One sees the laryngoscope attached to the support resting on the platform above the patient's chest. The laser wave guide is visible leading down and attached to the microscope. The surgeon sits with his arms supported on wide armrests while he manipulates the tissues with instruments held in his left hand, while guiding the laser beam with his right.

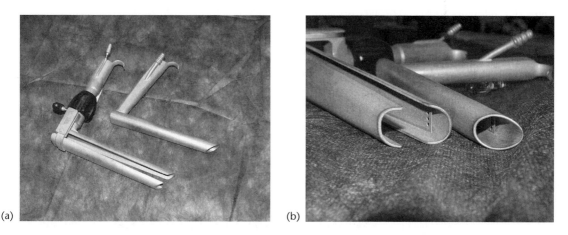

(a)   (b)

Figure 10.6 Laryngoscopes used for laser surgery of the oropharynx and larynx. Closed or distendable models are available. A suction channel is integrated into the body of the laryngoscope for removing the smoke plume from the operation site. (a) Distendable (right) and closed (left) laryngoscopes. The suction connectors are clearly visible. (b) View into the distal opening of the laryngoscopes showing the openings of the suction channels.

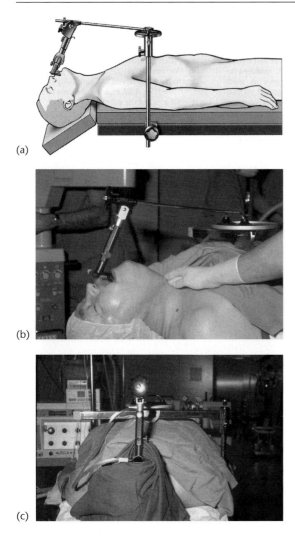

(a)

(b)

(c)

Figure 10.7 Patient with laryngoscope and chest support.

position giving the best visualization of the operating site (Figure 10.7).

When the CO_2 laser is being used, the laser beam is guided by mirrors in an articulated metal tube that is attached to the operating microscope where the invisible beam from the CO_2 laser is focussed together with the visible pilot beam from the helium–neon laser. The light of the Nd–YAG laser is applied with a flexible waveguide that can be introduced through a specially designed rhinoscope or bronchoscope.

Technical complications

The properties that make the laser beam a useful tool in surgery are those that also make it a risk for patient

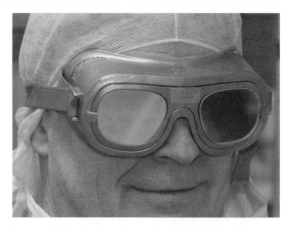

Figure 10.8 Safety goggles must either reflect or absorb the wavelength of the laser light in use.

and operating room (OR) personnel alike. The risks are so great that they are regulated by national agencies such as the British Standards Institute (BS IEC 60825-8:1999) or the American National Standards Institute (ANSI Z136.3-1988). These institutions have published guidelines that must be observed whenever surgical lasers are used.[8,9] Most other countries will have similar regulations. Not only the direct beam is dangerous but also stray rays reflected from metal surfaces. Even these can cause serious eye injuries, and all OR personnel must wear safety goggles with lenses that absorb light at the wavelength of the laser beam (Figure 10.8). Any glass or plastic lens, but not contact lenses, will absorb the far-infrared light of the CO_2 laser beam. The green-tinted lenses required for the Nd–YAG laser and the amber-orange lenses for use with the argon laser alter colour perception and make visual detection of cyanosis difficult. But there are special clear lenses available with a coating that absorbs the near-infrared wavelength of the Nd–YAG laser beam. The patient's eye must be taped shut and the eyelids protected by moistened gauze pads. Wet cloth should be applied to the exposed portions of the patient's face to prevent burns from reflected beams.

Direct hits with the laser beam can ignite flammable material and vaporize non-flammable material. How this affects the choice of endotracheal tube is described in detail below.

The beam of the CO_2 laser vaporizes tissue and produces a plume of smoke and fine particles. This plume has a disagreeable odour and can induce unpleasant subjective symptoms in sensitive individuals. The particles are in the size range of 0.1–0.8 μm[10] and can thus be transported and deposited in the alveoli. Smoke from the plume was

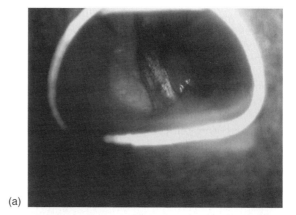

(a)

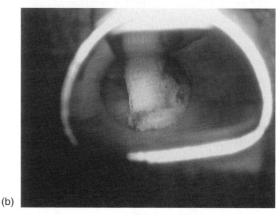

(b)

Figure 10.9 Pictures of endotracheal tube in position with wet swabs protecting cuff.

found to reduce mucociliary clearance and cause severe inflammation.[11] The condensate in the laser plume from the vaporization of 1 g of tissue has a mutagenic potential comparable with that of smoking three to six cigarettes.[12]

Although there is a theoretical possibility that the laser plume might act as a vector for viral infection, there is currently no consensus whether the smoke plume from vaporized papilloma tissue contains infectious virus particles or not.[13–15] There is also some evidence showing that bacteria can be spread in the plume.[16,17] Lacking firm evidence that the plume is innocuous, one should treat it as infectious and take measures to protect both patient and personnel. Removal of the fumes from the operation site with an effective exhaust system is the best way to prevent contamination of the workspace air.[18] OR personnel can be further protected with special face masks that filter out virus-sized particles.

Managing the airway

Airway management is the main concern in laser surgery of the upper aerodigestive tract, particularly for surgery of the larynx. It is even more critical for surgery in the trachea itself. The undisputed, hands-down winner for best protection of the airway against aspiration and best control of ventilation is endotracheal intubation with a cuffed tube. However, the method does have the drawback of occupying the same space as that in which the surgeon intends to operate (Figure 10.9). Some have tried to avoid this problem by using inhalational anaesthesia in a spontaneously breathing patient. There is no foreign object

in the way, but the airway is unprotected, the surgeon is exposed to appreciable concentrations of the anaesthetic and, in addition, has to work on a moving target. Other approaches that avoid the use of an endotracheal tube are to operate in apnoea or to use a jet ventilation technique. In the following sections we shall present each technique and describe in detail their advantages and disadvantages.

Apnoeic techniques

The technically least sophisticated method of resolving the competition between anaesthetist and surgeon for airway supremacy during laser surgery is to use the apnoea technique. In this technique, ventilation is interrupted periodically to give the surgeon access to the surgical site. The method is particularly useful in children and for subglottic or tracheal operations.[19,20] The anaesthetic of choice is a total intravenous regimen. Anaesthesia is induced and the patient's lungs are ventilated by bag and mask. When the plane of anaesthesia and the degree of neuromuscular relaxation are sufficiently deep, the surgeon exposes the vocal cords with the operating laryngoscope and introduces an endotracheal tube through its lumen into the trachea under direct vision. One should use the largest possible tube since obstruction of surgical vision is not an issue. The lungs are ventilated until end-tidal CO_2 is in the range of 35–40 mmHg. The inspiratory O_2 fraction is increased to obtain an O_2 saturation of 100%. This is not always possible in the patient population presenting for laser surgery of the laryngeal cancer, with their usual history of excessive smoking and chronic obstructive lung disease (COLD). However, even in these patients it is nearly always possible to bring the pulse oximetric O_2 saturation up to at least 97%. There is a theoretical risk that even moist tissue can ignite in a 100% O_2 atmosphere if it dries out and chars, but even if minute fragments do catch fire there is no risk of sustained combustion.

When the anaesthetist is satisfied that the ventilatory preparations of the patient are adequate, the surgeon removes the endotracheal tube and commences surgery. Apnoea can be maintained for up to 4 or 5 min before O_2 saturation begins to fall from a baseline of 100%. During this period arterial CO_2 will increase by about 10–20 mmHg. The permissible apnoea period is, of course, shorter in patients with relevant pulmonary pathology, diminished functional residual capacity (FRC) and baseline O_2 saturation under 100%. Apnoea should be terminated as soon as O_2 saturation begins to fall, or at an O_2 saturation of 90–95% at the lowest, since the drop will continue for a while even after ventilation is resumed. At the end of apnoea, the surgeon reinserts the endotracheal tube and the anaesthetist ventilates the lungs to remove the accumulated CO_2. This will take a few minutes, and O_2 saturation will usually have returned to baseline values long before end-tidal CO_2 has been brought down below 40 mmHg.

Endotracheal intubation

Endotracheal intubation is indubitably the best method for protecting the airway from the laser plume as well as from foreign material such as blood, secretions and bits of resected tissue. This is our method of choice as shall be described in more detail in the section on anaesthetic management. The method does have its drawback, though. One of these is that the endotracheal tube can impair access to the surgical site. This problem can be minimized by using a small calibre tube. A second drawback is that the endotracheal tube can be set on fire by a carelessly fired laser beam with catastrophic consequences (Figure 10.10).

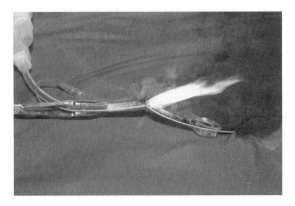

Figure 10.10 Picture of "blow-torch" flame from tube.

Older surveys give an incidence of this complication of 0.14–1.5% of all cases.[21–23] A 1984 survey of laser-related complications showed that endotracheal tube fires accounted for 41% of all perioperative complications.[24] In a study during the 2-year period from 1989 to 1990, only 14% of the 21 complications reported to the US Food and Drug Administration (FDA) were due to airway fires.[25] This may have been due to a change in the choice of endotracheal tube material or to greater care being taken to prevent the laser beam from hitting and igniting the tubes. Although there is great potential for serious consequences of endotracheal tube fires,[26,27] correct handling of the complication can avert major harm from the patient.[22,26]

The risk of an airway fire depends to a large extent on the material of the endotracheal tube and on modifications to its surface. Since there is no material that is truly flame resistant in a laser beam, what matters is how long it takes for the tube material to ignite, what minimum O_2 concentration is necessary for sustained combustion, how fast the material will burn and if the combustion products are noxious or toxic. These questions have been the subject of a large number of studies.

Polyvinyl chloride (PVC) has largely replaced red rubber as the material of most modern endotracheal tubes. Unfortunately, PVC strongly absorbs long-wave infrared light and is easily ignited by the far-infrared beams of the CO_2 laser.[28] It is much more susceptible to ignition by the laser than the red rubber of older endotracheal tubes.[29] On burning, PVC produces toxic fumes such as hydrochloric acid and vinyl chloride as well as carbonaceous deposits that can cause severe pulmonary damage. Ignition of intraluminal ("blow-torch") fires in unprotected PVC tubing occurs within less than 3 s of irradiation with a

Table 10.2 Characteristics of typical tube materials

	PVC	Red rubber	Silicone
Flammability index in O_2 (minimum O_2 concentration for sustained combustion)	26.3%	17.6%	18.9%
Flammability index in N_2O (minimum N_2O concentration for sustained combustion)	45.6%	37.4%	41.4%
Typical ignition times with CO_2 laser (at 15 W)	3 s	25 s	20 s
Combustion residue	Hydrochloric acid, Vinyl chloride, Carbonaceous ash	Carbonaceous ash	Silica ash

perpendicular, continuous narrow beam of CO_2 laser light at 15 W.[30] Under the same conditions, conventional red rubber tubing starts to burn on the surface after approximately 12 s of exposure, but a blow-torch flame does not occur until after 25 s.[30] Untreated silicone ignites more readily than red rubber.[31]

Clear PVC is transparent to visible and near-infrared light and is therefore little affected by Nd–YAG, argon or diode lasers *in vitro* as long as the lettering or barium stripe is not hit.[32] However, even a thin film of mucus or blood on the outer surface of the tube changes the absorption characteristics dramatically, rendering the material easily ignited by the Nd–YAG laser beam.[33] Controlled studies of the effects of the near-infrared light from the Nd–YAG laser on common endotracheal tube material have shown that all materials are vulnerable, although there are differences in the energy and duration of exposure required for combustion.[32] In a comparative study in dogs, PVC tubing was the first to ignite, causing extensive bronchial deposits of soot with significant mucosal ulceration and bronchial inflammation. Red rubber tubing was ignited less readily and the combustion products were less noxious than were those of PVC. Silicone tubing was slightly more resistant to ignition but produced large amounts of white silica ash.[34]

The composition of the respiratory gas mixture, particularly the O_2 content, greatly affects the combustibility of the tubing material. The index of flammability is the minimum inspired O_2 concentration necessary to maintain combustion of the material. This index is actually the highest for PVC, which requires an O_2 concentration of at least 26% for sustained combustion as opposed to 19% for silicone and 17% for red rubber. Table 10.2 gives a summary of the most common materials used in the manufacture of endotracheal tubes and their characteristics.

These materials also burn in N_2O without O_2; the flammability index for N_2O is 46% for PVC and about 40% for silicone and red rubber.[35] For this reason, N_2O is not recommended in laser surgery, since its addition to the respiratory gas mixture is just as hazardous as increasing the O_2 concentration. This implies that anaesthesia machines that can add only N_2O and not air to the inspiratory gas mixture are not suitable for use in laser surgery of the upper aerodigestive tract. The use of PEEP may reduce the risk of blow-torch flames in endotracheal tubes.[36]

Some studies recommend substituting helium for nitrogen in the respiratory gas mixture, showing that it delays the ignition of the endotracheal tube in the laser beam at low beam intensities.[37,38] They also recommend helium for patients with impaired pulmonary ventilation due to its lower viscosity and thus better flow characteristics.[39,40] However, at energies of more than 10 W, ignition is delayed by only a few seconds and the O_2 flammability index is improved by only 1–2%.[41] The appreciably higher costs and logistic difficulties far outweigh the slight advantages that helium might offer.

Note   Keep inspiratory O_2 concentration under 25%

Modern volatile anaesthetics do not burn at the concentrations used for maintenance of anaesthesia, but they could be ignited at concentrations seen during mask induction. Isoflurane burns at 7.0%, enflurane at 5.75% and halothane at 4.75%.[42] In fact, 2% halothane was shown to reduce the time to ignition of PVC tubes in 40% O_2 by almost 40%.[37] Even in normal concentrations, volatile anaesthetics might be broken down by the intense heat of the laser beam into potentially toxic pyrolysis products.

Protecting against endotracheal tube fires

Modifying standard endotracheal tubes

Some anaesthetists recommend wrapping the endotracheal tube with metal taping to reduce the risk of ignition by the laser beam.[22,29] This measure can significantly prolong the time that the tube can be subjected to a direct hit with the laser beam before it ignites. When wrapping the tube one must take great care to ensure that the tape lies flat on the tube and that there are no wrinkles. The tape must be wrapped with the edges overlapping to avoid any gaps though which the tube material would be vulnerable to ignition. Before using a tube modified in this manner, one would have to subject a prepared sample to the laser beam, since the degree of protection conferred by the wrapping is largely dependent on the type of tape used.[43]

Although wrapping with a suitable metal tape can protect the tube, the procedure has a number of drawbacks and we do not recommend it. The layer of tape increases the diameter of the tube by up to 2 mm, increases its stiffness, reducing its usefulness for endolaryngeal surgery, and the sharp edges of the tape increase the likelihood of mucosal damage. The shiny tape carries the risk of reflective damage.[44] The foil may unwrap during surgery either as a result of being hit by the laser beam or simply because the adhesive was faulty and this can cause airway obstruction or difficult extubation.[45] Most manufacturers of metal tape discourage the use of their products for medical purposes. In a number of countries, altering an endotracheal tube in such a manner will invalidate the licence leaving the anaesthetist solely responsible for complications and with little defence against litigation for laryngotracheal injuries.

Special purpose endotracheal tubes

Endotracheal tube manufacturers have marketed a number of tubes designed to confer a degree of resistance to laser-ignited airway fire. Nearly all of these tubes have flammable components that can ignite if the tubes are not used according to the manufacturers' guidelines and if specific warnings and precautions are not followed. The individual models are described below while Table 10.3 gives an overview of their properties. A major drawback is that these special purpose endotracheal tubes are at least 10 times more expensive than normal tubes.

The obvious solution to the problem of flammability is to manufacture the endotracheal tubes from metal.

Table 10.3 Special endotracheal tubes for laser surgery

Trade name	Manufacturer	Tube material	Inside diameter (mm)	Remarks
Laser-Flex with double cuff uncuffed	Mallinckrodt (Nellcor)	Flexible stainless steel, cuff is PVC	4.5; 5.0; 5.5; 6.0 3.0; 3.5; 4.0	For CO_2 and KTP lasers; can be ignited
Lasertubus	Rüsch	Latex coated with Merocel® (PVA) foam on silver foil	4.0–6.0 in 1 mm increments	For CO_2, Nd–YAG and argon lasers; two separate cuffs, one inside the other
Laser Trach	Kendall	Copper wrapped red rubber		For CO_2 and KTP lasers
Fome-Cuf	Bivona Medical (now Smith-Portex Group)	Silicone	3.0–7.0 in 1 mm increments	For CO_2 laser
Laser-Shield II	Medtronic-Xomed	Reflective aluminium wrap with smooth teflon overwrap	4.0–8.5 in 0.5 mm increments	For CO_2 and KTP lasers; dry methylene blue in cuff dyes inflation fluid
Laser-Shield	Medtronic-Xomed	Silicone with aluminium-filled outer layer		No longer manufactured
Norton Tube		Stainless steel		No longer manufactured, but since reusable some may still be in use

The first flexible metal endotracheal tube was described by Norton.[46] This tube was constructed of a metal spiral, and although it was not airtight, it did have the advantage of being non-flammable. Lacking a cuff, a tracheal seal could be obtained by packing with wet surgical swabs. This tube is no longer on the market, but since it was reusable some specimens might still be in service. Its heir on the market is the Laser-Flex® tube (Mallinckrodt-Nellcor), which is an air-tight corrugated spiral of matte-finished stainless steel with a PVC Murphy eye tip. It is designed for use with the CO_2 or KTP lasers,[47] but not with Nd–YAG lasers. The larger sizes have a double cuff and there is an uncuffed version for use in small children. In the double cuff model, the proximal cuff protects the distal cuff, which can maintain the tracheal seal, even if the proximal cuff is punctured. The tube can be ignited, and blood on the outer surface greatly increases the risk of combustion.[48] Metal tubes are thick walled and take up more room than standard endotracheal tubes of the same internal diameter. This can be a problem for surgery of the vocal cords or the subglottic region. Metal tubes, even when they do not ignite, can be heated by the laser beam and cause conductive thermal damage to adjacent tissue.

There are commercially available endotracheal tubes with a flame-retardant coating. These do not give total protection against laser-ignited airway fires but some do reduce the risk of immediate ignition by a short accidental hit with the laser beam. The Laser-Shield® (Medtronic-Xomed) was a silicone tube with an aluminium-filled silicone outer layer licensed for use with the CO_2 laser. It gave a slight but inconsistent protection against direct hits,[28,30] and it has since been replaced by the Laser-Shield II® which is a silicone tube wrapped with aluminium and coated with teflon. This model is intended for use with CO_2 and KTP lasers. This is essentially a commercial version of the homemade tape wrapped endotracheal tube with the advantages of a smooth, atraumatic outer coating and official stamp of approval. It retards the occurrence of blow-torch flames, even when coated with blood,[48] but does not completely prevent them, since the silicone inner material will ignite once the metal wrapping is breached by the laser beam. Ignition of the teflon surface itself can yield toxic fluorinated pyrolysis products while the aluminium wrapping can possibly become dislodged and cause airway occlusion.

The Laser Trach® tube (Kendall-Sheridan) is another commercially available, tape wrapped tube. It is manufactured from red rubber with a copper foil wrapping covered with an overwrap of fabric, and is meant to be used with CO_2 and KTP lasers. The outer wrap of fabric is soaked with water or saline prior to and during use and the pledgets supplied with the tube can be soaked in water or saline and placed around the cuff to give additional protection. This tube properly prepared can withstand a continuous 40 W CO_2 laser beam for more than 1 min without igniting, and the time to ignition by continuous contact irradiation at 40 W with an Nd–YAG laser was increased threefold to 18 s.[49] The Lasertubus® (Rüsch), intended for use with CO_2, argon or Nd–YAG lasers, takes a different approach to protecting the endotracheal tube from ignition. It is made of white rubber with two cuffs, one within the other, so that when the outer one is hit, the inner cuff can still maintain a tight tracheal seal. The surface of the tube is covered with a sponge-like polyvinyl alcohol coating (Merocel®) over a metal foil base. The coating can be soaked with saline or water to prevent ignition. This coating material is non-reflective which prevents beam deflection with subsequent damage to other structures.

The Fome-Cuf® (Bivona Medical Technologies) is an endotracheal tube that was designed with not so much flame resistance as cuff deflation and airway leakage after cuff puncture in mind. This is an important consideration, since cuff deflation will permit O_2-rich gas to circulate in the operative site and increase the risk of sustained combustion. The Fome-Cuf® consists of an aluminium wrapped silicone tube with a foam-filled cuff and is intended for use with CO_2 lasers. The cuff is self-inflating much like a modern ground pad for hikers and retains its size even if the cuff shell is penetrated. Since the cuff must be actively evacuated in order to properly remove the tube, damage to the shell can render this almost impossible. The cuff will then have to be drawn through the larynx in the "inflated" state. The outer surface of the tube shaft is flammable but a study showed that no blow-torch flame occurred.[50]

Jet ventilation

Basics

A number of anaesthetists advocate the use of jet ventilation for laser surgery of the larynx and lower airways. They see its advantages in the minimal obstruction of surgical access due to airway instrumentation and lack of flammable material within range of the laser beam. Proponents of the technique also like to stress the point that mean intrapulmonary pressure is lower with jet ventilation than with intermittent positive-pressure ventilation,[51] thus placing less strain on anastomoses or fistulae. The claim that there is less circulatory impairment, however, is probably unfounded.[52]

In jet ventilation, a narrow, high-velocity "jet" of gas is injected into the trachea to inflate the lungs. The basic technique was introduced in the 1960s, yet the term itself was not used in the literature until 1974.[53] The method gained popularity during the 1970s and was propagated as a "tubeless" method of ventilation for surgery of the larynx, trachea or bronchi in which a blocked endotracheal tube might impede or completely obstruct access to the operation site.[54–56] This is particularly the case for endotracheal or endobronchial surgery.[57–61] Paediatric laryngeal and tracheal surgery is an important domain for jet ventilation due to the small calibre of the airways.[62–65] The indication for its use in laryngeal surgery in adults, on the other hand, is less compelling.

The gas jet is applied through a narrow cannula whose tip can be placed either above the vocal cords (supraglottic) or below them (infraglottic). The supraglottic cannula is frequently incorporated into the laryngoscope. A transtracheal approach can also be employed using a curved cannula inserted through the cricothyroid membrane into the trachea[66] (Figure 10.11). Transtracheal jet ventilation has been advocated as a measure of last resort when confronted with a "cannot intubate, cannot ventilate" situation.[67] The basic principles are the same for each approach .

In the initial technique, the jet was applied at a low frequency under manual or mechanical control and ventilation was monitored by observing chest excursions.[69,70] Although this technique is still employed,[71,72] it was largely supplanted by high-frequency jet ventilation (HFJV) in the late 1970s.[73] The respiratory frequency in HFJV is typically between 60 and 150 per min (1–2.5 Hz), with frequencies up to 600 per min (10 Hz) occasionally being used. The driving pressure used in HFJV is much higher than that used in conventional intermittent pressure ventilation and is in the range of 80–450 kPa (0.8–4.5 bar). The typical jetted tidal volume in HFJV is around 2–3 ml kg^{-1}. Since this is no larger than anatomical dead space, mechanisms other than mass gas flow must act to effect CO_2 elimination. One of these is the Venturi effect in which a high-velocity stream of air entrains ambient air into its flow, so that the actual volume of moving gas is higher than that passing through the cannula.[74] This is caused both by the lower pressure surrounding the jet (Bernoulli's law) and also by the friction of the jet passing through the surrounding air. Just how effective the Venturi effect is, depends to a large extent on where the tip of the jet cannula is located and on the jet velocity.[74–76] By applying a constant so-called bias flow past the jet opening, one can control the composition of the gas entering the bronchi. The actual amount of entrained gas reaching the alveoli depends on the magnitude of backflow or bypass.[76,77] This latter factor is important

if one intends to give inhalational anaesthesia through a bias flow attachment.

A number of problems and difficulties are associated with the use of jet ventilation, and these might be partly responsible for its still remaining a technique

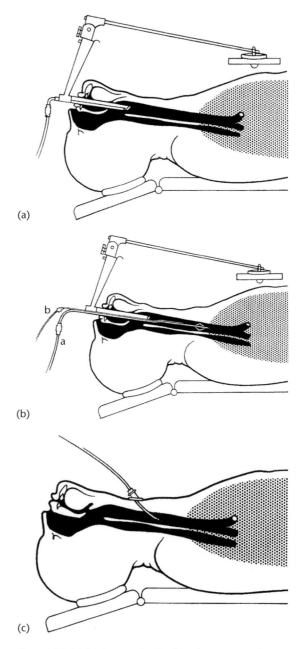

(a)

(b)

(c)

Figure 10.11 Various methods of applying jet ventilation. (a) Supraglottic jet integrated into the laryngoscope. (b) Infraglottic placement of the tip of the cannula. (c) Transtracheal introduction of jet cannula. (Modified from Ref [68].)

for enthusiasts. Some of these are of a technical nature. The gas stream is cold and dry and can damage the bronchial epithelium,[78] but some jet ventilators are equipped to moisten and heat the air jet, alleviating this problem. The narrow jet is itself capable of causing appreciable tissue damage if it impinges directly on the mucosa; a problem arising with infraglottic placement of the tip of the cannula. Excessive end-expiratory intrapulmonary pressure can build up since it is difficult to measure true airway pressures (P_{AW}). Modern jet ventilators have provisions for pressure monitoring and cut-off features designed to protect against barotrauma (see below), but sensor placement is crucial. Pressure recordings will be too low if the sensor is positioned too close to the jet orifice.

One main difficulty with jet ventilation is inefficient CO_2 elimination.[51,79] The patients most prone to this problem are male, overweight and those with pre-existing chronic obstructive or restrictive pulmonary pathologies.[80–82] This almost perfectly describes the clientele presenting for laser surgery of tumours of the upper aerodigestive tract. Complicating the fact that CO_2 elimination is impaired is the difficulty encountered in monitoring arterial CO_2 tension. In a refinement of HFJV, two frequencies are combined, one around 600 per min and a lower one of *ca.* 15–20 per min.[83] This is believed to counteract the problems with CO_2 elimination inherent in HFJV and to reduce the incidence and severity of O_2 desaturation.[84]

Technical aspects

There are a large number of commercially available jet ventilators, many of which are used predominantly in intensive care. Development is still in flux and models appear and disappear again with a certain regularity.[85] An HFJV presently in use in Europe is the Monsoon® (Acutronic Medical Systems, Switzerland) that replaces its predecessor, the AMS1000. This ventilator complies with regulations for medical equipment and is approved for clinical use (FDA approved). One can set ventilatory frequency, inspiratory time, driving pressure, inspired O_2 concentration, P_{AW} limits (peak inspiratory and end-expiratory) and humidification. P_{AW} is monitored through a separate line and gas flow is automatically shut down if pressure limits

are exceeded. These are features that any ventilator intended for use in laser surgery should have.

In an emergency situation, low-frequency jet ventilation can essentially be performed with a manually controlled injector connected to an appropriate cannula, either translaryngeal or transtracheal, and transtracheal cannulae for emergency jet ventilation are commercially available. Ventilation is monitored visually by observing thorax excursions. This method has a high-risk potential and should only be used when endotracheal intubation is not an option and an approved ventilator is not available.

As mentioned above, the tip of the jet cannula can be placed either below or above the level of the vocal cords. Although the supraglottic position gives better oxygenation and visualization, it leaves the airway completely unprotected. Its use is recommended only for diagnostic laryngoscopy, for the removal of foreign material from the trachea and bronchi and perhaps for laser vaporization of minute vocal cord and vocal fold processes. Cannulae for supraglottic jetting can either be integrated into the laryngoscope or can be attached to it by clamps.

Laser surgery of any extent should be performed with infraglottic jet position to avoid aspiration (see below). A frequently used, commercially available tube for infraglottic jetting is the Hunsaker Mon-Jet® (Medtronic-Xomed) (Figure 10.12). This tube has distal spacing vanes to prevent mucosal damage by centring the tip. It has an integrated second lumen for monitoring P_{AW} and CO_2. The Hi-Lo® jet tube (Mallinckrodt-Nellcor) is essentially only a normal, unblocked endotracheal tube with separate lines for jetting and monitoring integrated into the wall.

Initial ventilator settings would be 100% O_2 with a driving pressure of 150–200 kPa (1.5–2.0 bar) at a frequency of 100–150 cycles min^{-1} and an inspiratory time of 50%. The peak inspiratory pressure limit would be set to 40 mbar and maximum end-expiratory pressure to 15 mbar. In a patient with normal pulmonary compliance, these settings would give a jetted gas volume of 20 l min^{-1} and a tidal volume of approximately 135 ml with a peak pressure under 25 mbar and an end-expiratory pressure under 6 mbar. For slender

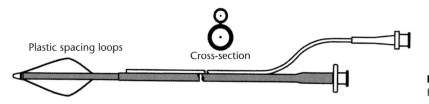

Plastic spacing loops

Cross-section

Figure 10.12 Diagram of Hunsaker Mon-Jet tube.

Table 10.4 Effects of ventilator settings on blood gases

Parameter	P_aO_2	P_aCO_2
Increase F_IO_2	↑↑↑	No change
Increase driving pressure	↑↑	↓↓↓
Increase ventilatory frequency	↑	↑
Increase inspiration time	↑	No change

↑ indicates increase; ↓ indicates decrease.

Table 10.5 Suggested anaesthetic for microlaryngo-scopic laser surgery

TIVA with propofol and remifentanil	
Propofol or	Infusion rate 5–6 mg kg^{-1} h^{-1} targeted effect-site concentration 2.0–2.5 µg ml^{-1}
Remifentanil then	1 µg kg^{-1} slow bolus injection, 0.2–0.3 µg kg^{-1} min^{-1} 1 µg kg^{-1} bolus at signs of insufficient analgesia
Balanced anaesthesia with isoflurane or desflurane with remifentanil	
Volatile	0.5 MAC end-expiratory concentration
Remifentanil then	1 µg kg^{-1} slow bolus injection 0.2–0.3 µg kg^{-1} min^{-1} 1 µg kg^{-1} bolus at signs of insufficient analgesia

patients and children one would reduce the driving pressure to 60–140 kPa (0.6–1.4 bar), while one would increase it to 350 kPa (3.5 bar) for obese patients or those with chronic obstructive pulmonary disease, if one actually intended to use HFJV in the latter. To avoid the risk of fire, the inspired O_2 concentration is reduced as low as possible to maintain pulse oximetric saturation between 97% and 99%.

Changing the ventilator settings will alter both oxygenation and CO_2 elimination (Table 10.4). Increasing F_IO_2 in the jetted gas as well as in the bias flow will increase arterial O_2 tension but have no effect on arterial CO_2. Increasing driving pressure or ventilatory frequency will increase partial pressure of O_2 in arterial blood (P_aO_2) and usually decrease partial pressure of CO_2 in arterial blood (P_aCO_2), but CO_2 elimination is impaired when the higher pressures and frequencies cause dynamic hyperinflation (intrinsic PEEP).[80,86]

P_{AW} depends on the rate of gas entrainment and the cross section of the expiratory pathway.[75,87] At a constant insufflation rate, any reduction of the cross section of the exhaust route, whether due to secretions, surgical instruments or laryngospasm, will cause an immediate rise in P_{AW}.[88–90] With older equipment lacking P_{AW} monitoring and automatic over-pressure gas cut-off, this can cause barotrauma (see below).

Severe impairment of airflow and a reduction of airway cross section by more than 80% are considered absolute contraindications for jet ventilation.[91] Obstructive and restrictive lung disorders are relative contraindications.[81]

For further details on the use of jet ventilation the reader is referred to journal reviews (e.g. Refs [68,92] or to the European Society of Jet Ventilation (www.esjv.org)).

Anaesthetic management for jet ventilation

Careful patient selection is important for jet ventilation. Contraindications must be observed and cannula position should be decided on in collaboration with the surgeon. Atropine or glycopyrrolate should be given preoperatively to reduce salivation and to blunt vagal reflexes.

Total intravenous anaesthesia (TIVA) is the method of choice for jet ventilation. For laser surgery we use a combination of propofol and remifentanil (see Table 10.5), although other combinations have been described in the past.[62,93–95] Adequate neuromuscular relaxation guided by relaxometry is required, particularly when the jet is located infraglottically, since glottic motion or laryngospasm can interfere with surgery and can lead to excessive intrathoracic pressure with its associated complications.[96] A neuromuscular blocker with a short recovery time such as mivacurium is recommended even for longer operations. Repetitive doses of 0.1 mg kg^{-1} mivacurium every 8–10 min usually give sufficient relaxation while still allowing rapid recovery.

Pulse oximetry and arterial CO_2 monitoring are mandatory during jet ventilation since arterial O_2 desaturation can occur despite an outward appearance of adequate ventilation, and CO_2 elimination can change rapidly.[62,97,98] Capnometry can be greatly inaccurate and usually underestimates the true value. This problem can be avoided by using transcutaneous or continuous intra-arterial CO_2 monitoring (see Chapter 4). One can also obtain fairly accurate end-tidal CO_2 values by periodically interrupting the jet to allow complete expiration of alveolar air.

Emergence from anaesthesia is managed by gradually reducing jet support of ventilation and allowing the patient to breathe spontaneously. The jet is shut off and the cannula removed when respiration is adequate.

Alternatively, one can remove the cannula and ventilate by mask and bag until the patient resumes breathing.

Risks and complications of jet ventilation

Even enthusiasts recognize that transtracheal jet ventilation is an unsafe technique in inexperienced hands. Jet ventilation for laser surgery has a higher incidence of complications than endotracheal intubation. In a study of 15,701 patients, the incidence of ventilation-related complications in jet-ventilated patients was 0.58%, and three-fourths of these were life threatening. Patients ventilated with an endotracheal tube had a 0.36% incidence of ventilation-related complications, only one-half of which were serious.[26]

Barotrauma is a complication of jet ventilation that can cause various degrees of airway rupture resulting in pneumothorax, pneumomediastinum, subcutaneous emphysema or pneumopericardium.[64,99–102] Contributing factors for barotrauma are infraglottic position of the jet, either transtracheal or translaryngeal, and concurrent obstruction of airflow from the bronchial tree, for example due to laryngospasm.[89,96] In a study in 643 patients with transtracheal HFJV, arterial desaturation was not uncommon, subcutaneous emphysema occurred with an incidence of 8.4% (of which 30% also developed pneumomediastinum), and seven patients suffered a pneumothorax.[97] Other complications such as hypoventilation, hypoxaemia, abdominal distension and stomach rupture[99,103] are more typical for a supraglottic jet catheter with an incorrectly directed cannula.

Contrary to what one would expect, aspiration is not frequent in jet ventilation, at least not when the tip of the jet cannula is in an infraglottic position, either via a transtracheal or a translaryngeal approach and when the ventilatory frequency is high enough to induce a constant backflow.[104–106] With the jet cannula in a supraglottic position, however, aspiration is probably inevitable since the airways are open and the high-velocity air stream will entrain loose foreign matter and fluids as well as vaporized material in the laser plume.

Airway fires also occur during jet ventilation[107] and these can sometimes have bizarre manifestations. In one memorable case, all required precautions including covering the patient's face with wet towels had been taken, yet the patient's moustache was set ablaze by a flame emanating from the surgeon's burning glove, passing through the O_2-rich atmosphere in the pharynx, then through the nasal passages, and causing second degree burns to the upper lip and nostrils.[108]

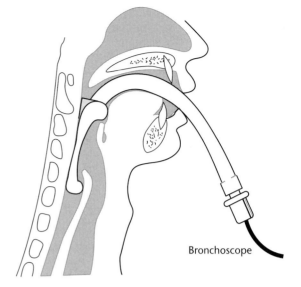

Figure 10.13 Diagram of bronchoscope being inserted through laryngeal mask airway.

Other methods of airway management

Laryngeal mask airway

The laryngeal mask and laser surgery of the airway might seem mutually exclusive concepts, since the former completely blocks the view of the latter. However, the laryngeal mask can be quite useful in conjunction with an Nd–YAG laser guided by a flexible bronchoscope for treatment of subglottic, tracheal or bronchial lesions.[109–111] Central tumourous airway obstruction is a typical indication for Nd–YAG surgery of the trachea or carina. The laryngeal mask allows laser treatment to proceed without having to interrupt ventilation. The laryngeal mask has the additional advantage that its connecting tube has a larger diameter than the standard endotracheal tube, leaving more space for the bronchoscope.

After the intubating laryngeal mask is introduced and positioned in the usual manner, a flexible bronchoscope is inserted through a ported connecting piece and advanced until the operation site is reached (Figure 10.13). The laser waveguide is then inserted through the biopsy channel and used to apply the laser beam.

Any laser plume will be forced into distal lung segment during inspiration, but this is not a risk unique to the laryngeal mask. There is also the risk that during resection of tracheal or bronchial tumours, fragments of the lesion will become dislodged and be carried into lower parts of the bronchial tree.

But then again, this is not a risk unique to the laryngeal mask. One must keep in mind that the surgical treatment of obstructive lesions of the central airways are usually desperate measures undertaken to prevent the patient from suffocating, and that the risk of laser plumes and tissue fragments are negligible in comparison. The use of the laryngeal mask certainly deserves careful consideration in these cases.

Cuirass ventilation

Cuirass ventilation works on essentially the same principle as the iron lung used in the times of polio epidemics.[112] In the modern version used for patients with various forms of respiratory failure,[113–115] the patient is no longer placed into a large iron tank but wears a plastic or metal cuirass resembling a knight's breastplate. It functions by applying negative pressure to the outside of the chest covered by the cuirass with a suction pump. This is then transmitted through the thorax and induces negative intrathoracic pressure as in normal inspiration.

Cuirass ventilation requires no endotracheal tube and is thus an obvious candidate for laser surgery of the larynx. Its main risk is that the airway is unprotected and open to the laser plume and foreign material. There is, however, no risk of barotrauma as in jet ventilation.

The reports on the use of cuirass ventilation for laser surgery have been encouraging,[116,117] but since the method requires equipment not routinely at the disposal of the anaesthetist, it remains the domain of specialists. The reader is refereed to the literature for further information.

Patients and preoperative assessment

The indications for laser surgery of the upper aerodigestive tract being so heterogeneous, ranging from resection of subglottic stenosis in the premature neonate or ablation of vocal fold nodules in singers to protracted hypopharyngeal resections in elderly patients with extensive co-morbidity, no universally applicable guidelines can be given for preoperative assessment and perioperative management.

Healthy patients presenting for resection of cysts, minor papillomas, tracheal webs, etc. can be treated as outpatients. However, the indication for a large percentage of the laser surgery of the upper aerodigestive tract is malignant disease, mainly squamous cell carcinomas. One must bear in mind that most of these carcinomas are closely associated with a history

of smoking and alcohol abuse,[118–120] both of which influence anaesthetic management as well as the probability and the nature of postoperative complications.[121–124] Patients with tumours of the larynx or hypopharynx are or were serious smokers looking back on a large number of pack-years. These patients will typically have COLD with wheezing and/or rhonchi and a productive cough. Due to the minimally invasive nature of the surgery, one would not be as strict in the preoperative optimization of the condition as one would be prior to abdominal surgery, but one must reckon with perioperative problems of ventilation and oxygenation. Heavy smokers develop tolerance to the analgesic effects of opioids and will require higher doses both for their anaesthetic as well as for postoperative analgesia.[125–127]

The patients are usually also more than just social drinkers and a glance at the red blood cell indices will probably reveal an erythrocyte morphology indicative of chronic alcohol consumption. Mean cell haemoglobin (MCH) and mean cell volume (MCV) will be in the high normal range or more likely pathologically elevated as a sign of alcohol-induced folic acid deficiency. Liver enzymes may also be elevated. Depending on the stage of the disease, chronic alcohol intake can induce tolerance to hypnotics,[128,129] or can increase central nervous system (CNS) sensitivity to their effects[130,131] and this must be taken into account. The direction and the magnitude of the change is difficult to determine beforehand, but clinical and laboratory evidence of more severe liver damage such as low serum albumin, coagulation defects, low plasma cholinesterase and ascites are usually signs of a patient with normal to lower anaesthetic requirements. Such patients can be exquisitely sensitive to the depressant effects of benzodiazepines and these should be avoided in the premedication.

Points to remember when evaluating patients with ear, nose and throat (ENT) tumours

- Airway can be compromised by tumour, visualization of glottis can be impaired, friable tumours bleed easily if touched. Refer to ENT records for description of extent and localization of tumour.
- Laryngoscopy and intubation may be impossible after prior radiation therapy. Check by palpating submental and neck tissues. If these are indurated consider awake fibre-optic intubation or preoperative tracheotomy in local anaesthesia.
- Probable history of alcohol abuse with altered response to hypnotics.
- Probable history of heavy smoking. Altered response to opioids, perioperative pulmonary complications likely.

Anaesthetic management

Laryngoscopy is one of the most stressful phases during anaesthesia, more so even than skin incision or intra-abdominal dissection. Since the surgeon's approach to the operation site for laser surgery of the upper aerodigestive tract is essentially unremitting laryngoscopy with a straight bladed laryngoscope, it is not hard to imagine that the patient will require a fairly deep plane of anaesthesia to tolerate it. On the other hand, when the surgeon has fired his final laser shot, he will pull out the laryngoscope and demand the next patient ready for surgery in 15 min at the latest. The choice of the anaesthetic must accommodate both of these constraining factors.

Anaesthetic

With modern anaesthetic drugs there are a number of ways to give deep anaesthesia with rapid recovery. In our experience, the optimal anaesthetic for laser surgery of the upper aerodigestive tract is a balanced technique combining a short-acting opioid with an intravenous hypnotic such as propofol or an inhalational agent such as isoflurane, sevoflurane or desflurane. We prefer remifentanil for the opioid, since its on–off kinetics more closely match the actual course of events in laser surgery than the alternatives alfentanil or sufentanil, particularly for prolonged operations such as resections for larynx cancer that can last for hours. The end of even such long procedures can come much more abruptly than in other types of minimally invasive surgery (Table 10.5).

For the routine patient, who has received an oral premedication with 7.5 mg midazolam or a similar drug before arriving in the OR, induction of anaesthesia is started with a bolus dose of remifentanil ($1 \mu g \, kg^{-1}$) followed by the induction dose of propofol ($1.5–2 \, mg \, kg^{-1}$) and starting the propofol infusion at an initial rate of $6–8 \, mg \, kg^{-1} h^{-1}$ ($100–133 \, \mu g \, kg^{-1} min^{-1}$). The remifentanil infusion is started at an initial rate of $0.2 \, \mu g \, kg^{-1} min^{-1}$. After about 5–10 min the infusion rate of propofol is reduced to about $5–6 \, mg \, kg^{-1} h^{-1}$ ($83–100 \, \mu g \, kg^{-1} min^{-1}$). This combination is usually adequate for the entire operation and the time from stopping the infusions of propofol and remifentanil until extubation is seldom longer than 5 min. If the patient shows signs of response to the surgical stimulation then one should give an additional injection of $0.5–1 \, \mu g \, kg^{-1}$ remifentanil and increase the infusion rate by $0.1 \, \mu g \, kg^{-1} min^{-1}$. Rarely does a patient require a rate of more than $0.3 \, \mu g \, kg^{-1} min^{-1}$. We try to keep the propofol infusion rate as low as possible while still assuring adequate hypnosis and treat somatic and autonomous responses with incremental doses of remifentanil, since propofol has a longer context-sensitive half time than remifentanil and increasing the dose of propofol will increase the time to extubation.

When using a target-controlled infusion (see Chapter 5) we set the targeted propofol plasma concentration at $4–5 \, \mu g \, ml^{-1}$ for about 2–3 min for induction and then reduce it to $2 \, \mu g \, ml^{-1}$ for maintenance. Studies in our institution with bispectral index (BIS) monitoring of depth of anaesthesia have shown that this is sufficient to provide an adequate level of hypnosis in the vast majority of patients. The infusion rate corresponding to this plasma concentration is initially about $6 \, mg \, kg^{-1} h^{-1}$ ($100 \, \mu g \, kg^{-1} min^{-1}$) and decreases over time to about $4.5 \, mg \, kg^{-1} h^{-1}$. Signs of sympathetic stimulation unresponsive to bolus injections of remifentanil are, of course, treated by increasing the target plasma concentration of propofol.

Contrary to theoretical considerations, maximal neuromuscular relaxation is usually only required for intubating the trachea and for the correct placement of the operating laryngoscope. Anaesthesia as described above is normally sufficient to prevent vocal cord motion, but additional relaxation is occasionally required. In our experience, a neuromuscular blocker such as rocuronium or cisatracurium at a dose of twice ED_{95} provides sufficient relaxation for most surgical procedures lasting from 60 to 90 min without leaving residual relaxation requiring reversal at the end. For shorter procedures we prefer mivacurium or even succinylcholine, depending on how long the operation is to last. For example, for removal of a solitary vocal cord cyst, a procedure of only a few minutes, we would induce anaesthesia when the surgical team is completely prepared and ready to go using succinylcholine with self-taming[132,133] for intubation and immobilization of the vocal cords. Not all consider self-taming an effective way to prevent postoperative muscle pain after succinylcholine,[134] but the alternative of using a pre-curarizing dose of a nondepolarizing relaxant would leave the patient with residual relaxation after such a short operation.

Ventilation

Our institution has been on the leading edge of major laser surgery of the upper airways for many years[5] and we have tried and tested virtually every method of airway management in an endeavour to find the optimal compromise between access for the surgeon and safety for the patient. We have finally opted for a stiff endotracheal tube made of PVC (MLT®, Mallinckrodt-Nellcor) with an inside diameter (ID) of 5 mm for the majority of adult patients. In selected cases, we use the apnoeic technique described above.

The choice of an endotracheal tube manufactured from the material most likely to catch fire if hit by the laser beam needs a bit of justification. The basis for the choice was essentially the external tube diameter and the fact that even metal tubes ignite if not properly protected. The outside diameter of the MLT® 5 mm ID tube is 6.9 mm as opposed to 7.5 mm for the Laser-Flex® tube, 8.0 mm for the Laser-Shield II® tube and 9.5 mm for the Rüsch Lasertubus with the same internal diameters. Reducing the ID exponentially increases the problems in maintaining adequate ventilation (see below), while a tube with a larger outside diameter will impair access to the subglottic space and the posterior larynx to a greater degree.

We insert the tube as far as possible into the trachea while maintaining equal bilateral breath sounds. In this position, the cuff is sometimes still visible in the depths of the trachea and thus vulnerable to being hit with the laser beam. The cuff is inflated with saline to prevent ignition, should it be hit despite all precautions[135] but we omit colouring the inflating fluid as recommended by some. The surgeon layers wet cotton pledgets over the cuff and the portion of the shaft of the tube that is visible beyond or adjacent to the laser target (Figure 10.9). This is also effective in preventing tube or cuff ignition, but the material must be remoistened frequently.[136] By far the best way to avoid laser-ignited airway fires is for the surgeon to exercise utmost care in the use of the laser. Shooting first and looking later is as out of place in laser surgery as in any other situation. However, there are reports of an endotracheal tube being ignited by sparks flying from the target tissue.[137] The inspired O_2 concentration must be kept at 25% or below to prevent catastrophic fires should the endotracheal tube be ignited despite all precautions.[35] In the past 15 years with several thousand patients, we have had only two incidences of airway fire, both of which were resolved with no residual damage to the patients. The management of airway fires is described in the section on Complications.

Solving the Hagen-Poisseuile equation for the driving pressure required to maintain constant flow

$$\Delta P = \frac{8 Q \eta L}{\pi r^4}$$

when changing the diameter of the tube, we find that the resistance to gas flow in the 5 mm ID endotracheal tube is more than five times that with the normally used 7.5 mm ID tube. Ventilatory management must

therefore be changed considerably to accommodate this more than 400% increase in airway resistance. Inspiratory tidal volume can be maintained fairly easily by increasing the maximum pressure setting on the ventilator. The ventilatory mode is changed from volume-controlled to pressure-controlled ventilation (PCV) and tidal volume is regulated by raising or lowering the maximum inspiratory pressure. One must keep in mind that during the short inspiration phase the pressure reading shown by the anaesthesia machine only reflects the pressure in the respiratory circuit and not that in the lungs. There is pressure gradient along the endotracheal tube and the pressure in the tube itself is considerably lower (Bernoulli effect). Expiration is passive, driven solely by the steadily decreasing gradient between intrapulmonary and breathing circuit pressures (external PEEP can be removed in order to maximize this gradient). Since the driving pressure during expiration is lower than that during inspiration, it will take longer for the inspiratory tidal volume to return through the endotracheal tube. This fact should be accommodated by increasing the inspiratory–expiratory ratio from the normal value of 1:1.5 to a ratio of 1:2.5 or even 1:3. At this I:E ratio, a respiratory rate of 10 per min should allow enough time for almost complete expiration. Monitoring expiratory flow is the best way to determine the appropriate respirator settings. Non-zero flow at the end of expiration indicates air trapping with positive end-expiratory intrapulmonary pressure (intrinsic PEEP). This can be beneficial if not excessive and makes external PEEP unnecessary. Spontaneous respiration through an endotracheal tube of this calibre is very strenuous and the patient should not be required to do so any longer than necessary.

Recovery and postoperative therapy

Recovery time from termination of the drug infusions to extubation is typically 5–10 min with the anaesthetic regimen described above. Emergence is smooth and bucking on the tube is rare. An audit of several hundred patients undergoing laser surgery of the upper aerodigestive tract in our institution showed that postoperative pain levels were only low to moderate. Our routine basic analgesic regimen sufficed for the majority of patients. We give either a diclofenac suppository (100 mg for adults or 1.5 mg kg^{-1} in patients under 50 kg) after induction of anaesthesia, or intravenous paracetamol (1000 mg in patients over 50 kg or otherwise 15 mg kg^{-1}) shortly before the end of surgery. Other non-opioid analgesics will probably work just as well if given early enough. Only 15% of the patients required additional analgesia with an opioid. More details are given in Chapter 7.

Some patients appear to have increased salivation postoperatively that may be a mucosal reaction to surgery but can also be simply due to difficulties in swallowing. There is no specific therapy. The early recovery period is otherwise usually uneventful and the patient can be discharged from the post-anaesthetic care unit to the ward within 30–60 min. Outpatients are usually fit for discharge home after approximately 60–90 min.

After extensive surgery of the larynx, hypopharynx or tongue, there is a risk of postoperative oedema and haemorrhage, and the surgeon might wish to leave the endotracheal tube in place and keep the patient sedated for the night. In this case, the narrow gauge laser tube should be replaced with a normal-sized nasotracheal or orotracheal tube to facilitate spontaneous breathing. Coughing or bucking on the tube must be avoided as this can cause bleeding or can force air through areas of the cricothyroid membrane penetrated by extensive laser resection causing subcutaneous emphysema (see below).

Typical laser surgical operations of the upper aerodigestive tract and their management are described in the following section.

Selected laser surgical operations

Benign lesions of the larynx

Typical congenital laryngeal lesions frequently requiring laser surgery are congenital laryngomalacia, cysts, laryngocele, haemangioma or stenosis. Acquired lesions are more common, and include vocal cord nodules, polyps or granulomas, papillomas, haemangiomas, keratosis, leucoplakia, laryngeal webs and stenoses, bilateral recurrent nerve palsy and Reinke's oedema. The CO_2 laser is used for the surgical treatment of these processes. Most of these operations are not very painful and a non-opioid analgesic administered early enough will usually suffice. Our standard drugs are either rectal diclofenac (1.5 mg kg^{-1}, maximum single dose 100 mg, t.i.d.) or intravenous paracetamol (1.5 mg kg^{-1}, maximum single dose 1000 mg every 6 h). Rectal diclofenac must be administered at least 45–60 min before the end of surgery while intravenous paracetamol can be given on emergence.

Vocal cord nodules, polyps, cysts, laryngoceles

The treatment of vocal cord nodules requires utmost care to avoid damaging healthy tissue, particularly the vocal ligament at the base of the lesion. The laser beam is focussed to a diameter of only 0.3–0.8 mm and moved by merely tenths of a millimetre to shave off the lesion. Obviously, the vocal cords must remain absolutely immobile. This is only possible using endotracheal intubation or with the apnoea technique. Supraglottic jetting is usually ruled out in any case by the moist gauze packed under the vocal folds to protect the trachea from the laser beam.

The trachea is intubated with a narrow (5 mm) stiff endotracheal tube that is carefully covered with wet swabs. Anaesthesia is performed as described above, using succinylcholine or mivacurium as the muscle relaxant of choice since this is a very short operation. The procedure for polyps, laryngoceles and cysts is essentially the same and as a rule there are no special perioperative risks to watch out for. Some patients present with polyps that are so large as to obstruct the view of the glottis. Symptoms such as severe dysphonia or dyspnoea, as well as the preoperative laryngoscopic findings will alert the anaesthetist. Intubation is usually not unduly difficult. The polyp is mobile and one can use a longer intubating stylet to push it aside and locate the glottis before inserting the endotracheal tube.

Reinke's oedema

Reinke's oedema is a bilateral condition caused by chronic inflammation due to smoking and voice abuse. Anaesthetic management is as described for vocal cord nodules, taking into consideration the fact that the prevalence of chronic obstructive pulmonary disease is usually higher in these patients. Glottic closure is impaired postoperatively due to the large amount of excess tissue that is resected. The patients are temporarily dysphonic, but this is a typical sequel to the operation and not intubation damage.

Chronic hyperplastic laryngitis

Chronic hyperplastic laryngitis is another smoking-related condition of the larynx that can also occur with occupational exposure to inhaled irritants. It is usually benign but can harbour precancerous areas and even microinvasive carcinoma. It affects the true and false vocal cords and epiglottis and is characterized by oedema, an increase in submucosal connective tissue and hyperplastic epithelial lining. Treatment consists in completely peeling-off the mucosa of the affected areas, literally stripping the endolarynx.

The trachea is intubated with a stiff endotracheal tube and anaesthesia is managed as described above. The tube is carefully covered with wet swabs to avoid it being hit by the laser beam. The operation lasts

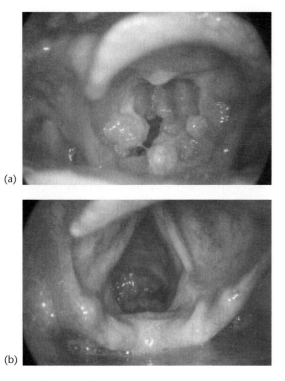

(a)

(b)

Figure 10.14 Pictures of larynx with massive papillomatosis. (a) glottic, (b) subglottic.

longer than, for example, the removal of vocal cord nodules and using a longer acting neuromuscular blocker such as vecuronium, atracurium or rocuronium for intubation will give adequate relaxation for the duration of the procedure. The endotracheal tube can be removed at the end of surgery without risk of airway occlusion due to oedema.

Laryngeal papillomatosis

Papillomas affect every age group from under 1 year to the elderly. Recurrent papillomatosis is an infectious viral disease caused by the human papilloma virus. Massive infestation can occlude the larynx or trachea and cause severe dyspnoea (Figure 10.14). There is no causal treatment, and repeated microsurgical ablation to maintain airway patency and improve vocal quality is the therapeutic mainstay.

Anaesthetic management is as described above with endotracheal intubation, even in children. The procedures are usually lengthy and the choice of neuromuscular blocker is left to the discretion of the anaesthetist. One chooses the size of endotracheal tube that allows optimal visualization and surgical access with a tolerable degree of ventilatory impairment. For adults this is usually a 5 mm stiff tube,

but we occasionally use one with a 4 mm ID. Except in cases with severe laryngeal obstruction, children can usually be intubated with the size normally used, although it is often better to choose one size smaller. The tube should be cuffed and the cuff should be inflated to seal the airway. The tube material must not be too pliable in order to prevent its being compressed by the laryngoscope; armoured tubes are a good choice. Infraglottic jet ventilation would be a possible alternative from a technical standpoint, but there is a risk that bits of infectious tissue or active virus in the laser plume might find their way into more distal parts of the airways. On the other hand, the endotracheal tube itself can transport infectious material and cause distal seeding.

Immediate extubation is always possible even after extensive operations. A single dose of a corticosteroid (e.g. 3 mg kg^{-1} prednisolone) might help to prevent mucosal oedema.

Capillary haemangiomas in infants

This lesion is usually localized in the posterior subglottis, usually unilaterally, but bilateral haemangiomas occur. The former is removed in a single session, while the latter are removed one side at a time with several weeks between operations to prevent postoperative stenosis from scarring and adhesion. The low power, precisely focussed laser beam coagulates the capillaries and there is little bleeding. Surgical access is sometimes obstructed by the endotracheal tube so that resection is performed in apnoea or with infraglottic jet ventilation: we prefer the apnoea method.

The standard anaesthetic regimen for laser surgery has to be modified for very young patients. For infants above the age of 3 months we use either TIVA with propofol and remifentanil, or a balanced technique with sevoflurane and remifentanil or alfentanil, while we only use the balanced technique in younger patients. Anaesthesia is induced either intravenously or by inhalation, the muscle relaxant is given and the patient is ventilated with bag and mask until it has taken full effect. The surgeon then inspects the trachea and main bronchi with a thin telescope. After further manual ventilation the surgeon exposes the larynx with the operating laryngoscope and inserts an endotracheal tube through the laryngoscope into the trachea. If surgical visualization is sufficient the operation is performed with the endotracheal tube in place. If the posterior subglottic area cannot be sufficiently exposed with the tube in place, the tube is removed and the operation carried out using the apnoea technique described above. The duration of each apnoea phase is, of course, much shorter than in adults. In very small children (newborns), the endotracheal tube is left in place for 1–2 days and intravenous corticosteroids are given.

Cavernous haemangiomas in adults

Anaesthetic management for the operation is very straightforward as described above with mandatory endotracheal intubation due to risk of bleeding. The only special feature of this operation is the propensity for haemorrhage from the large vessels. This can occur intraoperatively but also during the postoperative period. The patient should remain intubated until the following day and observed carefully for indications of secondary haemorrhage.

Bilateral recurrent nerve palsy

Bilateral recurrent nerve palsy causes dyspnoea that is occasionally so severe as to require tracheotomy. Operative enlargement of the glottis can alleviate the dyspnoea and allow the tracheostoma to be closed. Usually the posterior part of the vocal cords is resected (posterior cordectomy). The aim is to open the airway enough to give unobstructed breathing even under exertion, while keeping voice impairment to a minimum.

The anaesthetic management is as described above using mivacurium as the muscle relaxant of choice. The procedure is performed with endotracheal intubation. This is not difficult, even though the glottis is closed. However, the closed glottis precludes the use of jet ventilation. The endotracheal tube is protected from the laser beam by simply moving it ventrally out of the way and covering it with wet swabs. A prophylactic dose of prednisolone ($3–5\,mg\,kg^{-1}$) is given to prevent swelling and adhesions. Excessive formation of fibrin and granulation tissue in the resected slot can cause postoperative dyspnoea and require a second operation.

Stenosis of the larynx

There is a multitude of conditions causing stenosis of the larynx. One can be born with a congenital membranous stenosis of the anterior glottis (glottic web) (Figure 10.15). Intubation, even of short duration, can induce glottic or subglottic stenoses (Figures 10.16 and 10.17). Partial laryngectomy or radiation therapy for treatment of larynx cancer can cause glottic and supraglottic stenoses. Proliferative diseases, ingestion of caustic substances and burns are other causes, and that is not the end of the list.

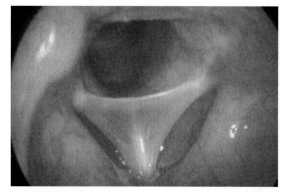

Figure 10.15 Glottic web.

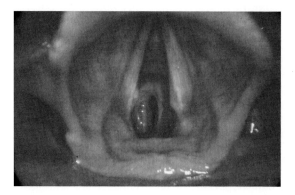

Figure 10.16 Stenosis after horizontal laryngectomy.

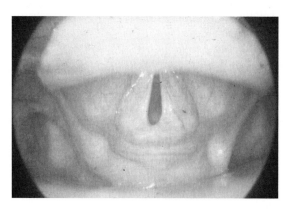

Figure 10.17 Stenosis after 40 min intubation.

Anaesthetic management can be complicated by the stenosis itself. If the lumen is wide enough, a slender endotracheal tube can be introduced into the trachea and the patient's lungs ventilated in the usual fashion. Frequently, however, the stenosis is so narrow that an endotracheal tube with the required internal diameter cannot be passed. In these cases we resort to a slight

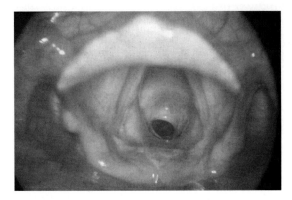

Figure 10.18 Picture of tracheal webs.

modification of the apnoea technique. In this method, the surgeon exposes the larynx with the operating laryngoscope and gently wedges the tip of a stiff endotracheal tube into the space above the stenosis and holds it in place. This is usually sufficient to give a good seal and to allow ventilation. The tube is then removed at intervals for surgery and replaced for further ventilation.

Infraglottic jetting could be an alternative method for ventilation if the jet tube does not fully occlude the remaining glottic lumen. The cross section of the expiratory airway is a main determinant of intrapulmonary pressure with jet ventilation, and is continuously changing during the operation. P_{AW} will have to be monitored carefully and driving pressure and expiration phase adapted to avoid barotrauma or hypoventilation.

Benign processes of the trachea

Typical tracheal processes are papillomatosis, fibromas, tracheal webs or granulation tissue and stenoses following long-term intubation. Many of these are amenable to laser surgery with CO_2, Nd–YAG or argon lasers (Figure 10.18).

We use the apnoea technique, but infraglottic jetting with the tip of the cannula distal to the operation site is an option if the tracheal lumen is wide enough to allow egress of insufflated air around the tube. For jet ventilation the O_2 concentration in the jetted air is limited to 30% or less.

Anaesthesia is induced as described and neuromuscular relaxation achieved using a relaxant with a duration of action appropriate for the length of the operation. The patient's lungs are ventilated by bag and mask until the muscles are completely relaxed and control of the airway then given to the surgeon. The surgeon often begins the procedure with endoscopy of trachea,

bronchi and oesophagus to assess the extent of the disease process. During tracheobronchoscopy the lungs can be ventilated by hand through the rigid bronchoscope. The surgeon then exposes the larynx and inserts the endotracheal tube into the trachea through the laryngoscope under direct vision. There are no restrictions on the type of tube that can be used since it is removed while the laser is being used. It is best to use the largest size that fits through the laryngoscope and into the trachea. This allows a large respiratory minute volume for rapid elimination of the CO_2 accumulating during the period of apnoea. The patient's lungs are ventilated with 100% O_2 for several minutes and the tube is then removed for surgery. Depending on the FRC of the patient's lungs, the apnoea period can last for 4–5 min. The tube is replaced when O_2 saturation begins to fall or at a SpO_2 of 90–95% at the latest. The lungs are ventilated for several minutes in order to eliminate the CO_2 that accumulated during apnoea. This is repeated until the operation is completed.

If jet ventilation is used, the jet tube can be inserted immediately after the surgeon has completed the tracheobronchoscopy. Ventilator settings will have to be adapted to give sufficient ventilation with acceptable P_{AW}. The O_2 concentration in the jet is set at 30% or less.

Benign processes of the nasal passages and the nasopharynx

Typical benign processes of this region treated by laser surgery are hypertrophied turbinates, septal spurs, polyps, cysts, papillomas, vascular lesions such as haemangiomas and choanal atresia. Most of these operations can be performed in local or topical anaesthesia on an outpatient basis. Those that require general anaesthesia can be handled in a normal fashion since there is little risk of damaging the orotracheal tube with the laser.

Opening of choanal atresia is another matter. The patients are newborns, perhaps even premature, and the condition has to be corrected rapidly, since newborns have trouble breathing through their mouths. Inhalational anaesthesia is used with an orotracheal tube. No special anaesthetic precautions related to the laser surgery need to be taken. The most serious risk is injury to the internal carotid artery if the surgeon works too far laterally.

Malignant diseases of the larynx and hypopharynx

Advances in laser surgery and in anaesthesia have made it possible to aim for curative surgical treatment of even extensive tumours of this region and to offer palliative surgery to the patient with inoperable disease that leaves the larynx and restores an unobstructed airway. Although the distinction between carcinoma of the larynx and hypopharynx is important from a surgical standpoint, anaesthetic management of the two does not differ greatly. The primary difference is that a standard-armoured endotracheal tube can be used for most pharyngeal tumours and that there is little risk of laser damage to the tube. Larynx carcinoma can range from a small cancerous lesion on the vocal cords to a bulky tumour causing dyspnoea. Surgical treatment of the former is hardly more invasive than for benign disorders of the vocal cords, and anaesthetic management is just as straightforward, with one caveat: due to its aetiology, patients presenting with cancer of the larynx frequently have concomitant pulmonary and cardiac disease. Larger tumours can make tracheal intubation difficult, due to both their size and their friability. Telltale signs of tumours of this size are inspiratory stridor, more than usual hoarseness or dysphagia. If at all possible, one should consult the rhinolaryngological report, which will include the findings of the preoperative laryngoscopic examination, perhaps even with photographic documentation. Very large tumours can completely block the view of the glottis and they can bleed profusely when touched (Figure 10.19). Or, they can narrow the glottis to such an extent that it is difficult to pass even the narrow laser tube. If the larynx is too obstructed or the risk of bleeding too great, the surgeon might elect to perform a preoperative tracheotomy in local anaesthesia. Hypopharyngeal carcinoma arises by definition outside the larynx but it can infiltrate laryngeal structures in advanced stages. One difference is the higher risk of severe intraoperative haemorrhage in laser surgery of hypopharyngeal tumours, particularly those involving the lateral wall of the piriform sinus.

Patients with prior radiotherapy of their tumour can be extremely difficult or even impossible to intubate. Radiation can indurate the soft tissues of the neck to such an extent that they are immobile and it is impossible to visualize the glottis. If the patient has a history of radiotherapy, one should actively search for induration by palpation and inspection, and discuss the possibility of awake fibre-optic intubation with the patient. Laser surgery itself sometimes proves impossible in these patients, since neuromuscular blockers do not relax the indurated tissues that prevent the surgeon from achieving the necessary exposure of the glottis.

The preoperative work-up of the patient presenting for laser surgery of the larynx or hypopharynx should

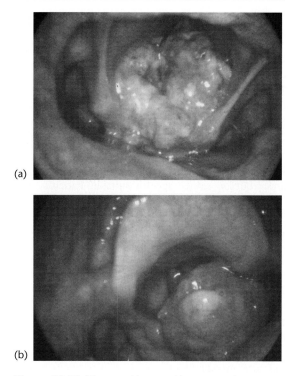

(a)

(b)

Figure 10.19 Pictures of larynx with gross carcinoma.

include a careful history with emphasis on cardiovascular and respiratory disease, particularly ischaemic heart disease, as well as drinking habits. Clinical and laboratory signs of alcohol abuse and hepatic insufficiency should be looked for. In patients with dyspnoea or even cyanosis, a preoperative lung function test and arterial blood gases will help to assess and manage the postoperative recovery period. Hypopharyngeal tumours can cause dysphagia and consequently malnutrition and dehydration.

The patients are usually given a total intravenous anaesthetic with remifentanil and propofol. Isoflurane is used as a hypnotic in place of propofol in patients with impaired liver function, particularly those with cirrhosis, since it maintains hepatic perfusion and does not impose a metabolic load on the organ. The propofol dose required for adequate hypnosis can be higher in these patients since alcohol induces cross tolerance. Patients with dysphagia have latent hypovolaemia and tend to develop relevant arterial hypotension after induction with normal doses of propofol. In these patients, the initial propofol dose is about $0.8\,\text{mg}\,\text{kg}^{-1}$ with additional injections. This is usually sufficient to induce loss of consciousness but not for adequate hypnosis. Additional doses of $0.5\,\text{mg}\,\text{kg}^{-1}$ are then given at

2-min intervals until the desired depth of hypnosis is achieved. When using target-controlled infusion the initial target concentration is set at $2.5–3.0\,\mu g\,ml^{-1}$. It takes approximately 5 min before an adequate level of sleep is reached but the incidence of hypotension is greatly reduced. Hypotension at induction is treated by infusing standard electrolyte solution, but blood pressure should be supported with vasoactive drugs to maintain coronary circulation until vascular filling is sufficient.

Rocuronium or cisatracurium are used for myorelaxation, but any similar agent is suitable. Patients with impaired liver function are at risk for prolonged action of mivacurium if they have reduced plasma cholinesterase activity. The patient's trachea is intubated with a 5 mm ID stiff endotracheal tube that is carefully protected from the laser beam with wet gauze. The settings on the ventilator must be altered as described above to accommodate the prolonged expiratory phase through the narrow tube.

Routine intraoperative monitoring consists of a continuous five-lead electrocardiogram (ECG), preferably with ST-segment analysis, non-invasive blood pressure measurements, pulse oximetric O_2 saturation and capnometry. A large bore peripheral venous catheter is sufficient for the operation itself, but arterial and central venous catheters might be warranted by pre-existing cardiovascular disease.

The recovery period is normally uneventful with no stridor or dyspnoea. Occasionally, after extensive resections, the surgeon might wish to leave the patient intubated, sedated and ventilated overnight if there is a risk of postoperative bleeding or airway obstruction. In this case, the narrow laser tube is replaced with the orotracheal tube normally used in the intensive care unit. Extubation of the spontaneously breathing only lightly sedated patient is then performed in the OR. If there is a risk of airway obstruction, extubation is performed in tracheotomy standby. A tube exchanger with an adapter for the ventilator can be passed through the endotracheal tube and left in the trachea as a guide, and as a means of insufflating O_2, in case bleeding necessitates reintubation (Figure 10.20).

Carcinomas of oral cavity and oropharynx

This region encompasses the lips, floor of mouth, buccal surfaces, palate, uvula posterior wall of oropharynx, tonsils and tongue. Surgery is straightforward, with the main risk being bleeding, particularly from large vessels adjacent to the lateral

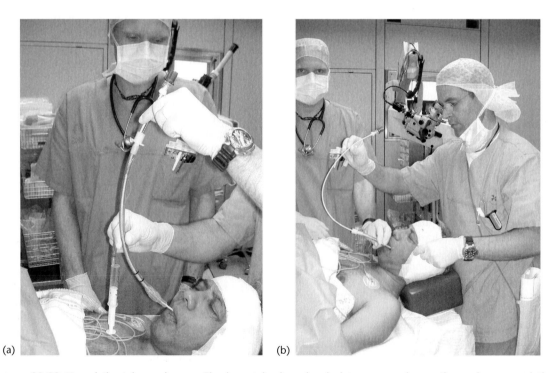

(a)   (b)

Figure 10.20 Use of the tube exchanger. The laser tube has already been removed over the exchanger and the larger armoured tube is being inserted.

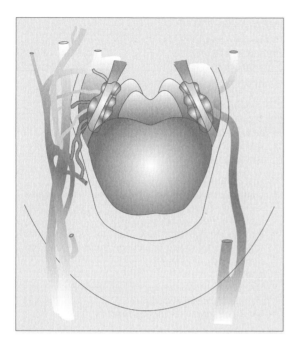

Figure 10.21 Large vessels in the vicinity of the lateral oropharynx. The internal carotid artery is occasionally directly adjacent to the tonsils and is easily injured.

oropharynx (Figure 10.21). There is no competition for the airway during laser surgery of this region, and the requirements for the endotracheal tube are relaxed. A standard diameter, armoured orotracheal or nasotracheal tube can be employed depending on the site of resection. Difficulties can arise if the tumour has infiltrated the cheek or the region around the temporomandibular joint causing trismus.

Nicotine and alcohol abuse are risk factors for these cancers as well, and the patient is likely to have concomitant cardiovascular and respiratory disease. Advanced malignancy impairs chewing and swallowing and the patient is likely to be malnourished and dehydrated. Anaesthetic management and precautions are the same as for laser surgery of tumours of the larynx and hypopharynx.

Complications

Fires

Laser beams can ignite nearly everything if they have enough power and impinge on the target for a sufficiently long time. The most susceptible materials in the OR are the surgical drapes, personnel clothing and plastic objects. These fires can endanger everyone including the patient. All personnel working in a laser

surgery OR should be aware of the potential danger and have been instructed in what to do should a fire breaks out. Fires of this type occur more often during laser surgery in ophthalmology and dermatology.

A laser-induced fire more typical for laser surgery of the upper aerodigestive tract occurs when combustible material is ignited in the patient's airways. The objects usually in the path of the laser beam are the endotracheal tube, surgical swabs and the surgeon's gloves. The airway tissue itself does not burn unless it has been dried and charred. The extent of the damage depends on the location and composition of the burning material and on the O_2 concentration in the ambient air. How seriously the patient is ultimately injured depends to a great extent on how rapidly the OR personnel responds and how the fire is managed.

Fire prevention is the most important single factor. This entails using flame-retardant materials wherever feasible, keeping the ambient O_2 concentration below the level required for sustained combustion and exerting utmost care when using the laser. The measures that can be taken to prevent endotracheal tube fires are described in detail above in the section on endotracheal intubation.

Should an airway fire occur despite all precautions, the primary objective is to keep the damage to the patient to a minimum: everything else is secondary to that goal. Quick, decisive action is important. Most fires are initially located on the outer surface of the endotracheal tube and cause local thermal destruction that is fairly limited in extent. However, if the fire is not extinguished immediately it will burn through the wall of the endotracheal tube, and the O_2-enriched gas mixture combined with the gas flow in the tube will give a blow-torch like flame blowing heat and toxic combustion products into the alveoli.

The airway fire protocol gives the sequence of actions to be taken. The surgeon, who will probably be the first to discover the flames, should immediately inform the anaesthetist while removing the burning material from the patient. The anaesthetist will discontinue ventilation and shut off the gas supply. The surgeon should remove the laryngoscope and any instruments and ready the patient for mask ventilation with 100% O_2. Direct laryngoscopy and rigid bronchoscopy is carried out to survey the extent of the damage and to remove any debris or foreign matter. Once the burning material has been removed, the airway secured and ventilation guaranteed the next steps can be instituted. The trachea should be reintubated and if damage is severe, a low tracheotomy might be indicated. Surgery should be brought to an end as rapidly as the operation permits. The patient should be closely monitored for at least 24 h with particular attention given to changes in oxygenation and ventilation.

Corticosteroids are frequently recommended as a measure to prevent or attenuate pulmonary damage.[138] Controlled studies in animals and a serendipitous clinical investigation in humans have shown, however, that they are of no benefit and that those with mineralocorticoid effects such as hydrocortisone may even increase mortality.[138–140] The so-called lazaroids (21-aminosteroids) have been shown to have a beneficial effect in the smoke inhalation injury model.[141] Tirilazar is a lazaroid that is on the market in some countries.

Subcutaneous emphysema

The cricothyroid membrane can be breached by the laser beam during surgery on the anterior portion of the larynx and the subglottis. Excessive P_{AW} will force air through the defect into extraluminal tissues and cause subcutaneous emphysema that can extend to the face and chest. The smaller the opening, the greater the risk of subcutaneous oedema, since the air forced into the tissues is trapped. Coughing and bucking on the tube are risk factors for this complication and the anaesthetist can be instrumental in preventing it. If the surgeon thinks that the patient might be at risk of subcutaneous emphysema, the ventral aspect of the throat should be compressed manually during extubation and effective antitussive measures should be instituted. A compression bandage is also sometimes applied by the surgeon.

In our experience, subcutaneous emphysema has never compromised respiration and has never required treatment.

Postoperative airway obstruction

As a rule, airway patency is better postoperatively than before surgery, since the obstructing tissue masses have been removed. Occasionally, however, postoperative oedema of the tongue or larynx can cause airway obstruction. The surgeon should alert the anaesthetist to this possibility and discuss the necessity of leaving the endotracheal tube in place postoperatively. Corticoids given early enough can sometimes prevent oedema. If postoperative stridor and dyspnoea are not too severe an initial therapeutic attempt can be made with nebulized epinephrine. Persisting or worsening dyspnoea and stridor should be evaluated by the surgeon and usually requires reintubation.

AIRWAY FIRE PROTOCOL

Immediate measures
- Anaesthetist:
  - Stop *all* gas flow
- Surgeon:
  - Remove burning material (endotracheal tube, pledgets, swabs, etc.)
  - Remove laryngoscope
- Extinguish fire with water or saline if still burning
- Ventilate with face mask (100% O_2 only if fire is extinguished)

Urgent measures
- Examine damaged endotracheal tube to determine if still intact. If not, search airways and oral cavity carefully for missing pieces
- Perform laryngoscopy and bronchoscopy to assess and document extent of damage and to remove foreign material if necessary
- Reintubate
- Consider bronchial lavage through flexible bronchoscope for tracheal involvement
- Terminate surgery as soon as feasible

Postoperative measures
- Chest X-ray
- Admit to intensive care unit for observation and treatment
- Provide respiratory therapy with supplementary O_2, mask continuous positive airway pressure (CPAP), nebulized epinephrine and other measures as deemed necessary
- Intubate and provide ventilatory support if required
- Antibiotics only for confirmed or suspected infection – not antibiotic prophylaxis
- Reassess tracheal damage at intervals by flexible bronchoscopy
- Corticoids not proven effective – administration discretionary

---

Arterial haemorrhage

The laser beam cannot seal blood vessels with a diameter of more than 0.5 mm. These will bleed and require ligation, clips or coagulation with the electrocauter. The tonsils and the lateral pharynx are in close proximity to the large vessels of the neck including the internal carotid artery (Figure 10.21). These can be perforated, slit or severed during laser surgery in this region. Injury to the carotid artery can cause severe bleeding requiring the concerted efforts of all attending personnel. The anaesthetist can assist the efforts of the surgeon by lowering the blood pressure and maintaining vascular filling with infusions. In intubated patients and with less severe haemorrhage, the bleeding is largely a surgical problem. However, in patients with jet ventilation or breathing spontaneously, enoral haemorrhage carries a high risk, if not certainty, of aspiration. Immediate efforts must be undertaken to secure the airway with an endotracheal tube. Occasionally, the bleeding cannot be staunched from enorally and the damaged vessel has to be approached through an external incision. Excessive pressure to the lateral pharynx to stop the bleeding during this period can actually compress the carotid artery to an extent that cerebral perfusion is compromised. In these cases, it is not advisable to lower the blood pressure, but instead to maintain or even increase it in order to preserve collateral perfusion.

Pneumothorax, pneumomediastinum, pneumopericardium

These conditions are not so much complications of laser surgery as of jet ventilation. One must be alert to the possibility of their occurring. Tension pneumothorax can occur bilaterally and requires immediate thoracocentesis. Pneumomediastinum does not usually cause acute symptoms.

Pneumopericardium can be life threatening and difficult to diagnose since the combination of symptoms – hypotension, tachycardia, elevated central venous pressure (CVP) – can be caused by more common complications such as pneumothorax and pulmonary embolism. Transthoracic or transoesophageal ultrasound will help in the diagnosis. Treatment of pneumopericardium requires some experience but is nevertheless relatively straightforward once the diagnosis is confirmed.

Venous gas embolism

The contact probe of the Nd–YAG laser uses a stream of gas to cool the sapphire probe tip. This has caused venous gas embolization in a number of cases of uterine surgery.[142] This complication has also be reported for Nd–YAG laser surgery of the trachea.[143,144] The complication is rare but potentially lethal and the anaesthetist must include it in the differential diagnosis of cardiovascular collapse during endotracheal surgery with a gas-cooled Nd–YAG laser.

Complications of laser surgery of the upper aerodigestive tract

- Subcutaneous emphysema
- Pneumothorax
- Pneumomediastinum
- Glottic oedema
- Arterial haemorrhage (e.g. carotid artery)
- Venous gas embolism
- Tracheo-oesophageal fistulae

References

1. Strong MS, Jako GJ. Laser surgery in the larynx. Early clinical experience with continuous CO_2 laser. *Ann Otol Rhinol Laryngol* 1972; **81**: 791–798.
2. Snow JC, Kripke BJ, Strong MS, Jako GJ, Meyer MR, Vaughan CW. Anesthesia for carbon dioxide laser microsurgery on the larynx and trachea. *Anesth Analg* 1974; **53**: 507–512.
3. Hunton J, Oswal VH. Anaesthetic management for carbon dioxide laser surgery in tracheobronchial lesions. *Anaesthesia* 1987; **42**: 1222–1225.
4. Vourc'h G, Tannieres ML, Freche C. Microlaryngeal surgery with the carbon dioxide laser: is the cuffed Carden tube really necessary? *Anaesthesia* 1980; **35**: 1019.
5. Steiner W, Ambrosch P. *Endoscopic Laser Surgery of the Upper Aerodigestive Tract: with Special Emphasis on Cancer Surgery*, 2nd edition. New York: Thieme Medical Publisher, 2001.
6. Davis RK (Ed.). *Lasers in Otolaryngology – Head and Neck Surgery*. Philadelphia: W.B. Saunders, 1990.
7. Niemz MH. *Laser–Tissue Interactions: Fundamentals and Applications*. New York: Springer Verlag, 2002.
8. American National Standards Institute. *American National Standard for the Safe Use of Lasers in Health Care Facilities (Z136.3-1988)*. New York: American National Standards Institute, 1988.
9. British Standards Institute. *Medical Laser Equipment BS IEC 60825-8:1999 Safety of Laser Products. Guidelines for the Safe Use of Medical Laser Equipment.* http://bsonline.techindex.co.uk.
10. Nezhat C, Winer WK, Nezhat F, Forrest D, Reeves WG. Smoke from laser surgery: is there a health hazard? *Laser Surg Med* 1987; **7**: 376–382.
11. Freitag L, Chapman GA, Sielczak M, Ahmed A, Russin D. Laser smoke effect on the bronchial system. *Laser Surg Med* 1987; **7**: 283–288.
12. Tomita Y, Mihashi S, Nagata K *et al.* Mutagenicity of smoke condensates induced by CO_2-laser irradiation and electrocauterization. *Mutat Res* 1981; **89**: 145–149.
13. Kunachak S, Sithisarn P, Kulapaditharom B. Are laryngeal papilloma virus-infected cells viable in the plume derived from a continuous mode carbon dioxide laser, and are they infectious? A preliminary report on one laser mode. *J Laryngol Otol* 1996; **110**: 1031–1033.
14. Garden JM, O'Banion KM, Shelnitz LS *et al.* Papillomavirus in the vapor of carbon dioxide laser-treated verrucae. *J Am Med Assoc* 1988; **259**: 1199–1202.
15. Ferenczy A, Bergeron C, Richart RM. Carbon dioxide laser energy disperses human papillomavirus deoxyribonucleic acid onto treatment fields. *Am J Obstet Gynecol* 1990; **163**: 1271–1274.
16. Byrne PO, Sisson PR, Oliver PD, Ingham HR. Carbon dioxide laser irradiation of bacterial targets in vitro. *J Hosp Infect* 1987; **9**: 265–273.
17. Walker NP, Matthews J, Newsom SW. Possible hazards from irradiation with the carbon dioxide laser. *Laser Surg Med* 1986; **6**: 84–86.
18. Ferenczy A, Bergeron C, Richart RM. Human papillomavirus DNA in CO_2 laser-generated plume of smoke

and its consequences to the surgeon. *Obstet Gynecol* 1990; **75**: 114–118.

19. Hawkins DB, Joseph MM. Avoiding a wrapped endotracheal tube in laser laryngeal surgery: experiences with apneic anesthesia and metal Laser-Flex endotracheal tubes. *Laryngoscope* 1990; **100**: 1283–1287.

20. Cohen SR, Herbert WI, Thompson JW. Anesthesia management of microlaryngeal laser surgery in children: apneic technique anesthesia. *Laryngoscope* 1988; **98**: 347–348.

21. Healy GB, Strong MS, Shapshay S, Vaughan C, Jako G. Complications of CO_2 laser surgery of the aerodigestive tract: experience of 4416 cases. *Otolaryngol Head Neck Surg* 1984; **92**: 13–18.

22. Snow JC, Norton ML, Saluja TS, Estanislao AF. Fire hazard during CO_2 laser microsurgery on the larynx and trachea. *Anesth Analg* 1976; **55**: 146–147.

23. Hermens JM, Bennett MJ, Hirshman CA. Anesthesia for laser surgery. *Anesth Analg* 1983; **62**: 218–229.

24. Fried MP. A survey of the complications of laser laryngoscopy. *Arch Otolaryngol* 1984; **110**: 31–34.

25. US Food and Drug Administration. Special report; laser safety. *Laser Nurs* 1990; **4**: 3–12.

26. Cozine K, Stone JG, Shulman S, Flaster ER. Ventilatory complications of carbon dioxide laser laryngeal surgery. *J Clin Anesth* 1991; **3**: 20–25.

27. Sosis MB. Airway fire during CO_2 laser surgery using a Xomed laser endotracheal tube. *Anesthesiology* 1990; **72**: 747–749.

28. Lai HC, Juang SE, Liu TJ, Ho WM. Fires of endotracheal tubes of three different materials during carbon dioxide laser surgery. *Acta Anaesthesiol Sin* 2002; **40**: 47–51.

29. Patel KF, Hicks JN. Prevention of fire hazards associated with use of carbon dioxide lasers. *Anesth Analg* 1981; **60**: 885–888.

30. Sosis MB, Dillon FX. A comparison of CO_2 laser ignition of the xomed, plastic, and rubber endotracheal tubes. *Anesth Analg* 1993; **76**: 391–393.

31. Ossoff RH. Laser safety in otolaryngology – head and neck surgery: anesthetic and educational considerations for laryngeal surgery. *Laryngoscope* 1989; **99**: 1–26.

32. Geffin B, Shapshay SM, Bellack GS, Hobin K, Setzer SE. Flammability of endotracheal tubes during Nd–YAG laser application in the airway. *Anesthesiology* 1986; **65**: 511–515.

33. Sosis MB, Dillon FX. Hazards of a new, clear, unmarked polyvinylchloride tracheal tube designed for use with the Nd–YAG laser. *J Clin Anesth* 1991; **3**: 358–360.

34. Ossoff RH, Duncavage JA, Eisenman TS, Karlan MS. Comparison of tracheal damage from laser-ignited endotracheal tube fires. *Ann Otol Rhinol Laryngol* 1983; **92**: 333–336.

35. Wolf GL, Simpson JI. Flammability of endotracheal tubes in oxygen and nitrous oxide enriched atmosphere. *Anesthesiology* 1987; **67**: 236–239.

36. Pashayan AG, SanGiovanni C, Davis LE. Positive end-expiratory pressure lowers the risk of laser-induced polyvinylchloride tracheal-tube fires. *Anesthesiology* 1993; **79**: 83–87.

37. Pashayan AG, Gravenstein JS. Helium retards endotracheal tube fires from carbon dioxide lasers. *Anesthesiology* 1985; **62**: 274–277.

38. AlHaddad S, Brenner J. Helium and lower oxygen concentration do not prolong tracheal tube ignition time during potassium titanyl phosphate laser use. *Anesthesiology* 1994; **80**: 936–938.

39. Jolliet P, Watremez C, Roeseler J *et al.* Comparative effects of helium–oxygen and external positive end-expiratory pressure on respiratory mechanics, gas exchange, and ventilation–perfusion relationships in mechanically ventilated patients with chronic obstructive pulmonary disease. *Intens Care Med* 2003; **29**: 1442–1450.

40. Guillemi S, Wright JL, Hogg JC, Wiggs BR, Macklem PT, Pare PD. Density dependence of pulmonary resistance: correlation with small airway pathology. *Eur Respir J* 1995; **8**: 789–794.

41. Simpson JI, Schiff GA, Wolf GL. The effect of helium on endotracheal tube flammability. *Anesthesiology* 1990; **73**: 538–540.

42. Leonard IE. The lower limits of flammability of halothane, enflurane, and isoflurane. *Anesth Analg* 1975; **54**: 238–240.

43. Sosis MB. Evaluation of five metallic tapes for protection of endotracheal tubes during CO_2 laser surgery. *Anesth Analg* 1989; **68**: 392–393.

44. Sosis M, Dillon F. Reflection of CO_2 laser radiation from laser-resistant endotracheal tubes. *Anesth Analg* 1991; **73**: 338–340.

45. Sprung J, Conley SF, Brown M. Unusual cause of difficult extubation. *Anesthesiology* 1991; **74**: 796–797.

46. Norton ML, de Vos P. New endotracheal tube for laser surgery of the larynx. *Ann Otol Rhinol Laryngol* 1978; **87**: 554–557.

47. Fried MP, Mallampati SR, Liu FC, Kaplan S, Caminear DS, Samonte BR. Laser resistant stainless steel endotracheal tube: experimental and clinical evaluation. *Laser Surg Med* 1991; **11**: 301–306.

48. Sosis MB, Pritikin JB, Calderelli DD. The effect of blood on laser-resistent endotracheal tube combustion. *Laryngoscope* 1994; **104**: 829–831.

49. Sosis MB, Braverman B, Calderelli DD. Evaluation of a new laser-resistant fabric and copper foil-wrapped endotracheal tube. *Laryngoscope* 1996; **106**: 842–844.

50. Sosis MB. What is the safest endotracheal tube for Nd–YAG laser surgery? A comparative study. *Anesth Analg* 1989; **69**: 802–804.

51. Lichtwarck-Aschoff M, Zimmermann GJ, Erhardt W. Reduced CO_2-elimination during combined high-frequency ventilation compared to conventional pressure-controlled ventilation in surfactant-deficient piglets. *Acta Anaesthesiol Scand* 1998; **42**: 335–342.

52. Spackman DR, Kellow N, White SA, Seed PT, Feneck RO. High frequency jet ventilation and gas trapping. *Br J Anaesth* 1999; **83**: 708–714.

53. el-Naggar M, Keh E, Stemmers A, Collins VJ. Jet ventilation for microlaryngoscopic procedures: a further simplified technic. *Anesth Analg* 1974; **53**: 797–804.

54. Klein JP, Sauvage JP, Desmonts JM. Value of jet ventilation during otorhinolaryngologic endoscopies practiced under general anesthesia. *Ann Anesthesiol Fr* 1976; **17**: 889–894.

55. Rioux J, Guerrier B, Cailar J. Ventilation by injection (jet ventilation) under general anesthesia for otorhinolaryngologic endoscopy. *Ann Anesthesiol Fr* 1975; **16**: 1J–9J.

56. Smith RB, Lindholm CE, Klain M. Jet ventilation for fiberoptic bronchoscopy under general anesthesia. *Acta Anaesthesiol Scand* 1976; **20**: 111–116.

57. Giunta F, Chiaranda M, Manani G, Giron GP. Clinical uses of high frequency jet ventilation in anaesthesia. *Br J Anaesth* 1989; **63(7 Suppl 1)**: 102s–106s.

58. Fischler M, Troche G, Guerin Y, Toty L, Vourc'h G. Development of anesthetic technics for resection-anastomosis of the trachea. *Ann Fr Anesth Reanim* 1988; **7**: 125–127.

59. Baraka A. Oxygen-jet ventilation during tracheal reconstruction in patients with tracheal stenosis. *Anesth Analg* 1977; **56**: 429–432.

60. Schneider M, Probst R. High frequency jet ventilation via a tracheoscope for endobronchial laser surgery. *Can J Anaesth* 1990; **37**: 372–376.

61. Macnaughton FI. Catheter inflation ventilation in tracheal stenosis. *Br J Anaesth* 1975; **47**: 1225–1227.

62. Männle C, Layer M, Vogt-Moykopf I, Becker HD, Zilow EP, Wiedemann K. High frequency jet ventilation during tracheal resection in children and infants. *Anasthesiol Intensivmed Notfallmed Schmerzther* 1997; **32**: 21–26.

63. Ihra G, Hieber C, Adel S, Kashanipour A, Aloy A. Tubeless combined high-frequency jet ventilation for laryngotracheal laser surgery in paediatric anaesthesia. *Acta Anaesthesiol Scand* 2000; **44**: 475–479.

64. Depierraz B, Ravussin P, Brossard E, Monnier P. Percutaneous transtracheal jet ventilation for paediatric endoscopic laser treatment of laryngeal and subglottic lesions. *Can J Anaesth* 1994; **41**: 1200–1207.

65. Remacle M, Bodart E, Lawson G, Minet M, Mayne A. Use of the CO_2-laser micropoint micromanipulator for the treatment of laryngomalacia. *Eur Arch Otorhinolaryngol* 1996; **253**: 401–404.

66. Ravussin P, Freeman J. A new transtracheal catheter for ventilation and resuscitation. *Can Anaesth Soc J* 1985; **32**: 60–64.

67. Benumof JL, Scheller MS. The importance of transtracheal jet ventilation in the management of the difficult airway. *Anesthesiology* 1989; **71**: 769–778.

68. Biro P, Wiedemann K. Jetventilation und Anästhesie für diagnostische und therapeutische Eingriffe an den Atemwegen. *Anaesthesist* 1999; **48**: 669–685.

69. Carden E, Galido J. Foot-pedal control of jet ventilation during bronchoscopy and microlaryngeal surgery. *Anesth Analg* 1975; **54**: 405–406.

70. Rontal E, Rontal M, Wenokur ME. Jet insufflation anesthesia for endolaryngeal laser surgery: a review of 318 consecutive cases. *Laryngoscope* 1985; **95**: 990–992.

71. Claes J, Vermeyen K, Van de Heyning PH, Boeckx E. Preglottic low-frequency venturi jet ventilation in laryngoscopic microsurgery in adults. The influence of inspiratory time and frequency of ventilation. *Clin Otolaryngol* 1989; **14**: 433–440.

72. Borland LM, Reilly JS. Jet ventilation for laser laryngeal surgery in children. Modification of the Saunders jet ventilation technique. *Int J Pediatr Otorhinolaryngol* 1987; **14**: 65–71.

73. Babinski M, Smith RB, Klain M. High-frequency jet ventilation for laryngoscopy. *Anesthesiology* 1980; **52**: 178–180.

74. Benhamou D, Ecoffey C, Rouby JJ, Spielvogel C, Viars P. High frequency jet ventilation: the influence of different methods of injection on respiratory parameters. *Br J Anaesth* 1987; **59**: 1257–1264.

75. Ng A, Russell WC, Harvey N, Thompson JP. Comparing methods of administering high-frequency jet ventilation in a model of laryngotracheal stenosis. *Anesth Analg* 2002; **95**: 764–769.

76. Tamsma TJ, Spoelstra AJ. Gas flow distribution and tidal volume during distal high frequency jet ventilation in dogs. *Acta Anaesthesiol Scand Suppl* 1989; **90**: 75–78.

77. Jones MJ, Mottram SD, Lin ES, Smith G. Measurement of entrainment ratio during high frequency jet ventilation. *Br J Anaesth* 1990; **65**: 197–203.

78. Ramanathan S, Arismendy J, Gandhi S, Chalon J, Turndorf H. Coaxial catheter for humidification during jet ventilation. *Anesth Analg* 1982; **61**: 689–692.

79. Capan LM, Ramanathan S, Sinha K, Turndorf H. Arterial to end-tidal CO_2 gradients during spontaneous breathing, intermittent positive-pressure ventilation and jet ventilation. *Crit Care Med* 1985; **13**: 810–813.

80. Rouby JJ, Simonneau G, Benhamou D *et al.* Factors influencing pulmonary volumes and CO_2 elimination during high-frequency jet ventilation. *Anesthesiology* 1985; **63**: 473–482.

81. Biro P, Eyrich G, Rohling RG. The efficiency of CO_2 elimination during high-frequency jet ventilation for laryngeal microsurgery. *Anesth Analg* 1998; **87**: 180–184.

82. Biro P, Layer M, Wiedemann K, Seifert B, Spahn DR. Carbon dioxide elimination during high-frequency jet ventilation for rigid bronchoscopy. *Br J Anaesth* 2000; **84**: 635–637.

83. Ihra G, Hieber C, Schabernig C *et al.* Supralaryngeal tubeless combined high-frequency jet ventilation for laser surgery of the larynx and trachea. *Br J Anaesth* 1999; **83**: 940–942.

84. Bacher A, Lang T, Weber J, Aloy A. Respiratory efficacy of subglottic low-frequency, subglottic combined-frequency, and supraglottic combined-frequency jet ventilation during microlaryngeal surgery. *Anesth Analg* 2000; **91**: 1506–1512.

85. Pillow JJ, Wilkinson MH, Neil HL, Ramsden CA. In vitro performance characteristics of high-frequency oscillatory ventilators. *Am J Respir Crit Care Med* 2001; **164(6)**: 1019–1024.

86. Korvenranta H, Carlo WA, Goldthwait Jr DA, Fanaroff AA. Carbon dioxide elimination during high-frequency jet ventilation. *J Pediatr* 1987; **111**: 107–113.

87. Baer GA. Effect of various tracheal diameter forms on airway pressure in experimental intratracheal injector ventilation. *Anaesthesist* 1985; **34**: 124–128.

88. Fischler M, Seigneur F, Bourreli B, Melchior JC, Lavaud C, Vourc'h G. Jet ventilation using low or high frequencies, during bronchoscopy. *Br J Anaesth* 1985; **57**: 382–388.

89. Craft TM, Chambers PH, Ward ME, Goat VA. Two cases of barotrauma associated with transtracheal jet ventilation. *Br J Anaesth* 1990; **64**: 524–527.

90. Biro P, Layer M, Becker HD *et al.* Influence of airway-occluding instruments on airway pressure during jet ventilation for rigid bronchoscopy. *Br J Anaesth* 2000; **85**: 462–465.

91. Ward KR, Menegazzi JJ, Yealy DM, Klain MM, Molner RL, Goode JS. Translaryngeal jet ventilation and end-tidal PCO_2 monitoring during varying degrees of upper airway obstruction. *Ann Emerg Med* 1991; **20**: 1193–1197.

92. Ihra G, Gockner G, Kashanipour A, Aloy A. High-frequency jet ventilation in European and North American institutions: developments and clinical practice. *Eur J Anaesthesiol* 2000; **17**: 418–430.

93. Mayne A, Joucken K, Collard E, Randour P. Intravenous infusion of propofol for induction and maintenance of anaesthesia during endoscopic carbon dioxide laser ENT procedures with high frequency jet ventilation. *Anaesthesia* 1988; **43(Suppl)**: 97–100.

94. Tolksdorf W, Kruschinski H, Pfeiffer J, Simon HB. Methohexital/alfentanil–thiopental/alfentanil for total intravenous anesthesia for direct laryngoscopy with 100% O_2 jet ventilation. *Anasthesiol Intensivther Notfallmed* 1988; **23**: 191–194.

95. Bacher A, Pichler K, Aloy A. Supraglottic combined frequency jet ventilation versus subglottic monofrequent jet ventilation in patients undergoing microlaryngeal surgery. *Anesth Analg* 2000; **90**: 460–465.

96. Schumacher P, Stotz G, Schneider M, Urwyler A. Laryngospasm during transtracheal high frequency jet ventilation. *Anaesthesia* 1992; **47**: 855–856.

97. Bourgain JL, Desruennes E, Fischler M, Ravussin P. Transtracheal high frequency jet ventilation for endoscopic airway surgery: a multicentre study. *Br J Anaesth* 2001; **87**: 870–875.

98. Fischler M. Anesthesia for tracheobronchial laser surgery. *Cah Anesthesiol* 1994; **42**: 99–101.

99. O'Sullivan TJ, Healy GB. Complications of Venturi jet ventilation during microlaryngeal surgery. *Arch Otolaryngol* 1985; **111**: 127–131.

100. Hardy MJ, Huard C, Lundblad TC. Bilateral tension pneumothorax during jet ventilation: a case report. *AANA J* 2000; **68**: 241–244.

101. Mikkelsen S, Knudsen KE. Pneumopericardium associated with high-frequency jet ventilation during laser surgery of the hypopharynx in a child. *Eur J Anaesthesiol* 1997; **14**: 659–661.

102. Gaitini LA, Fradis M, Vaida SJ, Somri M, Malatskey SH, Golz A. Pneumomediastinum due to Venturi jet ventilation used during microlaryngeal surgery in a previously neck-irradiated patient. *Ann Otol Rhinol Laryngol* 2000; **109**: 519–521.

103. Behne M, Klein G. Stomach rupture following normo-frequent jet ventilation. *Anaesthesist* 1987; **36**: 446–447.

104. Jawan B, Lee JH. Aspiration in transtracheal jet ventilation. *Acta Anaesthesiol Scand* 1996; **40**: 684–686.

105. Klain M, Keszler H, Stool S. Transtracheal high frequency jet ventilation prevents aspiration. *Crit Care Med* 1983; **11**: 170–172.

106. Yealy DM, Plewa MC, Reed JJ, Kaplan RM, Ilkhanipour K, Stewart RD. Manual translaryngeal jet ventilation and the risk of aspiration in a canine model. *Ann Emerg Med* 1990; **19**: 1238–1241.

107. Santos P, Ayuso A, Luis M, Martinez G, Sala X. Airway ignition during CO_2 laser laryngeal surgery and high frequency jet ventilation. *Eur J Anaesthesiol* 2000; **17**: 204–207.

108. Wegrzynowicz ES, Jensen NF, Pearson KS, Wachtel RE, Scamman FL. Airway fire during jet ventilation for laser excision of vocal cord papillomata. *Anesthesiology* 1992; **76**: 468–469.

109. Jameson JJ, Moses RD, Vellayappan U, Lathi KG. Use of the laryngeal mask airway for laser treatment of the subglottis. *Otolaryngol Head Neck Surg* 2000; **123**: 101–102.

110. Bishop P, Patel A. The intubating laryngeal mask and laser surgery. *Anaesthesia* 2003; **58**: 915–916.

111. Slinger P, Robinson R, Shennib H, Benumof JL, Eisenkraft JB. Case 6–1992. Alternative technique for laser resection of a carinal obstruction. *J Cardiothorac Vasc Anesth* 1992; **6**: 749–755.

112. Meyer JA. A practical mechanical respirator, 1929: the "iron lung". *Ann Thorac Surg* 1990; **50**: 490–493.

113. Goldstein RS, Molotiu N, Skrastins R *et al.* Reversal of sleep-induced hypoventilation and chronic respiratory failure by nocturnal negative pressure ventilation in patients with restrictive ventilatory impairment. *Am Rev Respir Dis* 1987; **135**: 1049–1055.

114. Howard RS, Wiles CM, Loh L. Respiratory complications and their management in motor neuron disease. *Brain* 1989; **112(Pt 5)**: 1155–1170.

115. Jackson M, Kinnear W, King M, Hockley S, Shneerson J. The effects of five years of nocturnal cuirass-assisted ventilation in chest wall disease. *Eur Respir J* 1993; **6**: 630–635.

116. Monks PS, Broomhead CJ, Dilkes MG, McKelvie P. The use of the Hayek oscillator during microlaryngeal surgery. *Anaesthesia* 1995; **50**: 865–869.

117. Broomhead CJ, Dilkes MG, Monks PS. Use of the Hayek oscillator in a case of failed fibreoptic intubation. *Br J Anaesth* 1995; **74**: 720–721.

118. Risch A, Ramroth H, Raedts V *et al.* Laryngeal cancer risk in Caucasians is associated with alcohol and tobacco consumption but not modified by genetic polymorphisms in class I alcohol dehydrogenases ADH1B and ADH1C, and glutathione-S-transferases GSTM1 and GSTT1. *Pharmacogenetics* 2003; **13**: 225–230.

119. MacFarlane GJ, MacFarlane TV, Lowenfels AB. The influence of alcohol consumption on worldwide trends in mortality from upper aerodigestive tract cancers in men. *J Epidemiol Commun Health* 1996; **50**: 636–639.

120. Lefebvre JL, Vankemmel B, Adenis L, Buisset E, Demaille A. Les carcinomes des voies aerodigestives superieures avant 40 ans (enfants exclus). A propos de 100 cas. *Ann Otolaryngol Chir Cervicofac* 1987; **104**: 89–92.

121. Tonnesen H, Kehlet H. Preoperative alcoholism and postoperative morbidity. *Br J Surg* 1999; **86**: 869–874.

122. Stopinski J, Staib I, Weissbach M. Do abuse of nicotine and alcohol have an effect on the incidence of postoperative bacterial infections?. *J Chir (Paris)* 1993; **130**: 422–425.

123. Moller AM, Maaloe R, Pedersen T. Postoperative intensive care admittance: the role of tobacco smoking. *Acta Anaesthesiol Scand* 2001; **45**: 345–348.

124. Myles PS, Iacono GA, Hunt JO *et al.* Risk of respiratory complications and wound infection in patients undergoing ambulatory surgery: smokers versus non-smokers. *Anesthesiology* 2002; **97**: 842–847.

125. Woodside JR. Female smokers have increased postoperative narcotic requirements. *J Addict Dis* 2000; **19**: 1–10.

126. Wewers ME, Dhatt RK, Snively TA, Tejwani GA. The effect of chronic administration of nicotine on antinociception, opioid receptor binding and met-enkelphalin levels in rats. *Brain Res* 1999; **822**: 107–113.

127. Tsui SL, Tong WN, Irwin M *et al.* The efficacy, applicability and side-effects of postoperative intravenous patient-controlled morphine analgesia: an audit of 1233 Chinese patients. *Anaesth Intens Care* 1996; **24**: 658–664.

128. Fassoulaki A, Farinotti R, Servin F, Desmonts JM. Chronic alcoholism increases the induction dose of propofol in humans. *Anesth Analg* 1993; **77**: 553–556.

129. Loft S, Jensen V, Rorsgaard S. Influence of moderate alcohol intake on wakening plasma thiopental concentration. *Acta Anaesthesiol Scand* 1983; **27**: 266–269.

130. Bakti G, Fisch HU, Karlaganis G, Minder C, Bircher J. Mechanism of the excessive sedative response of cirrhotics to benzodiazepines: model experiments with triazolam. *Hepatology* 1987; **7**: 629–638.

131. Servin F, Cockshott ID, Farinotti R, Haberer JP, Winckler C, Desmonts JM. Pharmacokinetics of propofol infusions in patients with cirrhosis. *Br J Anaesth* 1990; **65**: 177–183.

132. Strom J, Jansen F.C. Pain-reducing effect of self-taming suxamethonium. *Acta Anaesthesiol Scand* 1984; **28**: 40–43.

133. Wald-Oboussier G, Lohmann C, Viell B, Doehn M. "Self-taming": an alternative to the prevention of succinylcholine-induced pain. *Anaesthesist* 1987; **36**: 426–430.

134. Pace NL. Prevention of succinylcholine myalgias: a meta-analysis. *Anesth Analg* 1990; **70**: 477–483.

135. Sosis MB, Dillon FX. Saline-filled cuffs help prevent laser-induced polyvinylchloride endotracheal tube fires. *Anesth Analg* 1991; **72**: 187–189.

136. Sosis MB. Saline soaked pledgets prevent carbon dioxide laser-induced endotracheal tube cuff ignition. *J Clin Anesth* 1995; **7**: 395–397.

137. Hirshman CA, Smith J. Indirect ignition of the endotracheal tube during carbon dioxide laser surgery. *Arch Otolaryngol* 1980; **106**: 639–641.

138. Dressler DP, Skornik WA, Kupersmith S. Corticosteroid treatment of experimental smoke inhalation. *Ann Surg* 1976; **183**: 46–52.

139. Robinson NB, Hudson LD, Riem M *et al.* Steroid therapy following isolated smoke inhalation injury. *J Trauma* 1982; **22**: 876–879.

140. Nieman GF, Clark WR, Hakim T. Methylprednisolone does not protect the lung from inhalation injury. *Burns* 1991; **17**: 384–390.

141. Wang S, Lantz RC, Robledo RF, Breceda V, Hays AM, Witten ML. Early alterations of lung injury following acute smoke exposure and 21-aminosteroid treatment. *Toxicol Pathol* 1999; **27**: 334–341.

142. Baggish MS, Daniell JF. Catastrophic injury secondary to the use of coaxial gas-cooled fibers and artificial sapphire tips for intrauterine surgery. *Laser Surg Med* 1989; **9**: 581–584.

143. Peachey T, Eason J, Moxham J, Jarvis D, Driver M. Systemic air embolism during laser bronchoscopy. *Anaesthesia* 1988; **43**: 872–875.

144. Ross DJ, Mohsenifar Z, Potkin RT, Roston WL, Shapiro SM, Alexander JM. Pathogenesis of cerebral air embolism during neodymium–YAG laser photoresection. *Chest* 1988; **94**: 660–662.

Minimally invasive neurosurgery has seen a resurgence in popularity in recent years. Some of this enthusiasm is a semantic phenomenon, since a wide variety of minimally invasive operations, both intracranial and spinal, have been routine for years, if not decades. In fact, there is substantial evidence that minimally invasive neurosurgery has been performed on an outpatient basis for many centuries (Figure 11.1). One of the most frequently performed minimally invasive neurosurgical operations was introduced into clinical practice over a century ago by the Swiss physician Gottlieb Burkhardt. First used to alleviate the severe symptoms of schizophrenia, it became popular in the 1930s after the Portuguese neuropsychiatrist, Antonio Egas Moniz (awarded the 1949 Nobel prize for his work) described

his success in the treatment of patients with emotional disorders. In this procedure, a slender wire knife is inserted through small burr holes in the skull to sever the pathways connecting the frontal and prefrontal cortex to the thalamus. It gained notoriety through the efforts of Freeman and Watts, who performed the procedure indiscriminately on individuals with undesirable behaviour on an outpatient basis in their office. In its most ghastly form, known as the "ice-pick lobotomy", an ice-pick was driven through the roof of the orbits with a mallet under local anaesthesia, and flicked back and forth to sever the fibres.

Neurosurgical endoscopy is a technique that was introduced in the early 20th century, when open brain

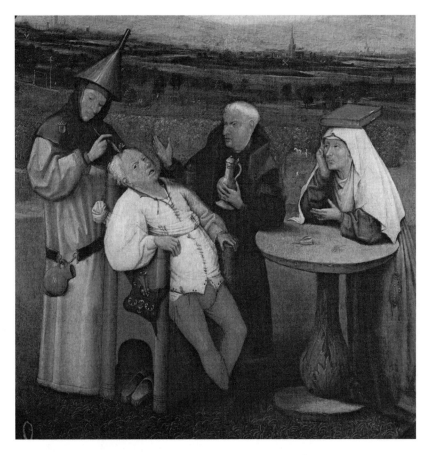

Figure 11.1 Patient being trepaned to remove the presumed cause of a behavioural abnormality. Details from "The Cure of Folly" or "The Stone Operation" by Hieronymus Bosch, 16th century. (Prado Museum, Madrid.)

surgery was associated with high mortality rates. As was the case in other surgical specialties, it was a urologist, Lespinasse, who performed the first endoscopic operation in neurosurgery. In 1910, he treated two children suffering from hydrocephalus, using a cystoscope to access and fulgurate the choroid plexus. One child died during the procedure while the other survived another 5 years. Dandy also used a cystoscope, renaming it "ventriculoscope", in the treatment of hydrocephalus. The method lost favour with the advent of the ventriculoperitoneal shunt, but the technique itself has profited greatly in recent years from innovations in optical instrumentation and video imaging technology. It now permits intraventricular operations, which would otherwise be impossible altogether or have an inacceptable mortality rate. Structures of the frontobasal brain can now be accessed through the sphenoid sinus, and no longer require a temporal or frontal craniotomy.

Microscopic lumbar disc surgery, in which the affected intervertebral space is approached through a small skin incision and a narrow channel opened with a speculum, has long since replaced the conventional operation that was associated with extensive tissue destruction. In other techniques, the spine is approached through the thorax, the peritoneum or through the retroperitoneum.

An exciting interdisciplinary development that has gained momentum during the past three decades has taken the patient out of the neurosurgical operating theatre and placed him under the fluoroscope in the radiology suite. Interventional neuroradiology using endovascular techniques and instrumentation for procedures ranging from superselective functional diagnosis to definitive treatment of arteriovenous malformations, cerebral aneurysms, carotid artery stenosis, occlusive cerebrovascular disease, and others that were previously only amenable to surgical therapy.

Transsphenoidal pituitary surgery

The anatomical localization and the physiological functions of the pituitary are the determinants of the difficulties associated with surgery on this tiny organ. The pituitary is located in close proximity to crucial neural and vascular structures. It lies in the hypophyseal fossa of the sphenoid bone, commonly referred to as the *sella turcica*, covered by the *diaphragma sellae*, and is connected to the hypothalamus by the pituitary stalk. The optic chasm lies superiorly and anteriorly to the pituitary stalk. The pituitary is surrounded laterally by the cavernous sinuses, which extend posteriorly into the petrosal sinus. The carotid arteries, and the oculomotor, trochlear, abducens and parts of the

trigeminal nerves pass through the cavernous sinuses on each side of the sella.

The pituitary gland is composed of an anterior part, the adenohypophysis, which accounts for most of its volume, and a posterior part, the neurohypophysis. The adenohypophysis is a plurihormonal endocrine organ made up of a variety of cell types. Somatotropes, which secrete growth hormone (GH), account for about half of the cell population of the adenohypophysis, and adrenocorticotropin hormone (ACTH) secreting corticotropes constitute another 20%. The latter also secrete β-endorphin. Of the remaining cells, prolactin (PRL) secreting lactotropes represent the largest fraction with about 20% of the gland, while gonadotropic-hormone (follicle stimulating harmone (FSH)/leutinizing harmone (LH)) and thyroid-stimulating hormone (TSH) producing cells make up the rest. Vasopressin (antidiuretic hormone (ADH)) is the primary hormone of the neurohypophysis. Tumours of the pituitary or of surrounding structures can either enhance or suppress the secretion of these hormones, and the patient can present with isolated or multiple hormonal abnormalities.

Tumours of the pituitary are nearly always benign adenomas that can arise from any of the cell types described above. Microadenomas with a diameter of less than 10 mm are quite frequent (20% of the population on autopsy), while macroadenomas (diameter >10 mm) are rare. The tumours are currently classified according to their secretory product (if any). The most common are prolactinomas and inactive null-cell adenomas, which each account for approximately 25%. ACTH-cell and GH-cell adenomas each represent about 15% of the pituitary tumours. Slightly more than half of the ACTH-cell tumours are endocrinologically active. Another 15% of all tumours secrete multiple hormones. Inactive adenomas can induce varying amounts of hypopituitarism by compression of the remaining gland or by interfering with the blood supply leading to infarction. Excessive hormone secretion causes typical clinical syndromes that can significantly influence anaesthetic management (Table 11.1).

Craniopharyngiomas are benign epithelial tumours commonly occurring in children. They are endocrinologically inactive and cause symptoms by local destruction or compression. The most common localization is the suprasellar cistern, but intrasellar tumours are also seen. Large lesions frequently erode the sella and contain calcifications either in or above the sella (Figure 11.2).

Approaching the patient with a pituitary tumour

The patient with a pituitary or hypothalamic lesion must have a careful preoperative endocrine evaluation

Table 11.1 Pituitary hormones and their effects relevant to anaesthesia and surgery

ACTH

Hypersecretion	Cushing syndrome, DM, immune suppression, hypertension, sodium retention, hypokalemia
Deficiency	Addison's disease, stress intolerance, cardiovascular instability

GH

Hypersecretion	Acromegaly (gigantism, if in children), cardiomegaly, cardiomyopathy, hypertension, DM, macroglossia, prognathism, enlargement of the mandible

TSH

Hypersecretion	Hyperthyroidism
Deficiency	Myxoedema, cardiac conduction defects, cardiomyopathy

Vasopressin (ADH)

Hypersecretion	Syndrome of inappropriate ADH secretion (SIADH)
Deficiency	DI

PRL, FSH/LH	Little relevance for anaesthesia

DM: diabetes mellitus; DI: diabetes insipidus.

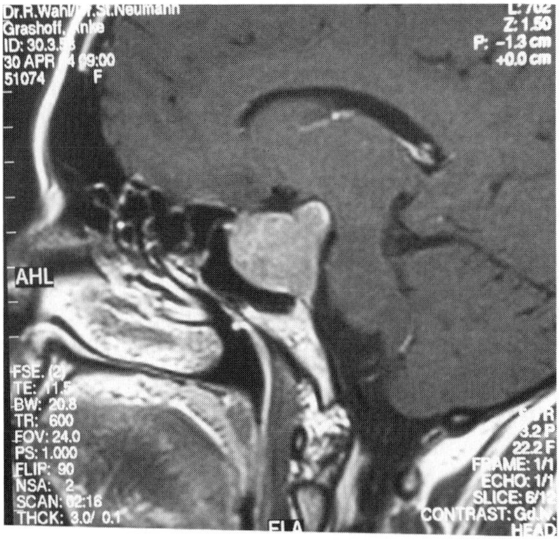

Figure 11.2 This magnetic resonance imaging (MRI) shows a large space-occupying lesion that has already destroyed the posterior part of the sella. This was a recurrent craniopharygeoma in a 49-year old female patient.

to recognize and minimize the potential for perioperative problems related to inadequate or excessive hormone secretion. Cortisol and thyroxin are the two most important hormones in this respect. Hypersecretion of these hormones is usually readily recognized by the clinical signs and symptoms of Cushing disease or hyperthyroidism. Pre-existing hypocortisolism or hypothyroidism are not apparent unless severe and long lasting, but can exacerbate acutely in the perioperative period with potentially catastrophic results. Fatigue, weakness, anorexia and hypotension in a patient with a sellar or suprasellar tumour should alert the anaesthetist to the possibility of these conditions, and prompt further evaluation, and possibly postponing surgery and instituting hormonal substitution therapy.

Patients with Cushing's disease may require antihypertensive medication, and diuretics (possibly in combination with aldosterone antagonists) to reduce sodium retention and alleviate hypokalemia. The DM of Cushing disease is due to the metabolic effects of cortisol and is not insulin dependent, and ketoacidosis is thus not a prime concern. Patients with hyperthyroidism due to excessive TSH secretion are not likely to develop a thyrotoxic crisis without the presence of autonomic thyroid adenomas. Severe symptoms of elevated levels of thyroid hormones may require preoperative thyrostatic treatment.

Over-secretion of GH causes arterial hypertension with cardiomyopathy that can cause perioperative circulatory problems. Macroglossia, prognathism and mandibular enlargement can interfere with endotracheal intubation.

Surgical complications include visual loss, vascular injuries, cranial nerve palsy, nasal bleeding, cerebrospinal fluid (CSF) leak and transient psychosis.

Anaesthetic management

The standard approach to the sella is currently via the transsphenoidal route (Figure 11.3). With this technique, first described by the Austrian rhinologist, Schloffer in 1907,[1] the surgeon accesses the sella through a submucous dissection of the nasal septum. The patient lies supine and the surgeon views the site through an operating microscope (Figure 11.4(a) and (b)).

Transsphenoidal operations are associated with minimal tissue destruction and a short period of wound closure. The anaesthetic technique for these procedures must take this into account, and allow for rapid emergence. Minimal invasiveness not withstanding, there is always the risk of major vascular damage in the vicinity of the sella, particularly with tumours with great lateral or vertical extent, and a large bore venous cannula should be inserted. The surgeon may request the anaesthetist to perform a Valsalva manoeuvre during the operation to cause suprasellar portions of the tumour to herniate through the *diaphragma sellae*.

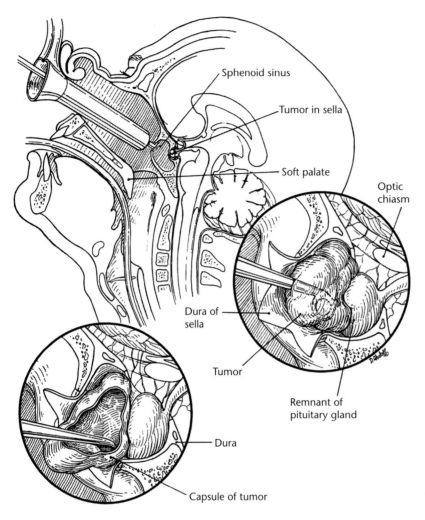

Figure 11.3 Diagram of the route by which the sella and its contents are accessed by the transsphenoidal approach.

Glucocorticoids are routinely administered to patients undergoing pituitary surgery to either treat pre-existing or prevent postoperative hypocortisolaemia. The corticoid hormone chosen for substitution therapy should replace both glucocorticoid and mineralocorticoid effects. Hydrocortisone is a logical choice, since it combines both. A standard therapeutic regimen that tends to over-substitute is to infuse 100 mg of hydrocortisone perioperatively and a further 100 mg during the first 24 postoperative hours. Further treatment is with an oral preparation. Some recommend methylprednisolone (40 mg IV) or dexamethasone (10 mg IV). These substances have purely glucocorticoid effects.

DI is a typical perioperative complication of pituitary surgery. Transient DI occurs in up to 20% of the patients, while permanent DI is less common with an incidence of around 2%. DI is manifested by large volumes of urine with low specific gravity. Care must be taken to replace fluid and electrolyte losses, particularly potassium. Severe polyuria should be treated with intravenous vasopressin or desmopressin.

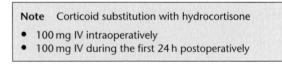

Note   Corticoid substitution with hydrocortisone
- 100 mg IV intraoperatively
- 100 mg IV during the first 24 h postoperatively

Neurosurgical endoscopy

After its slow start for the treatment of hydrocephalus early in the 20th century, endoscopic neurosurgery is now an established technique with a list of specific operations. Hydrocephalus is the most common indication, particularly that arising from aquaeductal

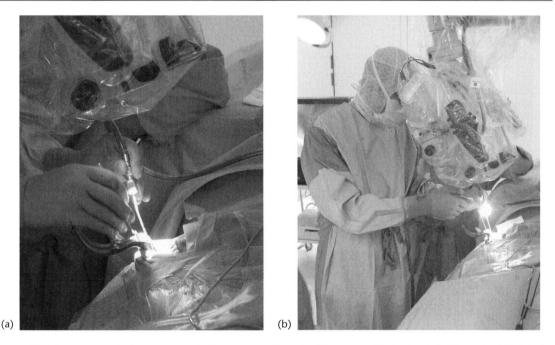

(a)   (b)

Figure 11.4 For microsurgical endoscopic pituitary surgery, the patient is supine with the head slightly reclined. This is the classical approach described by Cushing. The surgeon dissects a submucous path along the nasal septum and accesses the pituitary through the sphenoid sinus.

stenosis, or multiloculated hydrocephalus following infection. In the latter condition, CSF accumulates in non-communicating compartments separated by membranes. Among other standard indications are ventricular tumours including pineal tumours, and CSF drainage. Anaesthetic management for most minimally invasive neurosurgical procedures does not differ fundamentally from that for the conventional operations.

Endoscopic procedures in neurosurgery	
CSF diversion	Non-communicating hydrocephalus, multiloculated hydrocephalus
Cyst removal	Arachnoid cysts, colloid cysts
Intraventricular tumours	Pinealomas, ependymomas, cranio pharygiomas, etc. Stereotactic biopsy, excision

CSF diversion operations

Non-communicating hydrocephalus requires fluid diversion from the third ventricle. This is commonly done by implanting a ventricular shunt that drains into the peritoneum or the right atrium. Complications and the need for repeated operations increase the morbidity

of the patients. Relief is also possible in select patients by creating an opening in the floor of the third ventricle, which allows CSF to drain into the basal cisterns.[2] This operation, known as third ventriculostomy, was first performed in 1923 by Mixter,[3] shortly after the first attempts to treat hydrocephalus by fulgurating the choroid plexus.

The patient is positioned supine and a coronal burr hole is placed to allow access to the frontal horn of the lateral ventricle (Figure 11.5(a)). The endoscope is inserted and advanced to the third ventricle. The surgeon creates an opening in the floor of the ventricle distal to the mamillary bodies using the endoscope itself, a blunt instrument or a laser. The opening is dilated with a Fogarty catheter to stop venous bleeding. Acute increase of intracranial pressure can occur intra-operatively due to the infusion of irrigation fluid. Cardiovascular control centres are in immediate proximity to the third ventricle and acute complications, such as cardiac dysrhythmias, blood pressure swings, bradycardia and cardiac arrest, can occur when they are irritated.[4] The bradycardia that arises at the moment of perforation ceases when the surgeon either retracts the instrument or completes the perforation.[5] Postoperative complications include headache, high fever, short-term memory loss, inappropriate secretion of ADH (DI or water retention), cranial nerve palsy

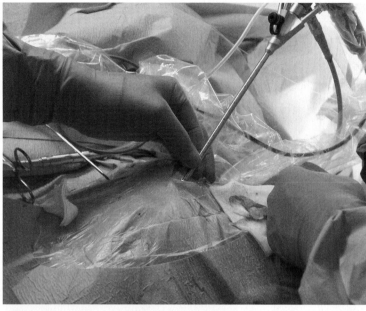

(a)

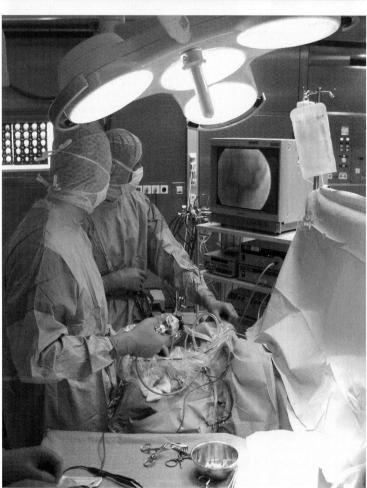

(b)

Figure 11.5 The rigid endoscope is introduced into the ventricle through a small skin incision and burr hole in the skull (a). The surgeon and the assistant follow the progress of the operation on the video monitor. A vascularized membrane is clearly visible on the screen in the picture (b).

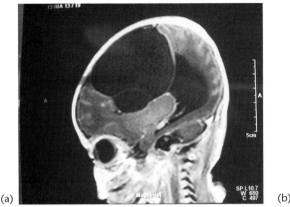 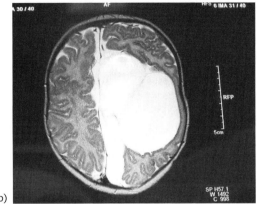

(a)   (b)

Figure 11.6 Computed tomography of an infant with a multiloculated hydrocephalus. Membranes are visible in both views. A venticuloperitoneal shunt operation had already been performed, but was ineffective, since the individual fluid-filled compartments did not communicate.

and transient confusion. Venous bleeding is usually easily controlled, but arterial haemorrhage may force abortion of the procedure and placement of an external ventricular drain.

Surgery for non-communicating hydrocephalus, frequently observed following intracranial infections, is aimed at opening connections in the membranes partitioning the fluid space and causing the multiloculated CSF accumulation (Figure 11.6). These membranes can be torn with grasping forceps inserted through the endoscope, or perforated using a laser. Holmium–yttrium–aluminium–garnet (YAG) lasers have been developed which have a wavelength highly absorbed by both water and haemoglobin and tissue. This wavelength reduces the risk of the laser beam injuring brain tissue after having penetrated the membrane. Acute increase of intracranial pressure can occur during these operations, but the cardiovascular derangement is less likely, since the walls of the third ventricle are not involved (Table 11.2).

Anaesthesia

Patients with hydrocephalus must be evaluated for hypovolaemia and electrolyte imbalance in the presence of vomiting and fluid restriction. Infants under 6 months of age usually do not require preoperative medication. A fully alert paediatric patient can be given an oral or rectal premedication with midazolam ($0.5\,mg\,kg^{-1}$ up to a maximum of 15 mg). Patients with increased intracerebral pressure or altered mental status should not have sedating medication.

Inhalational induction is an option for patients without increased intracranial pressure or vomiting. Intravenous induction should be preferred in all others. Induction

Table 11.2 Characteristic features and risks of specific neuroendoscopic procedures relevant to anaesthesia

Procedure	Features relevant to anaesthesia
CSF diversion	Increased ICP, obtunded sensorium, vomiting, haemorrhage, damage to basilar artery, damage to midbrain structures, cardiac dysrhythmias, cardiovascular instability with sudden changes in heart rate and blood pressure, disturbed ADH secretion with DI, ventriculitis, postoperative fever, temperature changes (use warmed irrigation fluid)
Intracranial cysts	Similar to above if intracranial pressure is elevated due to obstructed cerebrovascular fluid drainage
Biopsy, tumour removal	Damage to midbrain structures with cardiac dysrhythmias, abrupt intraoperative brady/tachycardia, hypo/hypertension, altered ADH secretion, haemorrhage from biopsy site

with propofol or barbiturate can decrease blood pressure, if given injudiciously, with possible impairment of cerebral perfusion pressure. Etomidate might be considered as alternative in the patient with circulatory compromise. Anaesthetic maintenance should not influence cerebral blood flow or intracranial pressure, and should give rapid awakening. Total intravenous anaesthesia (TIVA) with propofol and remifentanil, or a balanced technique with isoflurane, sevoflurane or desflurane are recommended, despite the somewhat higher costs for the drugs. Children require higher doses of anaesthetic drugs than adults. The infusion rate for propofol has to be increased by 50–100% above that for adults.[6,7] In our experience, remifentanil has to be given at a rate of at least $0.3–0.5\,\mu g\,kg^{-1}min^{-1}$, and propofol at a rate of at least $8–10\,mg\,kg^{-1}h^{-1}$. The age dependence of the MAC of volatile anaesthetics is a well-known fact. The use of propofol in children is considered controversial or even contraindicated by some.[8,9] The literature seems to show that there might be a slightly increased risk for children with severe bacterial infections and sepsis, or after prolonged infusions in an intensive care setting.[10] In our opinion and in our own experience, propofol can be safely used for anaesthesia in children observing the manufacturer's age restrictions. Deep relaxation is recommended to prevent even slightest movement.

Blood pressure and electrocardiogram (ECG) monitoring are crucial during endoscopic neurosurgical procedures due to the acute cardiovascular complications that can arise. Non-invasive blood pressure measurements can be difficult in small children, and direct arterial cannulation with invasive measurements can be indicated. This will also allow intermittent sampling for partial pressure of carbon dioxide in arterial blood (P_aCO_2) and haemoglobin determinations. Capnometry is essential to maintain a physiological arterial carbon dioxide (CO_2) tension; hypoventilation can cause hypercapnia with increased intracranial pressure, while hyperventilation directly reduces cerebral blood flow.

Interventional neuroradiology

The embolization of a cerebral arteriovenous malformation described by Luessenhop and Spence in 1960 was essentially the birth of interventional neuroradiology.[11] While they were initially performed without anaesthesiological assistance, they have become more and more complex, and anaesthetists are now present at most of them. The contribution of the anaesthetist to the success of the procedure ranges from simply aiding the patient to tolerate lying immobile for up to hours on end, to crucial blood pressure and blood gas manipulations, as well as managing arising complications. The interventions are inherently dangerous and the rate or major complications and death is around 1–2%.[12] Table 11.3 gives a short overview of common neuroradiological interventions with their particular demands on the anaesthetist and their inherent risks.

During the standard neuroradiological intervention, a 7.5 F introducer sheath is inserted into the femoral artery. A 7.0 F coaxial catheter is passed through the introducer sheath and positioned under fluoroscopic control in the carotid artery or vertebral artery. A thin, superselective catheter (1.5–2.5 F) is then advanced through this catheter into the cerebral arteries. Through this are passed the metal coils or balloons for obliterating aneurysms or the glue for closing arteriovenous malformations.

Simple procedures, such as percutaneous transluminal angioplasty and stenting of an occluded carotid artery can be performed in the spontaneously breathing patient under local anaesthesia, oral premedication and light supplemental intravenous sedation. Conscious sedation was the anaesthetic management of choice for nearly all neuroradiological interventions proposed by Young and Pile Spellman in their excellent 1994 review,[12] since it allows continuous neurological

Table 11.3 Interventional neuroradiological procedures and their risks and requirements relevant to anaesthesia (Adapted from Ref [12].)

Procedure	Features relevant to anaesthesia
Superselective anaesthesia functional examination (SAFE)	Performed prior to embolization to determine if catheter tip is not positioned too proximal, and if functional brain areas might be damaged
Therapeutic embolization	
Cerebral aneurysms	Rupture, deliberate hypo- or hypertension
Intracranial arteriovenous malformations	Deliberate hypotension, post-procedure NPPB
Extracranial arteriovenous malformations	Deliberate hypercapnia, post-procedure NPPB
Angioplasty and stenting of occluded carotids or other cerebral arteries	Cerebral ischaemia, deliberate hypertension concomitant ischaemic heart disease likely
Angioplasty of cerebral vasospasm following subarachnoid haemorrhage	Cerebral ischaemia, deliberate hypo- or hypertension
Intra-arterial chemotherapy	Airway swelling, intracranial hypertension

NPPB: oedema or haemorrhage in area, in which perfusion increases after the procedure "normal perfusion pressure breakthrough".

assessment of the patient. More recently, however, general anaesthesia with endotracheal intubation, deep relaxation and mechanical ventilation has gained favour during embolization of cerebral aneurysms or arteriovenous malformations.[13] The patient can remain immobile for longer periods, and manipulations such as deliberate hypotension or deliberate hypercapnia will not cause patient discomfort or induce vomiting.[14,15] Small children will nearly all require general anaesthesia. The choice of the general anaesthetic must be adapted to the patients' underlying and accompanying pathology. Patients with occlusive cerebrovascular disease are likely to have concomitant coronary artery disease and arterial hypertension, while those who have suffered subarachnoid bleeding from a ruptured intracranial aneurysm, might have an obtunded sensorium, elevated intracranial pressure and possibly vascular spasms with impaired cerebral perfusion. Mean arterial pressure (MAP) must be closely controlled and all measures that might increase intracranial pressure must be avoided. Recovery from general anaesthesia should be rapid in order to allow early postoperative neurological evaluation of the patient.

During preoperative assessment, the anaesthetist should make note of a history of coagulation disorders, protamine allergy, reactions to contrast medium, airway patency in the supine patient (important for conscious sedation), and the patient's ability to lie supine for several hours. Pre-existing arterial hypertension should be well controlled. Premedication usually consists of an anxiolytic such as midazolam. If deliberate hypotension is intended during the procedure, an oral beta-blocker such as atenolol or metoprolol might be given.

Neuroradiological interventions are not performed in the operation theatre, and the rooms are frequently not equipped with anaesthesia in mind. The anaesthetist must ensure that the minimum required equipment is immediately available in the room itself. This includes the anaesthesia machine with ventilator, a reliable oxygen (O_2) supply, suction, laryngoscopes, endotracheal tubes and everything else required for securing and maintaining the airway, syringe pumps, all necessary drugs, power lines with emergency circuits, defibrillator, etc.

Monitoring for intracerebral endovascular procedures consists of standard 5-lead ECG (preferably with ST segment analysis), two venous lines, pulse oximetry and capnometry. Blood pressure can be measured non-invasively in procedures unlikely to cause circulatory derangement or those not requiring deliberate hypo- or hypertension, but invasive monitoring is required in all other interventions. Patients with conscious sedation should be well protected against temperature loss, since shivering can interfere with imaging. Supplemental O_2 is administered to the spontaneously breathing patient through nasal prongs. End-tidal CO_2 partial pressure can be measured by inserting the collecting tube of an off-line capnometer alongside the nasal cannula. The capnometer reading will be lower than the actual arterial PCO_2, and for lengthy procedures an occasional blood gas sample should be drawn to assess the magnitude of the bias. One should consider inserting a urinary catheter for prolonged procedures, since the contrast medium acts as an osmotic diuretic. Central nervous system monitoring, such as processed electroencephalogram (EEG), somatosensory or acoustic evoked potentials, is implemented occasionally. In any event, the anaesthetist should be prepared to provide appropriate management and cardiovascular support in the event of potentially fatal ischaemic or haemorrhagic complications, which can occur in 1–8% of interventions.

Anaesthetic management

Conscious sedation

The goal of conscious sedation is to prevent anxiety, pain and discomfort, and to ensure the patient's immobility, while not appreciably interfering with respiration, airway patency, cardiovascular stability or with neurological assessment. A suitable technique combines the analgesic properties of a long-acting opioid such as fentanyl or sufentanil with a short-acting, easily titratable hypnotic such as propofol. The opioid is given after placing the venous cannula. There are some data that suggest that sufentanil might increase intracranial pressure (ICP) and lower cerebral perfusion pressure in patients with head injuries,[16,17] but other studies have contradicted these findings.[18,19] Sedation is induced by a small dose of propofol ($0.5\,\mu g\,kg^{-1}$) and maintained by the continuous infusion of propofol at an initial rate of $10–20\,\mu g\,kg^{1}\,min^{-1}$. The level of sedation is adjusted by increasing or decreasing the infusion rate. Other regimens are, of course, possible, and the anaesthetist should choose that with which he feels most competent.

Conscious sedation

- Oral premedication with midazolam (7.5 mg)
- Fentanyl ($2\,\mu g\,kg^{-1}$) or sufentanil ($0.2\,\mu g\,kg^{-1}$)
- Bolus dose of propofol ($0.5\,mg\,kg^{-1}$)

Then

- Continuous propofol infusion ($10–20\,\mu g\,kg^{-1}\,min^{-1}$); adjust as necessary
- Supplemental O_2 (2–4 l min^{-1}) via nasal prongs
- Pulse oximetric monitoring

General anaesthesia

TIVA with propofol and a suitable opioid maintains stable haemodynamics and has little effect on cerebral perfusion or intracranial pressure. Balanced anaesthesia with isoflurane or desflurane as the volatile component is equally suitable, if high end-expiratory concentrations are avoided. Suitable techniques are described in Chapter 5. Orotracheal intubation should be preferred over the nasotracheal route, since the complete anticoagulation required by most procedures could lead to significant bleeding from injured nasal mucosa.

General anaesthesia for interventional neuroradiology

- Oral premedication with midazolam (7.5 mg)
- TIVA with propofol and remifentanil or sufentanil (Chapter 5)
- Consider neuromuscular blockers to ensure an immobile patient

---

Blood pressure manipulations

Deliberate hypotension is primarily employed during neuroradiological interventions to reduce the blood flow through an arteriovenous malformation before injecting the glue to give it time to set. It need not be of long duration. The technique is not advisable during conscious sedation, since it may induce nausea and vomiting that can endanger the procedure and the patient.

A short-acting beta-adrenergic blocker (such as esmolol) or a combined alpha- and beta-blocker (such as labetolol) are good choices, since they do not affect cerebral perfusion as do nitroglycerine or sodium nitroprusside,[20] although these have been suggested for use during neuroradiological procedures.[21] Esmolol is given as an initial bolus injection of $1\,\text{mg}\,\text{kg}^{-1}$ followed by an infusion at an initial rate of $0.5\,\text{mg}\,\text{kg}^{-1}\text{min}^{-1}$. Labetolol can be added in small incremental injections if blood pressure is not reduced to the desired level, or if the infusion rate of esmolol is too high. Urapadil (10 mg increments) can be used if labetolol is not available.

Deliberate hypertension is occasionally required to provide collateral perfusion to ischaemic areas via the Willisan channels or through leptomeningeal pathways. Another indication is to maintain cerebral perfusion in patients with vasospasm. Phenylephrine is a first-line vasoconstrictor that is given in an initial dose of about $1\,\mu\text{g}\,\text{kg}^{-1}$ followed by an infusion titrated to increase blood pressure to about 30–50% above baseline. If ICP monitoring is in place, one aims at an MAP at least 60 mmHg above ICP. Norepinephrine infusions can also be given to provide the desired increase in blood pressure. One must begin carefully with a starting dose of 3–5 μg and then titrate the infusion to effect.

Blood pressure management during interventional neuroradiology

- Deliberate hypotension:
  - Consider premedication with beta-blocker
  - Induce hypotension with esmolol bolus injection ($1\,\text{mg}\,\text{kg}^{-1}$), followed by esmolol infusion starting at $0.5\,\text{mg}\,\text{kg}^{-1}\text{min}^{-1}$ and increased as needed
- If esmolol infusion is insufficient for adequate hypotension, or infusion rate too high add: labetolol (20 mg increments), if available; urapadil (10 mg increments) as alternative
  - Nitroglycerine and sodium nitroprusside increase cerebral blood flow
- Deliberate hypertension:
  - Phenylephrine bolus injection ($0.5–1\,\mu\text{g}\,\text{kg}^{-1}$) followed by infusion starting at $20\,\mu\text{g}\,\text{min}^{-1}$
  - Norepinephrine: bolus injection (5 μg) followed by infusion titrated to effect (start at *ca.* $5\,\mu\text{g}\,\text{min}^{-1}$)

Anticoagulation

The catheter and other introduced thrombogenic material can induce thrombus formation with distal thromboembolism and clot propagation. Some centres aim at preventing this by systemic anticoagulation with heparin, while others argue that anticoagulation increases the risk of intracranial haemorrhage. This is thus an issue that is at the discretion of the neuroradiologists. If heparin is used, protamine is frequently given at the end of the procedure to reverse the effects. The anaesthetist must be aware of the pulmonary and circulatory effects of protamine, as well as of its potential of causing allergic reactions.

References

1. Schloffer H. Erfolgreiche Operation eines Hypophysentumors auf nasalem Wege. *Wien Klin Wochenschr* 1907; **20**: 621.
2. Jones RF, Kwok BC, Stening WA *et al.* Neuroendoscopic third ventriculostomy. A practical alternative to extracranial shunts in non-communicating hydrocephalus. *Acta Neurochir Suppl* 1994; **61**: 79–83.
3. Mixter WJ. Ventriculoscopy and puncture of the third ventricle. *Boston Med Surg* 1923; **188**: 277–278.
4. Teo C, Rahman S, Boop FA *et al.* Complications of endoscopic neurosurgery. *Child Nerv Syst* 1996; **12**: 248–253.
5. El-Dawlatly AA, Murshid WR, Elshimy A, Magboul MA, Samarkandi A, Takrouri MS. The incidence of bradycardia during endoscopic third ventriculostomy. *Anesth Analg* 2000; **91**: 1142–1144.

6. Kataria BK, Ved SA, Nicodemus HF *et al.* The pharmacokinetics of propofol in children using three different data analysis approaches. *Anesthesiology* 1994; **80**: 104–122.

7. McFarlan CS, Anderson BJ, Short TG. The use of propofol infusions in paediatric anaesthesia. *Paediatr Anaesth* 1999; **9**: 209–216.

8. Bray RJ. Propofol infusion syndrome in children. *Paediatr Anaesth* 1998; **8**: 491–499.

9. Hatch D. Propofol in paediatric intensive care. *Br J Anaesth* 1997; **79**: 274–275.

10. Parke TJ, Stevens JE, Rice ASC *et al.* Metabolic acidosis and fatal myocardial failure after propofol infusion in children: five case reports. *Br Med J* 1992; **305**: 613–616.

11. Luessenhop AJ, Spence WT. Artificial embolization of cerebral arteries: report of use in a case or arteriovenous malformation. *J Am Med Assoc* 1960; **172**: 1153–1155.

12. Young WL, Pile Spellman J. Anesthetic considerations for interventional neuroradiology. *Anesthesiology* 1994; **80**: 427–456.

13. Debrun GM, Aletich VA, Thornton J *et al.* Techniques of coiling cerebral aneurysms. *Surg Neurol* 2000; **53**: 150–156.

14. Lai YC, Manninen PH. Anesthesia for cerebral aneurysms: a comparison between interventional neuroradiology and surgery. *Can J Anaesth* 2001; **48**: 391–395.

15. Munte S, Munte TF, Kuche H *et al.* General anesthesia for interventional neuroradiology: propofol versus isoflurane. *J Clin Anesth* 2001; **13**: 186–192.

16. Albanese J, Durbec O, Viviand X, Potie F, Alliez B, Martin C. Sufentanil increases intracranial pressure in patients with head trauma. *Anesthesiology* 1993; **79**: 493–497.

17. Sperry RJ, Bailey PL, Reichman MV, Peterson JC, Petersen PB, Pace NL. Fentanyl and sufentanil increase intracranial pressure in head trauma patients. *Anesthesiology* 1992; **77**: 416–420.

18. Werner C, Kochs E, Bause H, Hoffman WE, Schulte am Esch J. Effects of sufentanil on cerebral hemodynamics and intracranial pressure in patients with brain injury. *Anesthesiology* 1995; **83**: 721–726.

19. Lauer KK, Connolly LA, Schmeling WT. Opioid sedation does not alter intracranial pressure in head injured patients. *Can J Anaesth* 1997; **44**: 929–933.

20. Schroeder T, Schierbeck J, Howardy P, Knudsen I, Skafte-Holm P, Gefke K. Effect of labetolol on cerebral blood flow and middle cerebral arterial blood velocity in healthy volunteers. *Neurol Res* 1991; **13**: 10–12.

21. O'Mahony BJ, Bolsin SNC. Anaesthesia for closed embolisation of cerebral arteriovenous malformtations. *Anaesth Intens Care* 1988; **16**: 318–323.

INDEX

Note: page numbers in *italics* refer to figures and tables.